Evidence-Based Practices in Behavioral Health

Series editor

Nirbhay N. Singh, Medical College of Georgia, Augusta University, Augusta, USA

More information about this series at http://www.springer.com/series/11863

James K. Luiselli
Editor

Behavioral Health Promotion and Intervention in Intellectual and Developmental Disabilities

Springer

Editor
James K. Luiselli
North East Educational and Developmental
Support Center
Tewksbury, MA
USA

ISSN 2366-6013 ISSN 2366-6021 (electronic)
Evidence-Based Practices in Behavioral Health
ISBN 978-3-319-27295-5 ISBN 978-3-319-27297-9 (eBook)
DOI 10.1007/978-3-319-27297-9

Library of Congress Control Number: 2015957773

Printed on acid-free paper

This Springer imprint is published by SpringerNature
The registered company is Springer International Publishing AG Switzerland

Preface

Many children and adults with intellectual and developmental disabilities (IDDs) have serious health concerns that affect their learning, socialization, and quality of life. In recent years, there has been increased research attention toward treating individuals who have disease symptoms and chronic medical problems. Another vital concern is reducing health-risk factors and preventing onset of illnesses and other afflictions. Notably, the disciplines of applied behavior analysis (ABA) and more generally behavioral psychology have contributed greatly to health care for people with IDD. Behavioral methods are used in combination with traditional medicine and sometimes as a sole treatment agent. While early behavioral medicine applications were reported in the professional literature, there have been many new developments in theory, practice, and research.

This book addresses the contribution of behavioral psychology, applied behavior analysis, behavioral medicine, and cognitive–behavioral treatment to health issues among people who have IDD. It is intended as a contemporary synopsis and review of evidence-based procedures that have been extensively researched and translated into effective practices by multidisciplinary healthcare providers. From the perspective of tertiary prevention, chapters are included for treating health problems such as food refusal, sleep disorders, body-focused (tissue-damaging) repetitive behaviors, and rumination. A second emphasis of the book is on reducing risk factors that impose health concerns, for example, noncompliance with medical routines, maintaining personal hygiene, and substance abuse. Considering primary prevention, the book covers areas such as encouraging healthy lifestyles and increasing exercise—physical activity. In addition to highlighting these symptom-directed, risk reduction, and primary prevention interventions, chapters address consultation and training models for working successfully with physicians, nurses, parents, direct care practitioners, and ancillary healthcare professionals. In summary, my twofold purpose for the book has been to aggregate the most contemporary research on behavioral prevention and intervention for health issues among people with IDD, and to provide a research-to-practice translation so that practitioners can learn about and adopt the most effective and evidence-based methods.

I am most grateful to Springer Publishing for supporting the book, in particular Senior Editor for Behavioral Sciences, Judy Jones, and her outstanding editorial and production teams. Dr. Nirbhay N. Singh, a friend and most esteemed colleague, also helped me fashion the book. I wish to thank James M. Sperry, President–CEO of Clinical Solutions, Inc., and North East Educational and Developmental Support Center, for giving me the opportunity to join his organization of exemplary, respectful, and dedicated professionals—how wonderful to move on! Among many settings and locations that set the occasion for and reinforce my book writing and editing, I acknowledge Border Café, Burlington Mall, Carlisle Cranberry Bog, Dunkin' Donuts, Middlesex School, and Tufts University. In the end, the support, guidance, and humor of my wife, Dr. Tracy Evans Luiselli, and our children Gabrielle and Thomas, make it possible to keep everything in focus and to stay on a mindful path.

James K. Luiselli

Contents

About the Editor

James K. Luiselli is a clinical psychologist and Chief Clinical Officer at Clinical Solutions, Inc., Beverly, Massachusetts, and North East Educational and Developmental Support Center, Tewksbury, Massachusetts. Dr. Luiselli is a licensed psychologist, certified health service provider, diplomat in cognitive and behavioral psychology from the American Board of Professional Psychology (ABPP), and Board Certified Behavior Analyst (BCBA-D). He has held academic appointments at Harvard Medical School, Northeastern University, and Indiana State University. His primary interests include applied behavior analysis, cognitive–behavioral therapy, intellectual and developmental disabilities, high-risk clinical disorders, professional training, telehealth technology, organizational consultation, performance psychology, and research dissemination. Dr. Luiselli's publications include 13 books and approximately 50 book chapters and 275 journal articles. He serves as Associate Editor for the *Journal of Child & Family Studies* and *Behavior Analysis in Practice*, a Contributing Editor for *Child & Family Behavior Therapy*, and Editorial Board member for several other journals.

Contributors

Keith D. Allen Munroe-Meyer Institute for Genetics and Rehabilitation, University of Nebraska Medical Center, Omaha, USA

Megan St. Clair The Help Group, San Marino, USA

Robert Didden Radboud University Nijmegen, Nijmegen, The Netherlands

Neomi van Duijvenbode Radboud University Nijmegen, Nijmegen, The Netherlands

Kurt A. Freeman Division of Psychology, Institute on Development and Disability, Oregon Health and Science University, Portland, USA

Monica L. Garcia Center for Autism and Related Disorders, Woodland Hills, USA

Kimberly Guion Division of Psychology, Institute on Development and Disability, Oregon Health and Science University, Portland, USA

Sara Kupzyk Munroe-Meyer Institute for Genetics and Rehabilitation, University of Nebraska Medical Center, Omaha, USA

Giulio E. Lancioni Department of Neuroscience and Sense Organs, University of Bari, Bari, Italy

Joshua L. Lipschultz Florida Institute of Technology, Melbourne, FL, USA

James K. Luiselli Clinical Solutions, Inc., North East Educational and Developmental Support Center, Tewksbury, MA, USA

Jennifer M. Gillis Mattson Department of Psychology, Binghamton University, New York, NY, USA

Raymond G. Miltenberger University of South Florida, Tampa, FL, USA

Doretta Oliva Lega F. D'Oro Research Center, Osimo, Italy

Erin Olufs Division of Psychology, Institute on Development and Disability, Oregon Health and Science University, Portland, USA

Mark F. O'Reilly University of Texas at Austin, Austin, TX, USA

Meeta R. Patel Clinic 4 Kidz, Sausalito, USA

Kathryn M. Peterson Munroe-Meyer Institute, University of Nebraska Medical Center, Omaha, USA

Matthew Roth Auburn University, Auburn, USA

Melina Sevlever New York Presbyterian/Columbia University Medical Center, New York, USA

Jeff Sigafoos Victoria University of Wellington, Wellington, New Zealand

Nirbhay N. Singh Medical College of Georgia, Augusta University, Augusta, GA, USA

Claire A. Spieler University of South Florida, Tampa, FL, USA

Jonathan Tarbox FirstSteps for Kids, Hermosa Beach, CA, USA

Maria G. Valdovinos Psychology Department, Drake University, Des Moines, IA, USA

Joanneke VanDerNagel Radboud University Nijmegen, Nijmegen, The Netherlands

Valerie M. Volkert Munroe-Meyer Institute, University of Nebraska Medical Center, Omaha, USA; Marcus Autism Center, Emory University School of Medicine, Atlanta, GA, USA

David A. Wilder School of Behavior Analysis, Florida Institute of Technology, Melbourne, FL, USA; Florida Institute of Technology, Melbourne, FL, USA

Chapter 1
Health Conditions, Learning, and Behavior

Maria G. Valdovinos

Individuals with intellectual and developmental disabilities (IDD) often have co-morbid conditions or disorders (de Winter et al. 2011; Kidd et al. 2014; Ming et al. 2014). These conditions often present early in life (Schieve et al. 2012) but are also evident in later years. For example, research has demonstrated that individuals with IDD are at a greater risk for developing dementia than persons without disabilities (Cooper 1997). Common conditions include, but are not limited to: gastrointestinal issues, epilepsy, diabetes, sleep disorders, chronic pain, and neurocognitive disorders (e.g., dementia). If left untreated, these conditions can pose serious complications for overall health and functioning.

There is suggestion in the literature that co-morbid conditions are correlated with both age and severity of disability (Hermans and Evenhuis 2014). Thus, the older one becomes and/or the more severe the intellectual disability, the more likely one is to have multiple co-existing health conditions. Unfortunately, identifying chronic health conditions can prove to be challenging in the IDD population. This is, in part, attributed to communication deficits those with more severe and profound IDD may have. The more severe the disability, the less able one may be to self-report the ailments they are experiencing. And, unless the ailment is clearly identifiable as in some conditions (e.g., certain GI complaints, grand mal seizures, night-terrors), the more difficult identification of the condition becomes.

Managing these conditions is also not without challenges. For example, with regard to gastrointestinal issues (GI), prevalence of diarrhea, constipation, gaseousness, abdominal bloating, signs of abdominal discomfort, and food regurgitation in children with autism ranges from 48.8 (Galli-Carminati et al. 2006) to

M.G. Valdovinos (✉)
Psychology Department, Drake University, 2507 University Ave,
Des Moines, IA 50311, USA
e-mail: maria.valdovinos@drake.edu

J.K. Luiselli (ed.), *Behavioral Health Promotion and Intervention in Intellectual and Developmental Disabilities*, Evidence-Based Practices in Behavioral Health,
DOI 10.1007/978-3-319-27297-9_1

85.3 % (Horvath et al. 1999). Determining the cause of the condition and most effective course of treatment can be costly in terms of time and resources. And in some cases, such as chronic constipation, the course of treatment is focused on short-term outcomes (e.g., stool softeners) rather than longer-term management (e.g., diet, hydration, exercise).

In other conditions, such as neurocognitive disorders, communication and daily functioning increasingly become difficult. The mental deterioration experienced results in individuals becoming more reliant on their caretakers as they are less able to express their needs (Moss and Patel 1997). Indeed, any of the aforementioned conditions may impact one's experience with their environment, creating situations in which the interactions between behavior and the environment are altered in functional but undesired ways.

Another reason for identifying and managing these conditions is their relationship to challenging behaviors. Individuals with intellectual disabilities are often prescribed psychotropic medications to treat harmful or problematic behaviors (e.g., aggression, self-injury) (Aman and Singh 1988; Young and Hawkins 2002). These behaviors are important to address as they can functionally serve as barriers to independence, community living, least restrictive supports and achieving an optimal quality of life. However, in studies of longitudinal prescription patterns of psychoactive medication, it was found that roughly 60 % of the individuals surveyed were prescribed more than one psychotropic medication, with 24 % taking two medications, 15 % three medications, 7 % four medications, and 14 % five or more psychoactive medications (Lott et al. 2004). Despite the common use polypharmacy treatment, there is a paucity of literature supporting its effectiveness and limited research examining adverse effects (physiological and behavioral) that medication treatment may produce in individuals with IDD (Mayville 2007; Singh and Matson 2009). Indeed, there is evidence to suggest that medication side effects and effects produced by changes in medication may function as setting events for challenging behaviors (Rapp et al. 2007; Valdovinos et al. 2007, 2009).

Interaction Between Chronic Health Conditions and Challenging Behavior

There has long been an acknowledgement of the impact of environmental factors as motivators of challenging behaviors. What is becoming increasingly clear is that health conditions or biological factors also serve to motivate behavior (Langthorne et al. 2007). Whether these internally produced variables serve to occasion challenging behaviors or establish the consequences of said behaviors as stronger reinforcers has yet to be determined. What has been determined is that relationships exist between some chronic conditions and challenging behavior.

Gastrointestinal issues. As already discussed, many people with IDD experience gastrointestinal problems. Specifically, gastroesophageal reflux disease (GERD) is the most common experienced gastrointestinal issue experienced by the typically developing population with even greater incidence in those with IDD (Rada 2014). A very painful condition, GERD can be associated with self-injurious behavior (SIB). Thus, a connection between GERD, the pain it causes, and SIB has been made which suggests that SIB may intercept pain signals produced by GERD (Peebles and Price 2012). Although the concept of pain attenuation of SIB is not new (Symons 2002), others have suggested that although SIB may initially alleviate the pain associated with GERD or other gastrointestinal disorders (i.e., automatically reinforcing), it is likely that addressing the GERD as the sole method of treating SIB may not be sufficient (Swender et al. 2006). That is, once the health condition has been treated, there may be other contingencies maintaining challenging behaviors that need to be identified and addressed.

Chronic pain. The exact prevalence of chronic pain in the ID population is unknown because of previously cited communication difficulties and the possibility that people with IDD express pain differently than those without IDD (Courtemanche et al. 2012). As evidence of the difficulty in identification, the reported range of those with IDD who experience pain varies from approximately 18 % of adults who did not receive treatment for their pain (Boerlage et al. 2013) to 85 % of children with severe IDD (Breau et al. 2003b). Although evidence is limited, SIB may be one expression of or reaction to pain in those with severe and profound ID (e.g., Breau et al. 2003a; Peebles and Price 2012; Symons 2002; Symons and Danov 2005). Regardless of whether pain evokes SIB or SIB produces pain, there is support for conceptualizing pain as either a setting event or motivating operation for challenging behavior. For example, the existence of pain in a given area of the body can impact the topography of self-injury (e.g., head pain and head hitting or hair pulling) (Hartman et al. 2008) or escaping or avoiding situations/stimuli may become a more powerful motivator for challenging behavior (e.g., menstrual-associated pain establishes escape from some activities as reinforcing) (Carr et al. 2003).

Diabetes. Although, in general, there are no significant differences in obesity rates between those with and without IDD, researchers have found that a subset of the IDD population is more likely to be overweight than the general population (Stancliffe et al. 2011). Specifically, women, and those with Down syndrome, mild IDD, and living in community residential settings are more likely to be obese (Stancliffe et al. 2011). The obesity rates are of concern for many reasons but particularly because of the relationship between obesity, the factors that contribute to obesity, and Type 2 diabetes. Indeed this concern is compounded as individuals with IDD are more likely to develop Type 1 diabetes given the prevalence of genetic disorders within the population (Anwar et al. 1998; Taggart et al. 2013). Many of the antipsychotic medications prescribed to this population also have metabolic side effects associated with their use (e.g., olanzapine) (Musil et al. 2015). However, exact prevalence rates of diabetes within the ID population are not known, and estimates place the prevalence at approximately 8.6 % (McVilly et al. 2014). Given the many complications associated with diabetes there is evidence to suggest that diabetes and the associated symptoms can function as motivating operations. For example, Valdovinos and Weyand (2006) found that for one young girl with poorly regulated Type 1 diabetes, aggression and SIB were more likely to occur in demand situations when her blood glucose levels were outside of her normal range.

Allergic rhinitis and associated conditions. Allergic rhinitis, commonly known as allergies, often develops in childhood and is quite prevalent, with approximately 40 % of the pediatric population afflicted (Blaiss 2008). Allergies can impact many facets of life (e.g., sleep) and can cause several other health issues such as otitis media, sinusitis, and asthma. Furthermore, allergies have been reported to create anxiety or hyper-aroused physiological states (Gupta et al. 2006; Tonelli et al. 2009). All of the secondary conditions associated with allergies can function as setting events if left untreated or unmanaged. Considering otitis media, for example, research has demonstrated how a toddler, when otitis media was present, was more likely to engage in SIB in the presence of loud noise within various conditions of a functional assessment than when her ears were free of infection (O'Reilly 1997).

Seizure disorders. Seizure disorders are another common secondary condition found within the IDD population. Reported prevalence rates vary from 30 % to 50 %, with different rates associated with specific disorders (i.e., higher prevalence in those with autism than those with IDD alone) and an increased probability of a seizure disorder associated with level of IDD (i.e., more severe the disability the more likely the disorder) (Caplan and Austin 2000; Depositario-Cabacar and Zelleke 2010). Within recent years, greater attention has been focused on the relationship between seizure disorders and challenging behaviors. Specifically, a seizure disorder seems to account for the presence of challenging behaviors in individuals with ID (Smith and Matson 2010). Although causation has not been determined, additional research has found a temporal relationship between the occurrence of challenging behavior and seizure activity (Roberts et al. 2005). Interestingly, the antiepileptic medications commonly prescribed to treat seizure disorders in individuals with IDD often have psychoactive effects that subsequently impacts challenging behaviors as well as seizure activity (Coffey 2013). Treatment with antiepileptic medication is not without side effects and often these side effects necessitate changes in medication which may subsequently produce changes in seizure activity and challenging behaviors (Scheepers et al. 2004). Thus, both the seizure activity and the medications prescribed to reduce the activity warrant consideration in assessing treatments for challenging behavior.

Neurocognitive disorders. Consistent with the general population's increase in the prevalence of neurocognitive disorders, there is a corresponding elevation among people with IDD (Bishop et al. 2013; Cooper 1997). In particular, Alzheimer's disease is associated with general declines in health and physical functioning (Liu-Seifert et al. 2015). Medications may be prescribed to address and decrease the progression of cognitive and physical decline. Although it may seem that challenging behaviors associated with neurocognitive disorders may not be amendable via behavioral assessment and treatment, research with both the aging general population (Baker et al. 2006; Raetz et al. 2013) and IDD population (Millichap et al. 2003) suggests otherwise.

Sleep deprivation. People with IDD experience sleep difficulties such as night waking or broken sleep, early morning waking, difficulty in falling asleep, and lack of deep or REM sleep (Boyle et al. 2010; Didden et al. 2002). There are various biological contributors, including altered serotonin levels (Tordjman et al. 2013), sleep apnea, medication (Rapp et al. 2007), and pain (Breau and Camfield 2011), as well as environmentally influenced factors associated with daily schedules, activity level, lighting, and caregiver response (Figueiro et al. 2014; Mindell et al. 2015; Tatsumi et al. 2014). Regardless of the causes of the disruption in sleep, sleep deprivation has been found to also function as a variable that influences the likelihood of challenging behavior (Schwichtenberg et al. 2013; Symons et al. 2000), the frequency or rate of behavior (Kennedy and Meyer 1996), the topography of behavior (O'Reilly and Lancioni 2000) and the conditions under which challenging behavior is more likely to occur (O'Reilly 1995; O'Reilly and Lancioni 2000).

Psychotropic medication. In addition to the questions concerning the effectiveness of psychotropic medication for treating challenging behavior, there is uncertainty about the impact of known and unknown, short- and long-term adverse behavioral (Valdovinos and Kennedy 2004). Individuals diagnosed with IDD are just as likely, if not more so, to experience adverse side effects of psychotropic medication (Valdovinos et al. 2005). However, communication deficits make it difficult for people with IDD to report side effects. As well, diagnostic overshadowing decreases the likelihood even further that those side effects will be identified. Furthermore, there is evidence to suggest that the more medications one takes the greater the likelihood of experiencing more side effects (Sommi et al. 1998).

Missed identification of side effects is understandable because they can be subtle in presentation but have significant impacts on behavior. For example, risperidone has been known to produce muscle tension and headaches (Bryne et al. 2010). Stimulants, such as methylphenidate, may produce stomachaches, headaches, and irritable mood (Aman 1996; Karabekirogulu et al. 2008). What remains to be determined is how these side effects might impact the behavior these medications are prescribed to treat. Preliminary research, however, has found that medications can alter the severity of problem behaviors (i.e., SIB and aggression) (Matson et al. 2009); conditions under which challenging behavior is likely to occur (Crossland et al. 2003; Northup et al. 1999; Zarcone et al. 2004); and the effectiveness of reinforcers (Larue et al. 2008; Northup et al. 1997).

Assessment Methods for Diagnosis of Conditions

It is essential to determine if health conditions are present prior to addressing problematic behavior. Ruling out any existing health conditions before assessing environmental conditions that might account for challenging behavior is particularly crucial if the behavior appears suddenly or if there are sudden changes in topography, frequency, severity, or conditions under which behavior occurs. Some of the conditions discussed in this chapter may be identified via direct observation or clinical observation/examinations in the form of sleep studies, blood chemistry, and neuroimaging. However, isolating other conditions such as pain, neurocognitive disorders, and medication side effects may require an altogether different assessment, as reviewed below.

Assessing the presence of pain. The relationship between pain, challenging behavior, and pain expression is specific to the individual. Valid measures have been developed to identify the presence of pain in individuals with IDD, for example, the *Non-Communicating Children Pain Checklist and Non-Communicating Adult Pain Checklist* (Lotan et al. 2010; McGrath et al. 1998). Also, it is informative establish a baseline measure of pain (de Knegt et al. 2013) using an instrument such as the *Individualized Numeric Rating Scale* (Solodiuk et al. 2010). Once a baseline has been established, routine evaluations can be completed or evaluations can be done if changes in both challenging and adaptive behavior occur.

Assessing the presence of neurocognitive disorder. Assessing the presence of neurocognitive disorders is sometimes complicated by physicians or other professionals attributing symptoms to a person's intellectual disability instead of changes in mental status (Bishop et al. 2013;Prasher et al. 2007). This issue raises the importance of conducting baseline assessments in level of functioning while individuals with ID are not symptomatic. When baseline assessments are conducted, it is easier to track changes in behavior when neurocognitive disorders are suspected. Although many assessment tools are available for diagnosing Alzheimer's disease, not all are suitable for people with IDD. Routine assessments should target motor function and daily living skills, physical conditions, blood chemistry, hearing, vision, health, and psychiatric and neuropsychological status. It is further recommended that early screening and evaluation for neurocognitive disorders be conducted with adults who have Down syndrome as they are more likely to develop Alzheimer's disease (Prasher et al. 2007). Some standardized assessments that can be used include: *Adaptive Behavior Dementia Questionnaire* (Prasher 2009) and the *Dementia Screening Questionnaire for Individuals with Intellectual Disabilities* (Deb et al. 2007).

Assessing medication side effects. Many recommendations have been made to measure the impact of psychotropic medication on challenging behavior (Zarcone et al. 2008). Conversely, there is great difficulty in assessing the presence of medication side effects (Deb et al. 2009). As already stated, diagnosing biological variables is the first step in determining the etiology of challenging behavior and evaluating if medication side effects are impacting this behavior. This section addresses medication side effects broadly as many medications prescribed to those with ID produce side effects. For example, anticonvulsant medications have been found to more commonly impact affect, gait, and weight in individuals with ID (Sipes et al. 2011). Thus, biological measures include blood chemistry, urine analysis, and clinical indicators (Zarcone et al. 2008). The method for assessing the presence of side effects via direct observation are usually rating scales for specific side effects such as akathisia (*Abnormal Involuntary Movement Scale* [*AIMS*]) (Guy 1976) or broader side effects (e.g., *Matson Evaluation of Drug Side Effects Scale* [*MEDS*]) (Matson et al. 1998). Monitoring of side effects should occur while an individual is on a stable dose of medication and when medication dose and type changes.

Assessments to Determine the Impact of Health Condition on Challenging Behavior

Multiple assessment approaches can be used to determine the impact of identified health conditions on challenging behavior. For instance, monitoring the severity of symptoms, the frequency and severity of challenging behavior, and diurnal patterns can provide important information. Ultimately, however, determining how these health conditions impact the conditions under which challenging behaviors occur provide the greatest opportunity to reduce behavior and maximize one's quality of life.

Functional analysis. Conducting a functional analysis (FA) is one method for determining the causes of challenging behavior and subsequently developing the most appropriate behavioral intervention. An FA is an experimental assessment for identifying the "purpose" of challenging behavior by systematically presenting and removing conditions to mirror natural contingencies thought to maintain challenging behavior (Iwata et al. 1994). These manipulations test whether behavior is maintained by negative reinforcement, positive reinforcement, and/or automatic (non-socially mediated) reinforcement. Often, an interview is conducted prior to the FA to determine what variables may be controlling behavior. Typically, the FA includes alone, social attention, control, demand, and tangible conditions (Hanley et al. 2003). The *alone* condition is conducted to test for an automatic reinforcement hypothesis by observing an individual with social interaction and access to materials This condition is not conducted if the possibility of automatically maintained problem behavior is not likely (e.g., most aggression). The *social attention* condition assesses a social, positive reinforcement hypothesis. During these sessions, the individual has free access to items or toys that are moderately preferred and demands are withheld. Contingent on each occurrence of a targeted challenging behavior, a therapist provides attention to the individual. The *control* condition is conducted to serve as a means of diagnostic comparison. During these sessions, the individual has free access to several preferred toys and a therapist is present for the duration of the session while providing non-contingent attention and withholding demands. The *demand* condition assesses a social, negative reinforcement hypothesis: a therapist typically presents demands to the individual using a three-step hierarchical prompting sequence of verbal, gestural, and physical prompts. If the individual complies with the demand before the physical prompt (i.e., the third step of hierarchal prompting), the therapist provides contingent verbal praise. Contingent on the occurrence of challenging behavior, the therapist briefly withdraws demands. Finally, the *tangible* condition is conducted to test for a social, positive reinforcement hypothesis. Prior to the start of the session, the individual is provided access to a highly preferred item(s) and when the session begins, the therapist removes them.

Via an FA, one can also evaluate the potential impact that health conditions have on challenging behavior as well (O'Neill et al. 1997). These physiological variables are conceptualized as motivating operations, namely variables that impact the relative value of reinforcers by either increasing the effectiveness of a stimulus or decreasing the effectiveness of a stimulus as a reinforcer (Laraway et al. 2003; Michael 1982). By creating manipulations that directly impact or interact with the existing physiological state, one can test how this state influences the relationship between behavior and environment.

Functional analysis of biological setting events. First, functional assessment methodology can be used to determine the impact that *predictable* health events can have on behavior. For example, dysmenorrhea, a condition in which menstruation is accompanied by pain, is common in typically developing females at an estimated prevalence of 16–91 %. And 2–29 % of these females experiencing severe pain (Ju et al. 2014). Given the estimated prevalence, females diagnosed with ID are also likely to experience dysmenorrhea. Notably, Carr et al. (2003) provided a model for assessing the impact that pain associated with menstruation can have on problem behavior in women with IDD. Specifically, information regarding the health status and behavior of individuals was collected and this information in addition to data collected via direct observations was used to develop FA conditions. Researchers were able to determine how the pain experienced monthly impacted problem behavior during these activities.

Functional assessment methodology can also be used to discover *potential* biological events that may be impacting problem behavior. That is, when results of an FA suggest that problem behavior appears to be "automatically" maintained, an underlying health condition could be present and account for the indiscriminate results of the FA (Hanley et al. 2003). Carter (2005) conducted an FA for a young boy with a history of sinus infections who engaged in SIB. The initial FA results were undifferentiated, suggesting an automatic function; however, when the FA was repeated in the absence of a sinus infection, the result revealed near-zero rates of SIB. Indeed, it is possible that SIB was maintained by automatic reinforcement—manipulation of the pain associated with the sinus infection—a relationship discovered via the FA.

Furthermore, manipulations can be made to motivating operations within a functional analysis to target hypothesized underlying biological events. For example, research was conducted in which assessments were completed prior to and following meals for one child and the quantity of food eaten by another child were altered, both of whom presented with feeding problems and self-injury (Wacker et al. 1996). The results of this study provided the opportunity to evaluate how food satiation differentially impacted the rate of self-injury.

Functional analysis of medication effects. This FA methodology has also been employed to examine how individual medications impact the conditions under which challenging behavior occurs. For example, early studies evaluated the interactive effects between psychotropic medication treatment and behavioral interventions on problem behavior (Fisher et al. 1989) and how psychotropic medication could impact behavior hypothesized to be maintained by either multiple variables or via automatic reinforcement. The findings of this research suggested that psychotropic medication could have discriminate effects on both the conditions under which problem behavior occurred as well as the topography of behavior affected.

Since these first studies were published, more research has been conducted in the area. The impact of methylphenidate on responding within various tests of behavioral contingencies has been evaluated extensively (Northup et al. 1997, 1999; Larue et al. 2008). This line of research demonstrated that methylphenidate appears to alter the reinforcing magnitude of social positive reinforcement, specifically attention. For example, in one study, when children received methylphenidate they were more likely to choose playing with friends as an outcome for on-task behavior (i.e., math problem completion) than when they were taking a placebo (Northup et al. 1997). An additional study found that the rate of problem behaviors decreased more when methylphenidate (rather than placebo) was used in conjunction with verbal reprimands (rather than extinction) (Northup et al. 1999). Furthermore, researchers found that the dose of stimulant seemed to impact reinforcer magnitude differentially, that is to say, when participants were receiving a higher versus lower dose of medication, participants responded to gain access to social/play interaction rather than spend time alone or engaged in quiet activities (Larue et al. 2008).

In October of 2006, risperidone was approved by the Federal Drug Administration for the treatment of irritability associated with autism. This approval was granted, in part, based on a number of clinical trials of risperidone. Within one of these clinical trials, adjunctive research was conducted evaluating the functional effects of risperidone on problem behavior. Using a double-blind, placebo-controlled, crossover design, Zarcone et al. (2004) found that participants' problem behavior decreased discriminately only in demand conditions when receiving risperidone (Crosland et al. 2003). Zarcone et al. (2004) also found that for ten out of thirteen total participants, risperidone effectively reduced problem behavior. For three of these participants, risperidone discriminately decreased behaviors in the demand conditions. Overall, risperidone appears to have the greatest impact on those behaviors maintained by negative reinforcement. Incidentally, this finding is also supported by the basic literature in which rate of avoidance responding is suppressed in those animals given atypical antipsychotics (e.g., Arenas et al. 1999; Rodriguez 1992; Shannon et al. 1999).

The majority of research using FA methodology to evaluate medication effects has focused upon the impact of single medication use which provides great insight into how a specific medication can alter the behavior/environment relationship. However, the prescription practices in this population are complex. In most cases, people with IDD are prescribed multiple medications (Deb et al. 2015). And yet, only a few studies have been conducted to evaluate if and how modifying one of multiple medications can impact behavior function (e.g., Valdovinos et al. 2007, 2009). This line of research is valuable because the findings could reveal that any alterations in medication necessitate re-evaluation of behavior function and possibly other health conditions that might impact behavior. For example, recent research has demonstrated that rates of challenging behavior can rise after psychotropic medication changes but this increase in behavior can be temporary or can be mitigated by changes in other variables such as sleep (Rapp et al. 2007). Thus behavior monitoring needs to be continuous and expanded beyond the period of time after changes in medication are made.

Preference and reinforce assessments. Preference and reinforce assessments can provide valuable information when developing and implementing effective treatments. Furthermore, these assessments have been hypothesized to demonstrate how medications may alter the relative value of stimuli (Carlson et al. 2012). By extension, if medication effects on reinforcer value can be identified via preference or reinforcer assessments, it is conceivable that the effects other health conditions on preference and reinforcer value can also be assessed. For example, preliminary research on preferences in adults with neurocognitive disorders suggests that reinforcers can be identified using standard preference assessment procedures (Raetz et al. 2013). Furthermore, the outcomes from these preference assessments were used to successfully promote engagement in activities. For those health conditions that are recurring such as menstruation and ear infections, identifying changes in preferences or reinforcer magnitude may provide direction for antecedent modifications to address challenging behavior (e.g., offer access to different reinforcers during work completion, reduce noise levels).

As posited, although medication effects can function as motivating operations that ultimately impact the likelihood of behavior, behavior is dynamic and may change over time as a result of maturational changes, physiological conditions, physical environmental conditions, and contextual effects. For example, in the Larue et al. (2008) study, researchers discovered gradual changes in the selection of coupons traded for access to playtime with friends, alone playtime, or quiet time. These changes were then attributed to the different medication conditions assessed. It is unclear, however, if the changes observed in coupon selection were due solely to medication manipulations or to other factors such as the potential relationships that participants developed with the children with whom they played. Medication side effects are another potential variable that may account for any changes in the probability of behavior (Valdovinos and Kennedy 2004). For example, methylphenidate can suppress appetite and reduce the reinforcing magnitude of food. Despite intuitive speculation, empirical work needs to be undertaken to fully comprehend if and how medication side effects are altering the dimensions of the behaviors that these medications are prescribed to treat.

Treatment Recommendation of Challenging Behavior Associated with Health Conditions

When addressing challenging behavior, two general approaches can be taken and in instances where health conditions are also present. Finding effective ways to address the condition and the setting events they present is integral to reducing problem behavior and improving the quality of life of individuals with ID. These approaches involve either targeting the antecedents to problem behavior (i.e., setting events, motivating operations, discriminative stimuli) or manipulating consequences of problem behavior. Given that health conditions warrant treatment, antecedent-based interventions should be included as a part of the behavior plan. However, behaviors that occur in response to antecedent conditions can persist even when the health condition is remedied. Thus, understanding why and how a behavior developed and assessing possible contingencies for the behavior's maintenance is often necessary.

Antecedent-based interventions. Although recommended routine health checks are in place, research demonstrates that few providers actually completed the recommended checks for individuals with ID. For example, Teeluckdharry et al. (2013) found that only a third of psychiatrists monitored weight and blood sugar when prescribing antipsychotic medication to patients with IDD. Although formal methods for assessing side effects of psychotropic medications are limited, their presence has been found to impact the likelihood of and at times the severity of problem behavior (e.g., Matson et al. 2009; Valdovinos et al. 2005). Regardless of the medication status of an individual, routine blood work, urinalysis, weight, blood pressure, mammograms, and colonoscopies should be completed as indicated by the condition, age of the individual and identified risk factors. Caregivers can also conduct brief daily assessments of overall health. For example, checking temperature and pulse as well as the appearance of eyes, skin and throat, may lead to faster identification of illness that could impact behavior. Once health conditions are identified, they can be treated or managed as a part of antecedent-based intervention.

Antecedent-based approaches are valuable because by treating or managing the health condition, the potential motivating operation of the problem behavior is being addressed. Using the information gathered from assessments, including routine health assessments, physical sources of pain or discomfort can be addressed and any setting events or motivating operations for problem behavior can be treated.

Treating a health condition, however, is not the only available antecedent manipulation. Individuals with IDD can be taught to label their discomfort and either communicate the existence of a health condition to caregivers (e.g., Carr et al. 2003) or address the condition themselves. For example, in working with a child diagnosed with Williams syndrome and hyperacusis (a condition in which one is hypersensitive to sound), O'Reilly et al. (2000) were able to decrease problem behavior by having him wear earplugs to reduce noise level. Teaching individuals with IDD how to use smart technology to monitor health conditions, such as diabetes, has also been demonstrated to have positive effects in the prevention of more severe illness and can provide a method for communicating physical distress (Haymes et al. 2013).

Identifying and addressing common antecedents to challenging behavior can also be effective when addressing problems associated with neurocognitive decline. For example, pain, hunger, fatigue, and over or under-stimulation are setting events that can be anticipated to affect behavior From an intervention perspective, it is possible to reduce challenging behavior by scheduling daily routines with simple and visual prompts (Bayles and Kim 2003; Buchanan et al. 2011; Mace and Rabins 2011). Rarely, however, will antecedent procedures be the sole focus of an effective intervention. The best plans will be those that address both the environmental and biological contributors of behavior (Langthorne et al. 2007).

Consequence-based interventions. As already mentioned, once medical conditions have been addressed, the motivating operations for challenging behavior may have been eliminated but the behaviors persist albeit under different conditions. Thus, completing functional assessments during the presence of the medical condition and once the medical condition has been addressed are imperative for successful outcomes. Once the function of challenging behaviors has been identified, behavior support plans can be developed that address the behavior under both conditions. Successful plans will target any precursor behavior that may suggest presence of a medical condition, specify what the condition is, and instruct how to remediate the condition. Although research addressing the intersection between physiology and behavior is somewhat limited, addressing functional assessment outcomes provides the strongest basis for treatment.

With regard to chronic health conditions such as neurocognitive disorders, challenging behavior may become more severe or frequent due to declines in cognitive functioning and communication abilities. Despite the decline, consequence-based interventions can maintain daily living skills such as dressing, feeding, washing, and communication (Buchanan et al. 2011). Functionally-related interventions can also be developed to reduce challenging behavior associated with neurocognitive decline. For example, Baker et al. (2006) nearly eliminated escape-maintained aggression with non-contingent escape from bathroom routines. Although the participant in this study did not have IDD diagnosis, the results support similar functionally-derived interventions with this population.

With regard to stable medication use, research has also suggested that interventions can be designed to address changes in functional relations between behavior and the environment. The reality is that psychotropic medications are commonly used to address challenging behavior. However, changing challenging behavior with medication alone is one dimensional and a more preferred method is a balanced, interdisciplinary treatment approach, which integrates psychotropic medication and behavioral interventions (Hassiotis and Hall 2008; Huang et al. 2007). And although progress has been made in evaluating the effects that medication has on the functional relationship between behavior and reinforcers, there is limited research investigating combined behavioral and pharmacological treatment (Weeden et al. 2009). Understanding how function-based behavioral interventions and targeted medication prescription may interact could possibly improve the efficacy of combined treatments. For example, Dicesare et al. (2005) found that when one participant was taking methylphenidate rates of problem behavior decreased in conditions when attention was delivered contingently. Mace et al. (2009) also found that an alternate form of methylphenidate in conjunction with behavioral treatment decreased the rate of problem behavior in conditions where attention was manipulated.

Conclusion

Although this chapter addressed very specific medical conditions that can impact challenging behavior in people with IDD, it would be wrong to assume that there are no other conditions that could similarly impact behavior. Unfortunately, learning how to tact or identify alterations in one's physiology can be a difficult skill to teach. In the absence of this repertoire, the focus of any support plan should be to routinely screen all individuals with IDD for any detectable causes of distress such as tooth abscess, ear infection, sinus infection, hernias, and fractured/broken limbs. For more subtle conditions that may not be readily apparent (e.g., menstrual discomfort, headaches, gastrointestinal distress, neurocognitive decline), patterns of behavior should be evaluated. Identifying patterns should not be limited to challenging behavior; however, as changes in adaptive behavior could also suggest the presence of medical conditions. Monitoring eating habits, sleep, grooming, social interaction, and engagement in leisure/preferred activities may suggest the need for further evaluation of potential medical conditions. By addressing both biological and environmental stimuli affecting behavior, challenging behaviors can be better understood and addressed successfully.

References

Aman, M. G. (1996). Stimulant drugs in the developmental disabilities revisited. *Journal of Developmental and Physical Disabilities, 3*, 347–365.

Aman, M. G., & Singh, N. N. (1988). Patterns of drug use, methodological considerations, measurement techniques, and future trends. In M. G. Aman & N. N. Singh (Eds.), *Psychopharmacology of the developmental disabilities* (pp. 1–28). New Yok: Springer.

Anwar, A. J., Walker, J. D., & Frier, B. M. (1998). Type 1 diabetes metllitus and Down's syndrome: Prevalence, management and diabetic complications. *Diabetic Medicine, 15*, 160-163

Arenas, M. C., Vinader-Caerols, C., Monleón, S., Parra, A., & Simón, V. M. (1999). Dose dependency of sex differences in the effects of repeated haloperidol administration in avoidance conditioning in mice. *Pharmacology, Biochemistry, and Behavior, 62*, 703-709

Baker, J. C., Hanley, G. P., & Mathews, R. M. (2006). Staff-administered functional analysis and treatment of aggression by an elder with dementia. *Journal of Applied Behavior Analysis, 39*, 469–474.

Bayles, K. A., & Kim, E. S. (2003). Improving the functioning of individuals with Alzheimer's disease: Emergence of behavioral interventions. *Journal of Communication Disorders, 36*(5), 327–343.

Bishop, K. M., Robinson, L. M., & VanLare, S. (2013). Healthy aging for older adults with intellectual and developmental disabilities. *Journal of Psychosocial Nursing, 51*, 15–18.

Blaiss, M. S. (2008). Pediatric allergic rhinitis: Physical and mental complications. *Allergy and Asthma Proceedings, 29*, 1–6.

Boerlage, A. A., Valkenburg, A. J., Scherder, E. J. A., Steenhof, G., Effing, P., Tibboel, D., et al. (2013). Prevalence of pain in institutionalized adults with intellectual disabilities: A cross-sectional approach. *Research in Developmental Disabilities, 34*, 2399–2406.

Boyle, A., Melville, C., Morrison, J., Allan, L., Smiley, E., Espie, C. A., et al. (2010). A cohort study of the prevalence of sleep problems in adults with intellectual disabilities. *Journal of Sleep Research, 19*, 42–53.

Breau, L. M., & Camfield, C. S. (2011). Pain disrupts sleep in children and youth with intellectual and developmental disabilities. *Research in Developmental Disabilities, 32*, 2829–2840.
Breau, L. M., Camfield, C. S., McGrath, P. J., & Finley, G. A. (2003a). The incidence of pain in children with severe cognitive impairments. *Archives of Pediatric and Adolescent Medicine, 157,* 1219-1226.
Breau, L. M., Camfield, C. S., Symons, F. J., Bodfish, J. W., Mackay, A., Finley, G. A., et al. (2003b). Relation between pain and self-injurious behavior in nonverbal children with severe cognitive impairments. *Journal of Pediatrics, 142,* 498-503.
Buchanan, J. A., Christenson, A., Houlihan, D., & Ostrom, C. (2011). The role of behavior analysis in the rehabilitation of persons with dementia. *Behavior Therapy, 42*, 9–21.
Byrne, S., Walter, G., Hunt, G., Soh, N., Cleary, M., & Duffy, P., et al. (2010). Self-reported side effects in children and adolescents taking risperidone. *Australian Psychiatry, 18*, 42–45.
Caplan, R., & Austin, J. K. (2000). Behavioral aspects of epilepsy in children with mental retardation. *Mental Retardation and Developmental Disabilities Research Reviews, 6*, 293–299.
Carlson, G., Pokrzywinski, J., Uran, K., & Valdovinos, M. G. (2012). The use of reinforcer assessments in evaluating psychotropic medication effects. *Journal of Developmental and Physical Disabilities, 24*, 515–528.
Carr, E. G., Smith, C. E., Giancin, T. A., Whelan, B. M., & Pancari, J. (2003). Menstrual discomfort as a biological setting event for severe problem behavior: Assessment and intervention. *American Journal on Mental Retardation, 108*, 117–133.
Carter, S. L. (2005). An empirical analysis of the effects of a possible sinus infection and weighted vest on functional analysis outcomes of self-injury exhibited by a child with autism. *Journal of Early and Intensive Behavioral Intervention, 2*, 252–258.
Coffey, M. J. (2013). Resolution of self-injury with phenytoin in a man with autism and intellectual disability. *Journal of ECT, 29*, e12–e13.
Cooper, S. A. (1997). High prevalence of dementia among people with learning disabilities not attributable to Down's syndrome. *Psychological Medicine, 27*, 609–616.
Courtemanche, A., Schoeder, S., Sheldon, J., Sherman, J., & Fowler, A. (2012). Observing signs of pain in relation to self-injurious behaviour among individuals with intellectual and developmental disabilities. *Journal of Intellectual Disability Research, 56*, 501–515.
Crosland, K. A., Zarcone, J. R., Lindauer, S. E., Valdovinos, M. G., Zarcone, T. J., Hellings, J. A., et al. (2003). Use of functional analysis methodology in the evaluation of medication effects. *Journal of Autism and Developmental Disorders, 33*, 271–279.
de Knegt, N. C., Pieper, M. J. C., Lobbezoo, F., Schuengel, C., Evenhuis, H. M., Passchier, J., et al. (2013). Behavioral pain indicators in people with intellectual disabilities: A systematic review. *The Journal of Pain, 14*, 885–896.
de Winter, C. F., Jansen, A. A. C., & Evenhuis, H. M. (2011). Physical conditions and challenging behaviour in people with intellectual disability: A systematic review. *Journal of Intellectual Disability Research, 55*, 675–698.
Deb, S., Hare, M., Prior, L., & Bhaumik, S. (2007). Dementia screening questionnaire for individuals with intellectual disabilities (DSQIID). *British Journal of Psychiatry, 190*, 440–444.
Deb, S., Kwok, H., Bertelli, M., Salvador-Carulla, L., Bradley, E., Torr, J., et al. (2009). International guide to prescribing psychotropic medication for the management of problem behaviours in adults with intellectual disabilities. *World Psychiatry, 8*, 181–186.
Deb, S., Unwin, G., & Deb, T. (2015). Characteristics and the trajectory of psychotropic medication use in general and antipsychotics in particular among adults with an intellectual disability who exhibit aggressive behaviour. *Journal of Intellectual Disability Research, 59*(1), 11–25.
Despositario-Cabacaer, D. F. T., & Zelleke, T. G. (2010). Treatment of epilepsy in children with developmental disabilities. *Developmental Disability Research Reviews, 16*, 239–247.
Dicesare, A., McAdam, D. B., Toner, A., & Varrell, J. (2005). The effects of methylphenidate on a functional analysis of disruptive behavior: a replication and extension. *Journal of Applied Behavior Analysis, 38*, 125–128.

Didden, R., Korzilius, H., van Aperio, B., van Overloop, C., & de Vries, M. (2002). Sleep problems and daytime problem behaviours in children with intellectual disability. *Journal of Intellectual Disability Research, 46*, 537–547.

Figueiro, M. G., Plitnick, B., & Rea, M. S. (2014). The effects of chronotype, sleep schedule and light/dark pattern exposures on circadian phase. *Sleep Medicine, 15,* 1554-1564.

Fisher, W., Piazza, C. C., & Page, T. G. (1989). Assessing independent and interactive effects of behavioral and pharmacological interventions for a client with dual diagnosis. *Journal of Behavior Therapy and Experimental Psychiatry, 20*, 241–250.

Galli-Carminati, G., Chauvet, I., & Deriaz, N. (2006). Prevalence of gastrointestinal disorders in adult clients with pervasive developmental disorders. *Journal of Intellectual Disability Research, 50*, 711–718.

Gupta, S., Crawford, S. G., & Mitchell, I. (2006). Screening children with asthma for psychosocial adjustment problems: A tool for health care professionals. *Journal of Asthma, 43*, 543–548.

Guy W. (1976). *ECDEU Assessment Manual for Psychopharmacology* (pp. 534–537). Washington DC: US Department of Health, Education and Welfare.

Hanley, G. P., Iwata, B. A., & McCord, B. E. (2003). Functional analysis of problem behavior: A review. *Journal of Applied Behavior Analysis, 36*, 147–185.

Hartman, E. C., Gilles, E., McComas, J. J., Danov, S. E., & Symons, F. J. (2008). Clinical observation of self-injurious behavior correlated with changes in scalp morphology in a child with congenital hydropcephalus. *Journal of Child Neurology, 23*, 1062–1065.

Hassiotis, A. A., & Hall, I. (2008). Behavioural and cognitive-behavioural interventions for outwardly-directed aggressive behaviour in people with learning disabilities. *Cochrane Database of Systematic Reviews, 16*(3), CD003406.

Haymes, L. K., Storey, K., Maldonado, A., Post, M., & Montgomery, J. (2013). Using applied behavior analysis and smart technology for meeting the health needs of individuals with intellectual disabilities. *Developmental Neurorehabilitation*, early online, 1–13. doi:10.3109/17518423.2013.850750.

Hermans, H., & Evenhuis, H. M. (2014). Multimorbidity in older adults with intellectual disabilities. *Research in Developmental Disabilities, 35*, 776–783.

Horvath, K., Papadimitriou, J. C., Rabsztyn, A., Drachenberg, C., & Tildon, J. T. (1999). Gastrointestinal abnormalities in children with autistic disorder. *Journal of Pediatrics, 135*, 559–563.

Huang, W., O'Brien, H. R., Kalinowski, C. M., Vreeland, R. G., Kleinbub, L., & Hall, G. A. (2007). Multidisciplinary approach to optimizing pharmacological and behavioral interventions for person with developmental disabilities who are on psychotropic medications. *Journal of Developmental Physical Disabilities, 19*, 237–250.

Iwata, B. A., Dorsey, M. F., Slifer, K. J., Bauman, K. E., & Richman, G. S. (1994). Toward a functional analysis of self-injury. *Journal of Applied Behavior Analysis, 27*, 197–209.

Ju, H., Jones, M., & Mishra, G. (2014). The prevalence and risk factors of dysmenorrhea. *Epidemiology Reviews, 36*, 104–113.

Karabekirogulu, K., Yazgan, Y. M., & Dedeoglu, D. (2008). Can we predict short-term side effects of methylphenidate immediate-release? *International Journal of Psychiatry in Clinical Practice, 12*, 48–54.

Kennedy, C. H., & Meyer, K. A. (1996). Sleep deprivation, allergy symptoms, and negatively reinforced problem behavior. *Journal of Applied Behavior Analysis, 29*, 133–135.

Kidd, S. A., Lachiewicz, A., Barbouth, D., Blitz, R. K., Delahunty, C., McBrien, D., et al. (2014). Fragile X syndrome: A review of associated medical problems. *Pediatrics, 134*, 995–1005.

Langthorne, P., McGill, P., & O'Reilly, M. (2007). Incorporating "motivation" into the functional analysis of challenging behavior: On the interactive and integrative potential of the motivating operation. *Behavior Modification, 31*(4), 466–487.

Laraway, S., Snycerski, S., Michael, J., & Poling, A. (2003). Motivating operations and terms to describe them: Some further refinements. *Journal of Applied Behavior Analysis, 36*, 407–414.

Larue, R. H, Jr, Northup, J., Baumeister, A. A., Hawkins, M. F., Seale, L., Williams, T., et al. (2008). An evaluation of stimulant medication on the reinforcing effects of play. *Journal of Applied Behavior Analysis, 41*, 143–147.

Liu-Seifert, H., Siemers, E., Sundell, K., Price, K., Han, B., Selzler, K., et al. (2015). Cognitive and functional decline and their relationship in patients with mild Alzheimer's dementia. *Journal of Alzheimers Disease, 43*, 949–955.

Lotan, M., Moe-Nilssen, R., Ljunggren, A., & Strand, L. (2010). Measurement properties of the non-communicating adult pain checklist (NCAPC): A pain scale for adults with intellectual and developmental disabilities, scored in a clinical setting. *Research in Developmental Disabilities, 31*, 367–375.

Lott, I. T., McGregor, M., Engelman, L., Touchette, P., Tournay, A., Sandman, C., et al. (2004). Longitudinal prescribing patterns for psychoactive medications in community-based individuals with developmental disabilities: Utilization of pharmacy records. *Journal of Intellectual Disability Research, 48*(6), 563–571.

Mace, F. C., Prager, K. L., Thomas, K., Kochy, J., Dyer, T. J., Perry, L., et al. (2009). Effects of stimulant medication under varied motivational operations. *Journal of Applied Behavior Analysis, 42*, 177–183.

Mace, N. L., & Rabins, P. V. (2011). *The 36-hour day: A family guide to caring for people who have Alzheimer disease, related dementias, and memory loss* (5th ed.). Baltimore: John Hopkins University Press.

Matson, J. L., Fodstad, J. C., Rivet, T. T., & Rojahn, J. (2009). Behavioral and psychiatric differences in medication side effects in adults with severe intellectual disabilities. *Journal of Mental Health Research in Intellectual Disabilities, 2*, 261–278.

Matson, J. L., Mayville, E. A., Bielecki, J., Barnes, W. H., Bamburg, J. W., & Baglio, C. S. (1998). Reliability of the matson evaluation of drug side effects scale (MEDS). *Research in Developmental Disabilities, 19*, 501–506.

Mayville, E. A. (2007). Psychotropic medication effects and side effects. *International Review of Research in Mental Retardation, 34*, 227–251.

McGrath, P. J., Rosmus, C., Canfield, C., Campbell, M. A., & Hennigar, A. (1998). Behaviours caregivers use to determine pain in non-verbal, cognitively impaired individuals. *Developmental Medicine and Child Neurology, 40*, 340–343.

McVilly, K., McGillivray, J., Curtis, A., Lehmann, J., Morrish, L., & Speight, J. (2014). Diabetes in people with an intellectual disability: A systematic review of prevalence, incidence and impact. *Diabetic Medicine, 31*(8), 897–904.

Michael, J. (1982). Distinguishing between discriminative and motivational functions of stimuli. *Journal of the Experimental Analysis of Behavior, 37*, 149–155.

Millichap, D., Oliver, C., McQuillan, S., Kalsy, S., Lloyd, V., & Hall, S. (2003). Descriptive functional analysis of behavioral excess shown by adults with Down syndrome and dementia. *International Journal of Geriatric Psychiatry, 18*, 844–854.

Mindell, J. A., Li, A. M., Sadeh, A., Kwon, R. & Goh, D. Y. (2015). Bedtime routines for young children: A dose-dependent association with sleep outcomes. *Sleep, 38*, 717-722.

Ming, X., Brimacombe, M., Chaaban, J., Zimmerman-Bier, B., & Wagner, G. C. (2014). Autism spectrum disorders: Concurrent clinical disorders. *Journal of Child Neurology, 23*, 6–13.

Moss, S., & Patel, P. (1997). Dementia in older people with intellectual disability: Symptoms of physical and mental illness, and levels of adaptive behaviour. *Journal of Intellectual Disability Research, 41*(1), 60–69.

Musil, R., Obermeier, M., Russ, P., & Hamerle, M. (2015). Weight gain and antipsychotics: A drug safety review. *Expert Opinion on Drug Safety, 14*, 73–96.

Northup, J., Fusilier, I., Swanson, V., Huete, J., Bruce, T., Freeland, J., et al. (1999). Further analysis of the separate and interactive effects of methylphenidate and common classroom contingencies. *Journal of Applied Behavior Analysis, 32*, 35–50.

Northup, J., Fusilier, I., Swanson, V., Roane, H., & Borrero, J. (1997). An evaluation of methylphenidate as a potential establishing operation for some common classroom reinforcers. *Journal of Applied Behavior Analysis, 30*, 615–625.

O'Neill, R. E., Horner, R. H., Albin, R. W., Sprague, J. R., Storey, K., & Newton, J. S. (1997). *Functional Assessment and Program Development for Problem Behavior*. Pacific Grove, CA: Brooks/Cole Publishing.

O'Reilly, M. F. (1995). Functional analysis and treatment of escape-maintained aggression correlated with sleep deprivation. *Journal of Applied Behavior Analysis, 28*, 225–226.

O'Reilly, M. F. (1997). Functional analysis of episodic self-injury correlated with recurrent otitis media. *Journal of Applied Behavior Analysis, 30*, 165–167.

O'Reilly, M. F., Lacey, C., & Lancioni, G. (2000). Assessment of the influence of background noise on the escape-maintained problem behavior and pain behavior in a child with Williams syndrome. *Journal of Applied Behavior Analysis, 33*, 511–514.

O'Reilly, M. F., & Lancioni, G. (2000). Response covariation of escape-maintained aberrant behavior correlated with sleep deprivation. *Research in Developmental Disabilities, 21*, 125–136.

Peebles, K. A., & Price, T. J. (2012). Self-injurious behaviour in intellectual disability syndromes: Evidence for aberrant pain signalling as a contributing factor. *Journal of Intellectual Disability Research, 56*, 441–452.

Prasher, V. P. (2009). The adaptive behavior dementia questionnaire (ABDQ). In V. P. Prasher (Ed.), *Neuropsychological assessments of dementia in down syndrome and intellectual disabilities* (pp. 163–176). London: Springer.

Prasher, V., Percy, M., Jozsvai, E., Lovering, J. S., & Berg, J. M. (2007). Implications of Alzheimer's disease for people with Down syndrome and other intellectual disabilities. In I. Brown and M. Percy (Eds.), *A comprehensive guide to intellectual and developmental disabilities* (pp. 681-702). Baltimore, MD: Paul H. Brookes Publishing Co.

Rada, R. E. (2014). Dental erosion due to GERD in patients with developmental disabilities: Case theory. *Special Care in Dentistry, 34*, 7–11.

Raetz, P. B., LeBlanc, L. A., Baker, J. C., & Hilton, L. C. (2013). Utility of the multiple-stimulus without replacement procedure and stability of preferences of older adults with dementia. *Journal of Applied Behavior Analysis, 46*, 765–780.

Rapp, J. T., Swanson, G., & Dornbusch, K. (2007). Temporary increases in problem behavior and sleep disruption following decreases in medication: A descriptive analysis of conditional rates. *Behavior Modification, 31*, 825–846.

Roberts, C., Yoder, P. J., & Kennedy, C. H. (2005). Descriptive analysis of epileptic seizures and problem behavior in adults with developmental disabilities. *American Journal on Mental Retardation, 5*, 405–412.

Rodriguez, R. (1992). Effect of various psychotropic drugs on the performance of avoidance and escape behavior in rats. *Pharmacology, Biochemistry, and Behavior, 43*, 1155-1159.

Scheepers, B., Salahudeen, S., & Morelli, J. (2004). Two-year outcome audit in an adult learning disability population with refractory epilepsy. *Seizure, 13*, 529–533.

Schieve, L. A., Gonzalez, V., Boulet, S. L., Visser, S. N., Rice, C. E., Van Naarden Braun, K., et al. (2012). Concurrent medical conditions and health care use and needs among children with learning and behavioral developmental disabilities, national health interview survey, 2006–2010. *Research in Developmental Disabilities, 33*, 467–476.

Schwichtenberg AJ, Young GS, Hutman T, Iosif AM, Sigman M, Rogers SJ, Ozonoff S. (2013). Behavior and sleep problems in children with a family history of autism. *Autism Research, 6,* 169-176.

Singh, A. N., & Matson, J. L. (2009). An examination of psychotropic medication prescription practices for individuals with intellectual disabilities. *Journal of Developmental Physical Disabilities, 21*, 115–129.

Shannon, H. E., Hart, J. C., Bymaster, F. P., Calligaro, D. O., Delapp, N. W., Mitch, C. H., Ward, J. S., Fink-Jensen, A., Sauerberg, P., Jeppesen, L., Sheardown, M. J., & Swedberg, M. D. B. (1999). Muscarinic receptor agonists, like dopamine receptor antagonist antipsychotics, inhibit conditioned avoidance response in rats. *Journal of Pharmacology and Experimental Therapeutics, 290,* 901-907.

Sipes, M., Matson, J. L., Belva, B., Turygin, N., Kozlowski, A. M., & Horovitz, M. (2011). The relationship among side effects associated with anti-epileptic medications in those with intellectual disability. *Research in Developmental Disabilities, 32*, 1646–1651.

Smith, K. R. M., & Matson, J. L. (2010). Behavior problems: Differences among intellectually disabled adults with co-morbid autism spectrum disorders and epilepsy. *Research in Developmental Disabilities, 31*, 1062–1069.

Solodiuk, J. C., Scott-Sutherland, J., Meyers, M., Myette, B., Shusterman, C., Karian, V. E., et al. (2010). Validation of the individualized numeric rating scale (INRS): A pain assessment tool for nonverbal children with intellectual disability. *Pain, 150*, 231–236.

Sommi, R. W., Benefield, W. H., Curtis, J. L., Lott, R. S., Saklad, J. J., Wilson, J. (1998). Drug interactions psychtropic medications. In S. Reiss & M. G. Aman (Eds.), *Psychotropic medication and developmental disabilities: The international consensus handbook* (pp. 115–131). Columbus, OH: The Ohio State University.

Stancliffe, R. J., Lakin, K. C., Larson, S., Engler, J., Bershadsky, J., & Taub, S., et al. (2011). Overweight and obesity among adults with intellectual disabilities who use intellectual disability/developmental disability services in 20 U.S. states. *American Journal on Intellectual and Developmental Disabilities, 116*, 401–418.

Swender, S. L., Matson, J. L., Mayville, S. B., Gonzalez, M. L., & McDowell, D. (2006). A functional assessment of handmouthing among persons with severe and profound intellectual disability. *Journal of Intellectual and Developmental Disability, 31*, 95–100.

Symons, F. J. (2002). Pain and self-injury: Mechanisms and models. In S. Schroeder, T. Thompson & M. L. Oster-Granite (Eds.), *Self-injurious behavior: Genes, Brain, and Behavior* (pp. 223–234). Washington, D.C.: American Psychological Association.

Symons, F. J., & Danov, S. E. (2005). A prospective clinical analysis of pain behavior and self-injurious behavior. *Pain, 117*, 473–477.

Symons, F. J., Davis, M. L., & Thompson, T. (2000). Self-injurious behavior and sleep disturbance in adults with developmental disabilities. *Research in Developmental Disabilities, 21*, 115–123.

Taggart, L., Coates, V., & Tuesdale-Kennedy, M. (2013). Management and quality indicators of diabetes mellitus in people with developmental disabilities. *Journal of Intellectual Disability Research, 57*, 1152–1163.

Tatsumi, Y., Mohri, I., Shimizu, S., Tachibana, M., Ohno, Y., & Taniike, M. (2015). Daytime physical activity and sleep in pre-schoolers with developmental disorders. *Journal of Paediatric Child Health, 51*, 396-402.

Teeluckdharry, S., Sharma, S., O'Rourke, E., Tharian, P., Gondalekar, A., Nainar, F., et al. (2013). Monitoring metabolic side effects of atypical antipsychotics in people with an intellectual disability. *Journal of Intellectual Disability, 17(3)*, 223–235.

Tonelli, L. H., Katz, M., Kovacsiscs, C. E., Gould, T. D., Joppy, B., Hoshino, A., et al. (2009). *Brain, Behavior, and Immunity, 23*, 784–793.

Tordjman, S., Najjar, I., Bellissant, E., Anderson, G. M., Barburoth, M., Cohen, D., et al. (2013). Advances in the research of melatonin in autism spectrum disorders:Literature review and new perspectives. *International Journal of Molecular Sciences, 14*, 20508-20542.

Valdovinos, M. G., Caruso, M., Roberts, C., Kim, G., & Kennedy, C. H. (2005). Medical and behavioral symptoms as potential medication side effects in adults with developmental disabilities. *American Journal on Mental Retardation, 110*, 164–170.

Valdovinos, M. G., Ellringer, N. P., & Alexander, M. L. (2007). Changes in the rate of problem behavior associated with the removal of the antipsychotic medication quetiapine. *Mental Health Aspects of Developmental Disabilities, 10*, 64–67.

Valdovinos, M. G., & Kennedy, C. H. (2004). Behavior analytic conceptualization of psychotropic medication side effects. *The Behavior Analyst, 27*, 231–238.

Valdovinos, M. G., Nelson, S. M., Kuhle, J., & Dierks, A. M. (2009). Using analogue functional analysis to measure variations in problem behavior rate and function after psychotropic medication changes: A clinical demonstration. *Journal of Mental Health Research in Intellectual Disabilities, 2*, 279–293.

Valdovinos, M. G., & Weyand, D. (2006). Blood glucose levels and problem behavior. *Research in Developmental Disabilities, 27*, 227–231.

Wacker, D. P., Harding, J., Cooper, L. J., Derby, K. M., Peck, S., Asmus, J., et al. (1996). The effects of meal schedule and quantity on problematic behavior. *Journal of Applied Behavior Analysis, 29*, 79–87.

Weeden, M., Ehrhardt, K., & Poling, A. (2009). Conspicuous by their absence: Studies comparing and combining risperidone and applied behavior analysis to reduce challenging behavior in children with autism. *Research in Austism Spectrum Disorders, 3*, 905–912.

Young, A. T., & Hawkins, J. (2002). Psychotropic medication prescriptions: An analysis of the reasons people with mental retardation are prescribed psychotropic medication. *Journal of Developmental and Physical Disabilities, 14*, 129–142.

Zarcone, J. R., Lindauer, S. L., Morse, P. S., Crosland, K. A., Valdovinos, M. G., McKerchar, T. L., et al. (2004). Effects of risperidone on destructive behavior of persons with developmental disabilities: III. Functional analysis. *American Journal on Mental Retardation, 109*, 310–321.

Zarcone, J. R., Napolitano, D., & Valdovinos, M. G. (2008). Measurement of problem behaviour during medication evaluations. *Journal of Intellectual Disability Research, 52*, 1015–1028.

Chapter 2
Compliance with Medical Routines

Keith D. Allen and Sara Kupzyk

Compliance with medical routines is an important part of basic health care for everyone, but especially individuals with intellectual and developmental disabilities (IDD). Compliance with medical routines may be especially important for individuals with IDD because, as a group, individuals with IDD have poorer health than those in the general population; a problem that tends to be more pronounced in individuals with severe disabilities (Janicki et al. 1999). While poorer health results from a complex combination of variables, including genetics, income, and isolation, the lack of compliance with medical routines is a significant factor (Krahn et al. 2006). So, while many diseases and illnesses are preventable or treatable, the benefits only accrue if patients cooperate with the procedures involved in the delivery of medical care.

Perhaps the factor most responsible for noncompliance is the fear generated by common medical procedures. Routine health care can require patients to tolerate a wide variety of medical procedures of varying degrees of invasiveness. For example, routine health care procedures can range from the relatively mild intrusions of blood pressure cuffs, pill swallowing, temperature taking, and throat swabs to more invasive procedures such as blood draws, immunization injections, tooth extractions, and biopsies. Many of these routine medical procedures can be distressing and can generate considerable fear and anxiety in anyone, even when the procedures themselves are not a threat in any biological sense (O'Hare et al. 1989). Compounding this problem is the fact that individuals with IDD have been found to endorse a greater number and intensity of fears than normative samples

K.D. Allen (✉) · S. Kupzyk
Munroe-Meyer Institute for Genetics and Rehabilitation, University of Nebraska Medical Center, Omaha, USA
e-mail: kdallen@unmc.edu

J.K. Luiselli (ed.), *Behavioral Health Promotion and Intervention in Intellectual and Developmental Disabilities*, Evidence-Based Practices in Behavioral Health,
DOI 10.1007/978-3-319-27297-9_2

(Knapp et al. 1992). For example, individuals with Autism Spectrum Disorders exhibit higher rates of medical fears than typically developing individuals, with almost a third of individuals with IDD showing marked avoidance and total noncompliance with even the most basic medical exams (Gillis et al. 2009). In addition, the more intense and unfamiliar the sensory experiences associated with those medical procedures, the more intense are the avoidance and noncompliance exhibited by those with IDD. Indeed, the literature is replete with evidence of compliance problems during relatively common medical procedures such as physical examinations (Gillis et al. 2009), blood draws (Grider et al. 2012), immunizations (Wolff and Symons 2012), and nebulizer treatments (Reimers et al. 1988). However, the list also includes compliance problems with less common but critical health care routines such as cleaning of central lines (McComas et al. 1998), blood tests (Slifer et al. 2011), EEG evaluations (DeMore et al. 2009), blood transfusions (Gorski and Westbrook 2002), and catheterization (Gorski et al. 2004).

The fact that routine medical procedures might generate fear and anxiety should not be surprising. Many fears of medical procedures are developmentally appropriate. For example, typical young children exhibit fears of unusual or unfamiliar stimuli or loud or sudden noises. They also exhibit predictable fears associated with strangers, separation, loss of support, masks and dark (e.g., Silverman 2011). By school age, typical children show developmentally appropriate fears of bodily injury, blood and injections (Gullone 2005). Now consider that many medical and dental procedures have precisely these features. Dentists wear masks and use equipment that makes loud and sudden noises. Nurses are often strangers who draw blood. Imaging technicians typically ask that patients enter dark rooms, then lay back and wait alone for periods of time. Most, if not all of these procedures also include sensory experiences that are unusual, unfamiliar, and often uncomfortable. That anyone might wish to escape or avoid these situations is both logical and predictable.

Conceptually, we understand that many fear behaviors are respondent events; unconditioned responses elicited by unconditioned stimuli in the environment. Unconditioned stimuli may include the prick of a needle during an immunization injection, loud noises or vibrations from dental instruments, or placement in an isolated, confined space like an MRI scanner. The unconditioned responses can include mild, nonintrusive sweating, heart palpitations, rigidity, shallow breathing, and nausea or more disruptive behaviors such flinching, fainting and vomiting. The disruptions are compounded when many of the previously nonthreatening sights and sounds of the heath care environment (e.g., the sight of a nurse, the clothes he wears, the room where services are provided, etc.), through repeated pairing with unpleasant events, gradually become conditioned stimuli that elicit similar fear responses. Higher order conditioning can eventually result in more and more previously neutral stimuli that can elicit fears that are also referred to as conditioned emotional responses.

Conditioned emotional responses can also be strengthened and maintained by their consequences because these emotional responses often allow the individual to escape or avoid contact with threatening or feared events. That is, the escape or avoidance of contact with feared medical routines reinforces noncompliance, even though at times, the escape and avoidance are temporary at best. These behaviors can include a range of verbal and physical protests. The intensity of these protests can range from mild delay tactics to severe aggression. Verbal protests often include crying, moaning, complaining and requests for termination. Physical protests can involve physically blocking or pushing away health care providers and their equipment and may involve running away. More severe protests can include biting, hitting, and kicking. Unfortunately, here again because of repeated pairings with unpleasant events, previously neutral stimuli can acquire the ability to evoke noncompliant behaviors that, in the past, have produced escape or avoidance.

It is these escape and avoidance behaviors in particular that are at the heart of most noncompliance and have the potential to severely impact health outcomes. First, these disruptive avoidance behaviors can create risks of injury to everyone involved, leading health care providers to rely on restrictive means of gaining compliance (e.g., sedation or restraint). Many of these passive restraint procedures can themselves increase risks for serious and dangerous health complications (e.g., over sedation). Second the challenges associated with trying to manage disruptive behaviors can deter heath providers from a willingness to provide services in the first place, reducing access to care (Lennox and Kerr 1997). Third, caregivers may elect to avoid some preventive or elective health care procedures because of the physical risks and emotional embarrassment experienced when dealing with noncompliance. Finally, noncompliance can interfere with the full completion of procedures and disrupt a provider's concentration, thereby diminish the quality of care being delivered. As a result of these complications associated with noncompliance with medical routines, even a minor illness could create functional impairments and subsequent declines in health, resulting in increased dependency on others for care (Rimmer 1999).

Ultimately, the noncompliance with basic health care can have profound effects on very specific aspects of long term health and well-being. For example, individuals with IDD have been found to have significantly more unmet dental oral health needs such as fewer restored or repaired teeth and more missing or decayed teeth than in normative samples (Cumella et al. 2000; McKinney et al. 2014). Unmet oral health needs have also been strongly linked to respiratory disease (Azarpazhooh and Leake 2006) as well as to systemic conditions such as coronary heart disease and stroke (Seymour et al. 2007). These poorer health outcomes are attributable in large part to both inadequate hygiene and preventive care, inadequacies that are generally rooted in the avoidance of and noncompliance with the sensory and procedural demands of simple tasks like taking x-rays and cleaning teeth as well as more invasive ones like drilling and filling (Lewis et al. 2002).

Long term health risks from noncompliance are also found in the complications that follow failed MRIs. Recent studies of aging diseases have found that over a third of the individuals with IDD would not cooperate enough to generate quality imaging, even with sedation (Prasher et al. 2003). Common problems included refusal to go into the scanner and refusal to stay in the scanner for fear of being left alone in confined spaces. Perhaps more important, of those individuals who required sedation to complete the imagining studies, one in five experienced serious and dangerous complications from sedation that required emergency intervention. Thus, poor compliance has been a major factor limiting the use of MRIs with IDD and ultimately limiting what is known about aging diseases in this population.

Conceptual Considerations

Treatment of medical noncompliance should be developed with consideration that the noncompliance has both respondent and operant components. Interestingly, although consequences are typically considered to be the "mainsprings of behavior control" (Brady 1978, p. v), the conceptual analysis would suggest that the focus of treatment for medical noncompliance should center on its central respondent conditioning characteristics. Treatment begins by arranging for respondent extinction of the fear responses. To do so, stimuli that have been conditioned in the past to elicit fear responses and escape behavior are now repeatedly presented to the individual (in vivo exposure) in a hierarchy from least feared to most feared. The hierarchy is arranged so that less salient stimuli are presented first so that the initial exposures do not elicit fear or evoke avoidance behavior. The salience of a stimulus can be varied for example, by size of the stimulus, distance from the stimulus, and/or duration of exposure. Then the salience of the stimulus exposures can be increased slowly so as not to elicit fear and avoidance responding.

This *graduated exposure* can be enhanced or strengthened to the extent that the feared stimuli are gradually presented while the individual is relaxed. This requires either teaching a relaxation response (e.g., progressive muscle relaxation) or eliciting one by presenting stimuli that previously have been associated with being relaxed, such as watching movies, holding a favorite blanket, or listening to music. This process of pairing relaxation with graduated exposure can result in counter-conditioning, in which previously feared stimuli eventually come to elicit less intense fear responses and instead may even elicit pleasant responses.

Graduated exposure can also be enhanced or strengthened by considering the operant characteristics of the disruptive noncompliance behaviors. That is, many disruptive noncompliant behaviors are maintained by escape and avoidance of the planned medical routines behaviors, even if only temporary. As a result, one might consider strategies that prevent escape or avoidance (i.e., escape extinction). However, escape extinction procedures themselves can be predicted to evoke "bursts" of escape behavior, escalating in intensity, that further increase risks of harm to individuals with IDD and their caregivers or medical providers.

As an alternative to escape extinction, practitioners have typically developed approaches that emphasize reinforcement of cooperative behaviors (i.e., sitting or lying still and quiet), that are incompatible with noncompliance with medical routines (i.e., DRI procedures). These behaviors are initially reinforced in the presence of the least threatening or least feared stimuli associated with the medical routine to minimize the likelihood that escape behaviors are evoked and maximize the likelihood of success in exhibiting the desired behaviors. Gradually then, the more threatening, fearful, or uncomfortable aspects of a medical routine are "faded in", but only after the individual has experienced success (i.e., accessed reinforcement) for tolerating less threatening, less aversive conditions.

Note that the core feature of these enhanced approaches always involves the individual experiencing graduated, in vivo exposure to feared stimuli resulting, hypothetically, in respondent extinction. The addition of a relaxation response focuses additionally on counterconditioning. Here, the point of emphasis is on the individual being relaxed ***before*** the gradual presentation of the feared stimuli and then maintaining relaxation during the presentations. This particular form of graduated exposure is commonly called systematic desensitization (King et al. 2005). In contrast, the addition of a positive consequence focuses additionally on operant reinforcement of incompatible behaviors. Here, the point of emphasis is on delivering reinforcement ***after*** the presentation of the fear stimuli contingent on the individual exhibiting cooperative behaviors.

Research Findings

An evidence-based practice always begins with a review of the empirical research findings on the best available treatments. Doing so promotes effective practice, improves patient outcomes, and enhances public health (APA 2006). In order to evaluate the research findings on interventions to address noncompliance with medical routines in the IDD population, we looked at two relatively recent reviews of the literature regarding treatment of fears and/or phobias. Both were designed to critically evaluate the literature and determine which treatments, if any, met criteria for classification as "well-established" or "probably efficacious" treatments (Chambless and Ollendick 2001).

In their review of the literature on treatment of phobic responses in typically developing children (e.g., fear of dogs, flying, dark, snakes, tests, etc.), Davis and Ollendick (2005) identified two well-established treatments. The first treatment, what they called "reinforced practice", is an operant procedure involving repeated, controlled, graduated exposures after which the phobic individual receives reinforcement for not engaging in avoidance behavior. The second well-established treatment, called "participant modeling," involves having an individual watch a model interact with feared stimuli with no aversive outcome, purportedly resulting in vicarious extinction of the phobic responses in the observer who then must approach and interact with the phobic stimuli themselves. Davis and Ollendick (2005) also found systematic desensitization to be probably efficacious for treatment of behavioral avoidance and subjective fear. Finally, they found cognitive behavior therapy, which focuses on changing cognitions, to also be probably efficacious in typically developing children.

In contrast to the review by Davis and Olendick, which focused on the treatment of phobic responses in typically developing children, Jennett and Hagopian (2008) focused their review more specifically on the empirical evidence for treatment of phobic responses in individuals with IDD. They found 12 well-controlled single case experimental studies demonstrating treatment efficacy with phobic avoidance responses to stimuli as wide ranging as stairs, dogs, swimming pools, animatronic objects, needles and dental exams. The treatments that were found efficacious were comprised of seven main components, including graduated exposure, contingent reinforcement, prompting, modeling, escape extinction, and use of distracting/relaxing stimuli. Graduated exposure was the only component used in all treatment packages. The authors concluded that behavioral treatment that focuses on learning principles and provides direct and graduated exposure is well established for treating phobic responses in individuals with IDD.

Because these reviews did not look specifically at phobic avoidance responses to medical procedures by individuals with IDD, we did an additional search of the literature. We were interested in any additional studies not covered in previous reviews that (1) targeted individuals with IDD who were resistant, avoidant, or noncompliant with (2) preventive, diagnostic, or treatment-related medical and/or dental procedures. As a result, we searched databases PubMed, Medline, and Psych Info using key words and combinations of key words that included terms such as medical or dental noncompliance, resistance, phobia, or avoidance as well as intellectual and/or developmental disability. Our goal was not to conduct a critical review of the studies, but to evaluate the extent to which studies targeting medical noncompliance in individuals with IDD were found to include the empirically supported approaches identified previously by critical reviews.

Our search identified 27 studies with participants with IDD (see Table 2.1), predominantly children, ranging in age from 22 months to 41 years old. Diagnoses included those with autism, mild to severe intellectual disabilities, and developmental delay. The routines that were addressed included dental exams and cleaning, pill swallowing, physical exams, nebulizer treatment, needle sticks, central line care, and wearing of positive airway pressure masks. The most common routines targeted for intervention involved dental exams and needle sticks.

Assessment components. Given that many individuals with IDD often have limited ability to report on private experiences such as fear or anxiety, all of the studies employed direct observations of behavior as the primary measure of treatment outcome. Typical "fear" behaviors that were measured included aggression, protests, refusals, screams, and turning away or running. The most common dependent variable was the percentage of steps completed within the medical/dental routine. In baseline, the researchers typically exposed participants to the medical/dental procedure that was targeted and then documented the frequency and/or intensity of avoidance behaviors as well as the number/percentage of steps completed in the routine. These initial observations were also critical in conducting a task analysis so that the therapists could understand what tasks were involved in completing each step of the routine in sequence and also for understanding which stimuli elicited the most intense avoidance and escape behaviors.

Table 2.1 Summary of studies identified

Author(s)	Medical/dental routine	Population	Study design	Treatment components	Treatment outcomes
Altabet (2002)	Dental exam and clean	63 adults	Control group design	Dist + GE + IM	Tx group completed more steps of routine. No differences in sedation or restraint
Beck et al. (2005)	Pill swallowing	8 children, 4–9 yrs	AB design with replication across participants	GE + Rfmt	7 of 8 participants were able to swallow target pill at end of treatment, 6 of 8 maintained success at home
Boj and Davila (1989)	Dental exam	28, 3–4 yrs	Matched control group design	VM	Tx group had higher heart rates and no differences in behavior or anxiety ratings
Cavalari et al. (2013)	Physical examination	16 year-old	Changing criterion	GE + Rfmt + IM	Participant was able to complete full exam by end of treatment
Conyers et al. (2004)	Dental exam	6 adult ages 33–54	Multiple baseline	GE + Rfmt + VM	VM was effective for 1 participant. All participants completed all 18 steps when desensitization package was implemented
Cuvo et al. (2010a)	Dental exam	5 children, 3–5 yrs	Multiple probe across participants	Dist + GE + Rfmt + VM + EE	Participants demonstrated compliance with the exams and showed maintenance of responding
Cuvo et al. (2010b)	Physical examination	6 children, 3-6 yrs	Multiple probe across participants	Dist + GE + Rfmt + VM + EE	Participants demonstrated compliance with the exams and showed maintenance of responding
Davit et al. (2011)	Venipuncture compliance	58 children, 0–21 yrs	Quasi-randomized trial	GE	All increased compliance with steps toward blood draw
DeMore et al. (2009)	Overnight EEG evaluation	17 children, 4–17 yrs	Case study	GE + Rfmt + IM + EE	9 tolerated all training steps and 15 (88 %) tolerated all 21 electrode placements for 9 h actual EEG

(continued)

Table 2.1 (continued)

Author(s)	Medical/dental routine	Population	Study design	Treatment components	Treatment outcomes
Ghuman et al. (2004)	Pill swallowing	4 children, 5–6 yrs	Case study	GE + Rfmt	Two learned to swallow targeted pills in 3 sessions; 1 in 5 sessions; 1 withdrew
Gillis et al. (2009)	Physical examination	18 children 2–13 yrs	Pre- post- design	GE + Rfmt + IM	15 of 18 participants met physical exam criterion after 25 sessions. Three took 38, 42, and 62 sessions to meet criterion
Gorski et al. (2004)	Dialysis, catheterization, medication refusal	3 boys, 10–14 yrs	Changing criterion	Dist + GE + BM + Rfmt	Increased compliance with specified tasks to 90–100 % completion
Grider et al. (2012)	Blood draw	21 year-old	ABCD—case study design	Dist + GE + Rfmt	Participant reached 100 % compliance after 27 exposure trials
Hagopian et al. (2001)	Blood-injury-injection	19 year-old male	Changing criterion	Dist + GE + Rfmt	The participant was able to sit unrestrained for blood draw procedure at the end of treatment
Isong et al. (2014)	Dental exam and cleaning	80, 7–17 yrs	Randomized controlled trial	VM versus Dist versus VM + Dist	No significant differences between groups, although Dist and Dist + video Modeling did show significant improvements within group
Luscre and Center (1996)	Dental exam	3 children, 6–9 yrs	Multiple baseline across participants	Dist + GE + IM + Rfmt	The participants showed and increased to 85–100 % steps completed in an analog and in vivo settings
Lunsky et al. (2003)	Breast, pelvic exams	22 women	Pre- post- assessments	Dist + GE	Participants showed improved knowledge, beliefs about coping
Maguire et al. (1996)	Dental procedures	4 adults	Multiple baseline across participants	GE + Rfmt	All participants showed an improvement in cooperation and decrease in resistance. Results maintained
McComas et al. (1998)	Central- venous line care	Infant, 22 mo	Multiple schedule design	BM + Rfmt + EE	The child was more compliant with the low-probability requests following high-probability requests

(continued)

Table 2.1 (continued)

Author(s)	Medical/dental routine	Population	Study design	Treatment components	Treatment outcomes
Orellana et al. (2014)	Dental exam	38 children and 34 adults	Pre post assessment	GE + VM	There were significantly more components completed post treatment
Reimers et al. (1988)	Nebulizer treatment	Child, 2 yrs	Case study: ABC design	GE + Rfmt + EE	The participant consistently wore mask for 20 min treatment and maintained for 3 months
Riviere et al. (2011)	Medical examination	2 children, 6–8 yrs	ABABCB	BM + Rfmt	Participants increased compliance with low-probability requests
Shabani and Fisher (2006)	Blood draw (needle phobia)	18 year-old	Variation of an ABAB reversal design	GE + Rfmt	The participant was able to complete blood sample procedures and the behavior generalized to other settings
Slifer et al. (2007)	Positive airway (PAP) mask	4 children, 3–5 yrs	Multiple baseline	Dist + GE + Rfmt + EE	All participants tolerated wearing the PAP during sleep
Slifer et al. (2008)	Electroencephalogram	7 children, 2–10 yrs	AB replicated across subjects	Dist + GE + Rfmt + EE	All participants showed 100 % compliance with EEG without restraint, anesthesia, or sedation
Slifer et al. (2011)	Needle sticks	8 children, 4–16 yrs	ABAB	Dist + GE + Rfmt + EE	Participants cooperated with real needlestick after 4–15 sessions
Wolff and Symons (2012)	Needle-to-skin contact	Adult male	Changing criterion	GE + Rfmt + EE	The participant was compliant with needle-to-skin contact

Note GE Graduated exposure, *Rfmt* Reinforcement, *Dist* Distraction/Relaxation, *BM* Behavioral momentum, *EE* Escape extinction, *VM* Video modeling, *IM* In vivo modeling

To assist in behavior measurement, some studies used the Brief Behavioral Distress Scale (Tucker et al. 2001), a tool that has demonstrated good reliability and validity. Observers record the essential steps of the medical/dental procedure and then record the occurrence and nonoccurrence of the clearly defined target behaviors (i.e., noninterfering distress behaviors, potentially interfering distress behaviors, interfering distress behaviors, and active coping response without verbal delay) for each step. A *Total Distress Score* and *Active Coping Response Score* are calculated, which allows for comparison across procedures that have varying numbers of steps.

Several studies also included structured rating scales during the behavioral assessment. For example, the Behavioral Observation Assessment (BOA; Gillis and Romanczyk, n.d.) is used to rate participant behaviors on a 7-point Likert scale, from negative/avoidant to positive/approach. The instrument also prompts observes to include information about the current treatment step and behaviors specific to each step. The tool is used for progress monitoring and treatment modifications. Some studies targeting dental exams or dental cleaning included the Frankl scale (Frankl et al. 1962), a 4 point Likert scale that is widely used throughout clinical dentistry to provide subjectively ratings of cooperation and compliance during treatment. Ratings from the Frankl Scale have been found to be highly correlated with independent, direct observations of escape and avoidance behaviors in children (Allen et al. 2003).

Treatment components. Across the 27 studies that were reviewed, the most common components used in treatment of fear avoidance and noncompliance with medical/dental routines in individuals with IDD were graduated exposure and contingent reinforcement.

Graduated exposure. All of the treatment interventions included some aspect of in vivo exposure to the feared/avoided stimuli and 23 of the 27 included some effort to conduct these exposures gradually. Note that the investigators used a wide array of labels for interventions that included core features of graduated exposure. Sometimes these labels were used interchangeably with the term graduated exposure (e.g., systematic desensitization, in vivo desensitization, contact desensitization, in vivo graduated exposure, fading, etc.) and sometimes these labels draw attention to the fact that the graduate exposure was preceded by efforts to elicit relaxation (e.g., counterconditioning) or was part of a treatment package (e.g., behavioral compliance training, reinforced practice, differential reinforcement, etc.).

A review of their procedures indicates that the gradual presentation of feared stimuli can be accomplished in a number of ways. The first is to simply present the stimuli in the order in which they will be encountered in the actual procedure or routine, but to conduct a thorough task analysis so that the steps can be broken down into substeps if necessary to promote success during exposures. The second approach is to reorder the stimuli into a fear hierarchy in which the steps that evoke the least avoidance responses are presented first, even if they are presented out of sequence, and the steps that evoke the most avoidance responding are saved for later. Regardless of which approach is used, steps in an exposure protocol can be sequenced based on dimensions such as duration of exposure to the stimulus, size of the stimulus, or distance from a stimulus (Jennett and Hagopian 2008). Over two thirds of the studies included actual exposure hierarchies to guide the steps and dimensions to be presented during the exposure.

Exposures sequenced according to task analysis. Cavalari et al. (2013) developed an exposure protocol that was sequenced according to the 12-steps of a typical routine medical examination for a 16 year-old female with autism. Compliance with the steps was evaluated during baseline by presenting each step in sequence until noncompliance was demonstrated. Exposures then followed the typical sequence but were "graduated" by requiring the patient to demonstrate repeated compliance with each step prior to advancing to the next step. In addition, substeps were created to increase compliance with what were observed in baseline to be more difficult steps (e.g., gradually increasing the time in contact with certain medical instruments).

Once graduated exposure begins, it may be necessary to revise the sequence of steps to promote compliance. For example, Grider et al. (2012) originally developed a 12-step exposure sequence of a blood draw routine, but the adult male with autism was unable to progress past the seventh step (i.e., exposure to syringe with needle). Therefore, a step in which the syringe was displayed without the needle attached was added to the exposure sequence. The addition of the step helped the participant to progress to the next planned step.

Time exposed to the stimulus. Reimers et al. (1988) implemented a hierarchy based on an increasing number of minutes of wearing a mask during nebulizer treatment. The child was required to meet the specified time criteria to gain access to a preferred edible. The first criterion was 3 s of mask wearing and the terminal criterion was 20 min, the amount of time needed to complete the nebulizer treatment. In the early steps of the hierarchy, small increases in the amount of time were required (e.g., 30 s to 1 min). As treatment progressed, larger increases in criteria were required (e.g., 5 min 30 s to 10 min 30 s).

Size of the stimulus. Beck et al. (2005) treated noncompliance with pill swallowing by gradually exposing children to pills of increasing size, beginning with a very tiny pill about the size of a cupcake sprinkle. They then used a hierarchy of nine mock pills of increasing size. The children started with the smallest size pill and progressed to the next pill size contingent on success with pill swallowing on two to three trials until they had reached the terminal pill size.

Distance from the stimulus. Shabani and Fisher (2006) gradually decreased the distance from a participant's index finger to a lancet device used to draw blood samples. Through an initial assessment, it was determined to start at a distance of 61 cm from the finger because the participant did not show signs of distress at this distance. After two to three successful trials (i.e., arm kept in designated location for blood draw), the experimenters moved to the next closer step and continued with closer and closer exposures at distances of 46, 31, 8, 5, 1 cm and finally an actual blood draw.

In one study treating needle phobia using a similar "fading in" graduated approach, Wolff and Symons (2012) found that a male with autism and IDD would not tolerate the needle moving closer than about 12 feet. At that point they introduced a "warning stimulus" to show the individual how long the exposure would last. In this case, the warning stimulus may actually have enhanced the salience of duration, making the exposure less aversive.

One challenge for any therapist implementing a treatment program involving graduated exposure with individuals with IDD is deciding when to progress to the next step in the hierarchy. Criteria established for moving to the next step varied in the studies reviewed. The majority of protocols required two to three trials of compliance/no disruptive behavior (e.g., Beck et al. 2005; Cuvo et al. 2010a, b; Wolff and Symons 2012) before moving to the next step. Others required that the participant appear relaxed or calm or comfortable with a step before progressing (e.g., Conyers et al. 2004; Slifer et al. 2011) and recommended moving back to a previous step to help a child feel comfortable if necessary (e.g., Davit et al. 2011). Some protocols required that the participant receive a neutral or positive rating on an assessment measure (Gillis et al. 2009) before progressing. Still others increased the demands on a scheduled basis, independent of how the participant performed or appeared (e.g., Gorski et al. 2004; McComas et al. 1998). For the remainder of the studies, the progression to the next step was unclear from the description of some of the treatments or more subjective. For example, Slifer et al. (2008), noted that the "pace was one that challenged and taught the child, but did not overly distress the child" and Slifer et al. (2007) reported only that the participants progressed gradually through the steps.

Contingent reinforcement. Eighty percent of studies included reinforcement contingent on desired behavior and usually in combination with graduated exposure. Only in two studies involving efforts to increase compliance with behavioral momentum was reinforcement used without graduated exposure. Reinforcement was delivered contingent upon appropriate approach behaviors, successful completion of a step, or compliance with substeps in the medical/dental routine. Caregiver interviews and preference assessments were often used to identify probable reinforcers (e.g., Cuvo et al. 2010b; Gillis et al. 2009). For example, Cuvo et al. (2010a, b) asked parents and the child's clinician to complete a questionnaire of the child's preferred items. The items were then presented in a brief paired stimulus preference assessment (Fisher et al. 1992) every 2 weeks to determine which items to use contingent on completion of steps.

Other researchers have used conditioned reinforcers, such as tokens or money to reinforce compliance. For example, Maguire et al. (1996), provided adult males with mild to severe intellectual disabilities specific praise and access to monetary compensation for demonstrating cooperative behavior during each 30 s segment of the dental treatment procedure. Hagopian et al. (2001) provided tokens contingent on compliance every 10 s (faded to 20 s) that could be exchanged following the session for preferred items.

Other treatment components. While 74 % of the studies used combinations of graduated exposure and contingent reinforcement, about 40 % of the studies included either in vivo or video modeling, distraction/relaxation procedures, or prompting procedures.

Modeling. When modeling was included in a treatment, whether in vivo modeling or video modeling, it was typically used as a supplement to graduated exposure and reinforcement. In most cases, it was a medical provider or a therapist who actually was performing as a model, in some cases modeling appropriate behavior while undergoing the entire routine and in other cases modeling acceptance of specific steps within a routine. For example, dentists often use a procedure call Tell-Show-Do (Orellana et al. 2014), in which they provide sensory and procedural information, show the instruments they will be using, and then model for their patients the acceptance of being touched by instruments like tooth explorers, mirrors, or drills. However, they do not typically model acceptance of every step in an exam, such as getting in the chair or accepting the light being turned on. In addition, this approach would also typically be combined with components like graduated exposures and contingent reinforcement (e.g., Maguire et al. 1996).

Several studies used a typically developing child as a model and video recorded the model successfully completing a medical/dental exam (Cuvo et al. 2010a, b). Parents were then given the video recording on a DVD and asked to have their child watch the video daily at home in preparation for exposure and reinforcement sessions in clinic.

Two studies have attempted to examine the efficacy of modeling alone to address medical/dental noncompliance. Conyers et al. (2004) found that watching a video of a well-known staff person undergoing each of the procedures in a dental exam did eliminate resistance in one adult with IDD, but two others showed no change in avoidance behavior until in vivo graduated exposure was introduced. Isong et al. (2014) also found that a group exposed to video modeling experienced no reductions in distress or noncompliance compared to a control group when undergoing preventive dental exams. This suggests that for some individuals, the vicarious exposure encountered with video modeling may not be enough. Luscre and Center (1996) also noted problems with ensuring that participants actually attended to a modeling video depicting a typical peer undergoing dental treatment.

Distraction/Relaxation. A number of investigators acknowledge the value of trying to elicit positive responses that can counter the fear responses that may be elicited during in vivo exposure (e.g., Luscre and Center 1996). For example, Slifer et al. (2007) included access to preferred activities during exposure trials of positive airway pressure mask wearing in order to produce an "emotional state that is incompatible with the anxiety (i.e., pleasure and relaxation)". This was hypothesized to inhibit the anxiety response typically elicited by the procedure. This type of counterconditioning can be achieved by providing the individual with noncontingent access to pleasurable stimuli that include things like movies, TV, toys, or music (e.g., Hagopian et al. 2001), but can also be achieved by teaching specific relaxation responses like progressive muscle relaxation or diaphragmatic breathing (Lunsky et al. 2003; Gorski et al. 2004). These efforts at distracting or relaxing are typically initiated before exposure trials begin and then continue during the exposure trials. Whether access to these pleasurable activities actually elicit relaxation or functioning as distractors (or both) is unknown. Grider et al. (2012) suggested that access to a preferred video during difficult steps in an exposure protocol involving blood draws helped to distract the participant from the blood draw procedure, making it easier to complete. However, it is equally possible that the preferred video also elicited a calm, relaxed response that also made the exposures easier to complete.

Prompts. Some protocols have included prompts to help evoke the desired calm and cooperative behaviors needed to complete the mental-dental routine. Cavalari et al. (2013) developed a social story to prompt desired behavior during a routine physical examination. The story was read to an adolescent with autism and IDD prior to each graduated exposure session to prompt compliance and was available throughout the day during breaks. Other investigators have included photographs depicting the steps in the procedure to prompt appropriate behavior (e.g., Orellana et al. 2014). Cuvo et al. (2010b), had a physician assistant show children with autism a picture of another child successfully tolerating each step in a physical exam as a visual prompt for appropriate behavior. If the child did not comply, the child was again prompted by presentation of the picture paired with a verbal direction.

Behavioral momentum. Two studies were found to forego the traditional exposure-based approaches to medical/dental noncompliance described previously and instead evaluated increasing compliance using behavioral momentum. In this approach, the probability of complying with demands associated with a medical routine (i.e., low probability requests) is increased by preceding those demands with a string of demands for compliance with very easy tasks (i.e., high probability requests). In both studies, the presentation of high probability requests just prior to the presentation of low probability requests resulted in increases in compliance in the medical routine for a toddler needing central venous line care (McComas et al. 1998), and for children with autism undergoing a physical exam (Riviere et al. 2011).

Managing noncompliance. Each of the components describe above are designed to reduce the probability of problem behaviors occurring from the outset and/or to reinforce more appropriate responding. Nevertheless, it is important to consider how one will respond to noncompliance when it does occur. Responses to noncompliance varied across the studies, but typically involved either (1) physically blocking escape attempts and physically guiding compliance (escape prevented), (2) taking brief breaks from trials, ignoring the problem behavior, and then continuing exposure trials (escape permitted for brief periods) or (3) ending exposure trials when problems occurred (escape permitted that day). The first approach, escape extinction, aims to further weaken undesirable behaviors by eliminating one of the primary consequences thought to be responsible for maintaining noncompliance. While the latter two approaches offer only temporary escape (because exposure trials ultimately begin again), even temporary escape or avoidance can help maintain fear and noncompliance (Allen and Wallace 2013). Regardless of the approach taken to address noncompliance, these procedures were never used in isolation, but were used in combination with efforts to reduce the probability of noncompliance while reinforcing incompatible alternatives.

Escape extinction. Escape extinction was used by about a third of the investigators as a component of their intervention package. For example, Reimers et al. (1988) added escape extinction after they found that their graduated exposure and contingent reinforcement decreased avoidance behaviors when a nebulizer mask was first presented to a toddler with a developmental delay, but did not increase the amount of time the child left a mask on for nebulizer treatment. When they added escape extinction (i.e., the child was no longer allowed to remove the mask), there was a gradual increase in mask wearing and he was eventually able to wear the mask for the duration of the treatment. The appropriate mask wearing maintained following treatment with caregivers only periodically providing praise for mask wearing. In another study evaluating procedures for teaching children with IDD to tolerate needle sticks necessary for immunizations and/or blood draws, the children were not permitted to escape or avoid any of the procedures via redirecting, blocking and physically guiding the children to stay in the situation and complete each exposure (Slifer et al. 2011).

Practice Recommendations

Recommendation 1: The results of a conceptual analysis of medical/dental noncompliance suggested that conditioning is responsible for previously neutral stimuli acquiring the ability to both elicit emotional responses and evoke avoidance behaviors. Thus, one could take a preventive approach to dealing with noncompliance by taking early steps prior to the emergence of problem behaviors to increase the probability that neutral stimuli in medical and dental settings are conditioned to elicit relaxed behavior and evoke approach responses (Table 2.2). So, for example, rather than waiting until children are sick or have a cavity to visit the pediatrician or dentist, respectively, one could recommend to parents and caregivers that they make planned "field trips" to those settings when children are well with the intention of making the trip highly reinforcing in the presence of stimuli that are likely neutral or of low stimulus salience. These trips could be and probably should be short; no more than 15 min. A trip to the dentist might include playing with preferred toys in the exam room, interacting with staff and professionals who do NOT have masks and gloves on, riding the chair up and down, exploring nooks and crannies with the dental mirror, shining the dental light at objects in the room and choosing from different color toothbrushes before going home. A trip to the pediatrician might involve playing with preferred toys in the exam room, interacting with a staff person or medical professional who has no equipment, masks or gloves on, reading a short book, playing with a toy stethoscope and eventually trying it out on a parent, receiving a preferred trinket or edible and going home. Subsequent trips might include gradual exposure to slightly more salient stimuli, but because these are conducted by parents and caregivers and not trained clinicians, it is best to place the emphasis on exposure to stimuli not likely to already

Table 2.2 Summary of recommendations

Preventing the need for treatment
1. Parents/caregivers gets permission to plan multiple 10 min "field trips" to medical/dental clinic
2. Providers are asked to approve visit with only relaxing and reinforcing activities
3. Parents request no exposure to masks, gowns, gloves, or typical medical/dental instruments
4. Parents bring preferred toys, activities, edibles with them
5. Emphasis on ending visit while individual is relaxed and enjoying themselves
Preparation for treatment of medical/dental noncompliance
1. Conduct a task analysis
2. Develop a fear hierarchy
3. Conduct no-treatment exposures; observe the intensity of behavior, features of most salient stimuli, and how far the client is able to progress
4. Revise the task analysis to include any necessary substeps
5. Conduct a preference assessment
Treatment of medical/dental noncompliance
1. Provide noncontingent access to some preferred items to distract/relax the individual
2. Use in vivo modeling of appropriate behavior
3. Begin graduated exposure and provide reinforcement for compliance
4. Progress to the next step when the individual has been compliant with the current step and appears relaxed
5. Back up to easier steps if necessary to establish success

be conditioned as aversive. Planning multiple trips with relaxed and reinforcing experiences will be important for increasing the probability that neutral or low salience stimuli acquire conditioned calming or reinforcing properties. Of course, medical/dental staff will not have much time to invest in these activities and it is important to know that medical and dental professionals are not typically paid for their time; they are paid for procedures that are performed. So, it may be necessary to be highly flexible about when these type of activities are planned; often at the end of the day or during periods of low clinical activity. However, it may be more important to find a medical or dental professional who is experienced or comfortable with individuals with disabilities and understands that these early investments of time on positive conditioning and reap benefits in terms of patient loyalty and in terms of the ability to provide quality care with minimal risk.

Recommendation 2: The result of the research review appear clear: those who are interested in an evidence-based approach to addressing noncompliance with medical or dental procedures will start with in vivo graduated exposure as the core component in their treatment protocol (Table 2.2). Of course, an evidence-based practice always takes into consideration the unique needs of the individual client as well as the expertise of the practitioner when developing a treatment protocol and, perhaps as a result, there are certainly examples (albeit few) within the literature where in vivo graduated exposure was not used. Determining how best to approach the exposures will likely first require conducting an initial task analysis to determine all of the steps that would typically be included in the medical or dental routine involved.

Once all of the steps have been identified, the client will likely need to undergo one or more no-treatment (baseline) exposures to each step in the routine to allow observations about the intensity of avoidance behavior associated with each stimulus and each step and to see which steps and stimuli the client can tolerate and which must be terminated because of noncompliance. Thus, even if an individual cannot tolerate, for example, the blood pressure cuff at the beginning of a physical exam, or cannot tolerate the x-ray at the beginning of a dental exam, the initial assessment would continue on with other planned steps to allow an assessment of behavior at each step in the routine. This will help determine where to begin with treatment as it may not be necessary to conduct exposure training with every step in a medical or dental routine if only certain steps are disrupted or terminated.

This initial observation should also help evaluate whether to create "substeps" for some routines (i.e., breaking some steps into smaller steps), and which features of relevant stimuli (e.g., distance, size, duration, or intensity of exposure) are most salient and most amenable to gradual presentation. Some studies include sample hierarchies for graduated exposure that are generic enough to be useful in many typical situations where noncompliance might appear in individuals with IDD, including dental exams (i.e., Altabet 2002; Cuvo et al. 2010a), physical exams (e.g., Cavalari et al. 2013), blood draw routines (e.g., Slifer et al. 2011; Grider et al. 2012) and pill swallowing (e.g., Beck et al. 2005).

Recommendation 3: Include a preference assessment during treatment development to identify tangible items and passive activities that can be used as reinforcers delivered contingent upon desired calm, "coping" behaviors after each exposure (Table 2.2). These may include edibles, music, videogames, TV, toys, and/or tokens/money that can be exchanged later. Consider making noncontingent access to some of these preferred items available just before each session of graduate exposures to distract/relax the individual before the exposures begin.

Recommendation 4: Consider including in vivo modeling by a parent or caregiver of appropriate behavior prior to or during graduated exposures. This approach is low cost and could be easily incorporated with minimal disruption to the routine. Note that modeling has been found ineffective as a lone intervention for dental routines.

Recommendation 5: Give careful consideration to how disruptive behavior will be addressed. Most researchers have demonstrated good success without including escape extinction, but doing so may require a more gradual approach to exposures that lengthens the course of treatment. Rejecting escape extinction may also reduce some risks of injury to the individual and the providers who might be asked to use physical guidance or blocking. However, it is important to assess the medical necessity of treatment to determine whether allowing escape from treatment presents its own risks.

Research Recommendations

Although the research literature shows considerable agreement about the key components of an effective intervention to address medical/dental noncompliance, there are important questions that remain unanswered about these components. The vast majority of the studies on medical/dental noncompliance have implemented treatment packages that include a variety of components, so the independent effects of the individual components or the summative effects of multiple components are not well known. These issues are important for the advancement of both science and practice. For example, evaluating the power of respondent extinction and counterconditioning alone are important for a science like applied behavior analysis that tends to emphasize the operant aspects of behavior change. But component analyses are also important for practitioners who may not have the time or resources to implement complex intervention packages; an approach that researchers sometimes rely on to maximize treatment outcomes.

Practitioners would also benefit from research that attempts to clarify the best criteria for deciding when to advance exposures. Most procedures required mastery (i.e., compliance) with the current step on two or three sessions before moving on to the next step, but focusing on compliance alone during exposures may lead to practitioners progressing when fear responses have not yet been extinguished. Yet it is unknown whether asking practitioners to continue with exposures until calm behavior is observed adds anything valuable to a protocol. Furthermore, it is not clear how best to operationalize "calm" or whether adding more objective measures of fear responses (e.g., heart rate) might be useful alternatives.

Perhaps not surprisingly, the majority of interventions targeting medical/dental noncompliance in individuals with IDD have been developed within the field of applied behavior analysis. As a result, the most well supported interventions have numerous features characteristic of applied behavior analysis; they tend to be explicitly behavioral, individualized, function-driven treatments evaluated within small n research studies that emphasize demonstrations of functional relations and internal validity. While this approach is highly valued within a natural science of behavior, interventions that are highly individualized do not lend themselves to wide dissemination or adoption, even within applied behavior analysis and certainly not within medical/dental clinics where these problems are typically first encountered. However, there are enough common elements to treating medical noncompliance that they could be standardized to create a manualized protocol. Randomized controlled trials could then provide additional demonstrations of generality of the intervention, something thought to be important to the dissemination of an intervention (Barlow et al. 2009).

References

Allen, K. D., Hutfless, S., & Larzelere, R. (2003). Evaluation of two predictors of child disruptive behavior during restorative dental treatment. *Journal of Dentistry for Children, 70*(3), 1–5.

Allen, K. D., & Wallace, D. W. (2013). Effectiveness of using noncontingent escape for general behavior management in a pediatric dental clinic. *Journal of Applied Behavior Analysis, 46*, 723–737. doi:10.1002/jaba.82

Altabet, S. C. (2002). Decreasing dental resistance among individuals with severe and profound mental retardation. *Journal of Developmental and Physical Disabilities, 14*, 297–305. doi:10.1023/A:1016032623478

APA. (2006). Evidence based practice in psychology. *American Psychologist, 61*(4), 271–285. doi:10.1037/0003-066X.61.4.271

Azarpazhooh, A., & Leake, J. L. (2006). Systematic review of the association between respiratory diseases and oral health. *Journal of Periodontology, 77*(9), 1465–1482. doi:10.1902/jop.2006.060010

Barlow, D., Nock, M., & Hersen, M. (2009). *Single-case experimental designs: Strategies for studying behavior change*. Boston: Pearson Education.

Beck, M. H., Cataldo, M., Slifer, K. J., Pulbrook, V., & Guhman, J. K. (2005). Teaching children with attention deficit hyperactivity disorder (ADHD) and autistic disorder (AD) how to swallow pills. *Clinical Pediatrics, 5*, 515–552. doi:10.1177/000992280504400608

Boj, J. R., & Davila, J. M. (1989). A study of behavior modification for developmentally disabled children. *Journal of Dentistry for Children, 56*, 452–457.

Brady, J. V., (1978). Foreward. In W. W. Henton & I. H. Iverson (Eds.), *Classical conditioning and operant conditioning*. (pp v–vii). New York: Springer.

Cavalari, R., DuBard, M., Luiselli, J. K., & Birtwell, K. (2013). Teaching an adolescent with Autism and intellectual disability to tolerate routine medical examination: Effects of a behavioral compliance training package. *Clinical Practice in Pediatric Psychology, 1*, 121–128. doi:10.1037/cpp0000013

Chambless, D. L., & Ollendick, T. H. (2001). Empirically supported psychological interventions: Controversies and evidence. *Annual Review of Psychology, 52*, 685–716.

Conyers, C., Miltenberger, R. G., Peterson, B., Gubin, A., Jurgens, M., Selders, A., et al. (2004). An evaluation of an in vivo desensitization and video modeling to increase compliance with dental procedures in persons with mental retardation. *Journal of Applied Behavior Analysis, 37*, 233–238. doi:10.1901/jaba.2004.37-233

Cumella, S., Ransford, N., Lyons, J., & Burnham, H. (2000). Needs for oral care among people with intellectual disability not in contact with community dental services. *Journal of Intellectual Disabilities Research, 44*, 45–52.

Cuvo, A. J., Godard, A., Huckfeldt, R., & DeMattei, R. (2010a). Training children with autism spectrum disorders to be compliant with an oral assessment. *Research in Autism Spectrum Disorders, 4*, 681–696. doi:10.1016/j.rasd.2010.01.007

Cuvo, A. J., Law Reagan, A., Ackerlund, J., Huckfeldt, R., & Kelly, C. (2010b). Training children with autism spectrum disorders to be compliant with a physical exam. *Research in Autism Spectrum Disorders, 4*, 168–185. doi:10.1016/j.rasd.2009.09.001

Davis, T. E., & Ollendick, T. H. (2005). Empirically supported treatments for specific phobia in children: Do efficacious treatments address the components of a phobic response? *Clinical Psychology: Science and Practice, 12*, 144–160. doi:10.1093/clipsy.bpi018

Davit, C. J., Hundley, R. J., Bacic, J. D., & Hanson, E. M. (2011). A pilot study to improve venipuncture compliance in children and adolescents with autism spectrum disorders. *Journal of Developmental and Behavioral Pediatrics, 32*, 521–525. doi:10.1097/DBP.0b013e3182245b09

DeMore, M., Cataldo, M., Tierney, E., & Slifer, K. (2009). Behavioral approaches to training developmentally disabled children for an overnight EEG procedure. *Journal of Developmental and Physical Disabilities, 21*, 245–251. doi:10.1007/s10882-009-9139-7

Fisher, W., Piazza, C. C., Bowman, L. G., Hagopian, L. P., Owens, J. C., & Slevin, I. (1992). A comparison of two approaches for identifying reinforcers for persons with severe and profound disabilities. *Journal of Applied Behavior Analysis, 25*, 491–498. doi:10.1901/jaba.1992.25-491

Frankl, S. N., Shiere, F. R., & Fogels, H. R. (1962). Should the parent remain with the child in the dental operatory? *Journal of Dentistry for Children, 29*, 150–163.

Gillis, J. M., Hammond Natof, T., Lockshin, S. B., & Romanczyk, R. G. (2009). Fear of routine physical exams in children with autism spectrum disorders: Prevalence and intervention effectiveness. *Focus on Autism and Other Developmental Disabilities, 24*, 156–168. doi:10.1177/1088357609338477

Gillis, J. M., & Romanczyk, R. G. (n.d.). Behavioral observation assessment. Unpublished survey. Gorski, J., Slifer, K. J., Kelly-Suttka, J., & Lowery, K. (2004). Behavioral interventions for pediatric patients' acute pain and anxiety: Improving health regimen compliance and outcome. *Children's Health Care, 33*, 1–20. doi: 10.1207/s15326888chc3301_1

Gorski, J., & Westbrook, A. C. (2002). Differential reinforcement to treat non-compliance in a pediatric patient with leukocyte adhesion deficiency. *Pediatric Rehabilitation, 5*, 29–35.

Gorski, J., Slifer, K., Kelly-Suttka, J., & Lowery, K (2004). Behavioral interventions for pediatric patients' acute pain and anxiety: Improving health regimen compliance and outcome. *Children's Health Care, 33*(1), 1–20.

Grider, B., Luiselli, J. K., & Turcotte-Shamski, W. (2012). Graduated exposure, positive reinforcement, and stimulus distraction in a compliance-with-blood-draw intervention for an adult with autism. *Clinical Case Studies, 11*, 253–260. doi:10.1177/1534650112448921

Gullone, E. (2005). The development of normal fear: A century of research. *Clinical Psychology Review, 20*, 429–451. doi:10.1016/S0272-7358(99)00034-3

Ghuman, J., Cataldo, M., Beck, M., & Slifer, K. (2004). Behavioral training for pill-swallowing difficulties in young children with autistic disorder. *Journal of Child and Adolescent Autistic Disorder, 14*(4), 601–611.

Hagopian, L. P., Crockett, J. L., & Keeney, K. M. (2001). Multicomponent treatment for blood-injury injection phobia in a young man with mental retardation. *Research in Developmental Disabilities, 21*, 141–149. doi:10.1016/S0891-4222(01)00063-4

Isong, I. A., Rao, S. R., Holifiedl, C., Iannuzzi, D., Hanson, E., & Ware, J., et al. (2014). Addressing dental fear in children with autism spectrum disorders: A randomized controlled pilot using electronic screen media. *Clinical Pediatrics, 53*, 230–237. doi:10.1177/0009922813517169

Janicki, M. P., Dalton, A. J., Henderson, C. M., & Davidson, P. W. (1999). Mortality and morbidity among adults with intellectual disability: Health services considerations. *Disability and Rehabilitation, 21*, 284–294.

Jennett, H. K., & Hagopian, L. P. (2008). Identifying empirically supported treatments for phobic avoidance in individuals with intellectual disabilities. *Behavior Therapy, 39*, 151–161. doi:10.1016/j.beth.2007.06.003

King, N. J., Muris, P., & Ollendick, T. H. (2005). Childhood fears and phobias: Assessment and treatment. *Child and Adolescent Mental Health, 10*, 50–56. doi:10.1111/j.1475-3588.2005.00118.x

Knapp, L. G., Barrett, R. P., Groden, G., & Groden, J. (1992). The nature and prevalence of fears in developmentally disabled children and adolescents: A preliminary investigation. *Journal of Developmental and Physical Disabilities, 4*, 195–203. doi:10.1007/BF01046964

Krahn, G., Hammond, L., & Turner, A. (2006). A cascade of disparities: Health and health care for people with intellectual disabilities. *Mental Retardation and Developmental Disabilities Research Reviews, 12*, 70–82. doi:10.1002/mrdd.20098

Lennox, N., & Kerr, M. (1997). Primary health care and people with an intellectual disability: The evidence base. *Journal of Intellectual Disability Research, 41*, 365–372. doi:10.1111/j.1365-2788.1997.tb00723.x

Lewis, M. A., Lewis, C. E., Leake, B., King, B. H., & Lindemann, R. (2002). The quality of health care for adults with developmental disabilities. *Public Health Reports, 117*, 174–184.

Lunsky, Y., Straiko, A., & Armstrong, S. (2003). Women be healthy: Evaluation of a women's health curriculum for women with intellectual disabilities. *Journal of Applied Research in Intellectual Disabilities, 16*, 247–253. doi:10.1046/j.1468-3148.2003.00160.x

Luscre, D. M., & Center, D. B. (1996). Procedures for reducing dental fear in children with autism. *Journal of Autism and Developmental Disorders, 26*, 547–556. doi:10.1007/BF02172275

Maguire, K. B., Lange, B., Scherling, M., & Grow, R. (1996). The use of rehearsal and positive reinforcement in the dental treatment of uncooperative patients with mental retardation. *Journal of Developmental and Physical Disabilities, 8*, 167–177. doi:10.1007/BF02578447

McComas, J. J., Wacker, D. P., & Cooper, L. J. (1998). Increasing compliance with medical procedures: Application of the high-probability request procedure to a toddler. *Journal of Applied Behavior Analysis, 31*, 287–290. doi:10.1901/jaba.1998.31-287

McKinney, C. M., Nelson, T., Scott, J., Heaton, L., Vaughn, M., & Lewis, C. (2014). Predictors of unmet dental need in children with autism spectrum disorder: Results from a national sample. *Academic Pediatrics, 14*, 624–631. doi:10.1016/j.acap.2014.06.023

O'Hare, M. W., Ghoneim, M. M., Hinrichs, J. V., Mehta, M. P., & Wright, E. J. (1989). Psychological consequences of surgery: Psychological preparation of mothers of preschool children. *Psychosomatic Medicine, 51*, 356–370.

Orellana, L. M., Martinez-Sanchis, S., & Silvestre, F. J. (2014). Training adults and children with an autism spectrum disorder to be compliant with a clinical dental assessment using a TEACCH-based approach. *Journal of Autism and Developmental Disorders, 44*, 776–785. doi:10.1007/s10803-013-1930-8

Prasher, V., Cumella, S., Natarajan, K., Rolfe, E., Shah, S., & Haque, M. S. (2003). Magnetic resonance imaging, down's syndrome and Alzheimer's disease: Research and clinical implications. *Journal of Intellectual Disability Research, 47*, 90–100. doi:10.1046/j.1365-2788.2003.00445.x

Reimers, T. M., Piazza, C. C., Fisher, W. W., Parrish, J. M., & Page, T. J. (1988). Enhancing child compliance with nebulized respiratory treatment. *Clinical Pediatrics, 27*, 605–608. doi:10.1177/000992288802701208

Rimmer, J. H. (1999). Health promotion for people with disabilities: Emerging paradigm shift from disability prevention to prevention of secondary conditions. *Physical Therapy, 79*, 495–502.

Riviere, V., Becquet, M., Peltret, E., Facon, B., & Darcheville, J. (2011). Increasing compliance with medical examination requests directed to children with autism: Effects of a high-probability request procedure. *Journal of Applied Behavior Analysis, 44*, 193–197. doi:10.1901/jaba.2011.44-193

Seymour, G. J., Ford, P. J., Cullinen, M. P., Leishman, S., & Yamazaki, K. (2007). Relationship between periodontal infections and systemic disease. *Clinical Microbiology & Infection, 13*, 3–10. doi:10.1111/j.1469-0691.2007.01798.x

Shabani, D. B., & Fisher, W. W. (2006). Stimulus fading and differential reinforcement for the treatment of needle phobia in a youth with autism. *Journal of Applied Behavior Analysis, 39*, 449–452. doi:10.1901/jaba.2006.30-05

Silverman, W. K. (2011). Fears and phobias. In G. Koocher & A. la Greca (Eds.), *The parents guide to psychological first aid* (pp. 231–238). Oxford: University Press.

Slifer, K. J., Avis, K. T., & Frutch, R. A. (2008). Behavioral intervention to increase compliance with electroencephalographic procedures in children with developmental disabilities. *Epilepsy & Behavior, 13*, 189–195. doi:10.1016/j.yebeh.2008.01.013

Slifer, K. J., Hankinson, J. C., Zettler, M. A., Frutchey, R. A., Hendricks, M. C., & Ward, C. M., et al. (2011). Distraction, exposure therapy, counterconditioning, and topical anesthetic for acute pain management during needle sticks in children with intellectual and developmental disabilities. *Clinical Pediatrics, 50*, 688–697. doi:10.1177/0009922811398959

Slifer, K. J., Kruglak, D., Benore, E., Bellipanni, K., Falk, L., Halbower, A. C., et al. (2007). Behavioral training for increasing preschool children's compliance with positive airway pressure: A preliminary study. *Behavioral Sleep Medicine, 5*, 147–175. doi:10.108/15402000701190671

Tucker, C. L., Slifer, K. J., & Dahlquist, L. M. (2001). Reliability and validity of the brief distress scale: A measure of children's distress during invasive medical procedures. *Journal of Pediatric Psychology, 26*, 513–523.

Wolff, J. J., & Symons, F. J. (2012). An evaluation of multi-component exposure treatment of needle phobia in an adult with autism and intellectual disability. *Journal of Applied Research in Intellectual Disabilities, 26*, 344–348. doi:10.1111/jar.12002

Chapter 3
Personal Hygiene

Jennifer M. Gillis Mattson, Matthew Roth and Melina Sevlever

Introduction

Personal hygiene is generally defined as encompassing multiple behaviors required to maintain a clean and healthy body in the context of both social norms as well as physical health. Personal hygiene is one of the most effective ways to prevent contracting and spreading illness and disease and is cited as one of the important areas for intervention for individuals with intellectual and developmental disabilities (IDD) (Myles 2005). With respect to behavioral health, establishment of personal hygiene skills leads to an improved quality of life, improved medical outcomes for an individual, and a reduction in disease incidence (Ersoy et al. 2009; Sheppard 2006). The level of independence in managing one's personal hygiene is an important factor in determining type of residential placement, in the development of social relationships and success in social contexts as well as vocational placements. In other words, personal hygiene promotes independence in addition to improving health outcomes. Noting that there are multiple personal hygiene skills that one learns across the lifespan, this chapter addresses grooming, oral hygiene and menstrual care.

J.M.G. Mattson (✉)
Department of Psychology, Binghamton University, New York, NY 13902-6000, USA
e-mail: jmattson@binghamton.edu

M. Roth
Auburn University, Auburn, USA

M. Sevlever
New York Presbyterian/Columbia University Medical Center, New York, USA

J.K. Luiselli (ed.), *Behavioral Health Promotion and Intervention in Intellectual and Developmental Disabilities*, Evidence-Based Practices in Behavioral Health,
DOI 10.1007/978-3-319-27297-9_3

Grooming is a daily self-care activity, involving multiple skills (e.g., hand washing, showering, shaving, hair care, and using health care products) that spans across the lifespan. Barriers to appropriate grooming in individuals with IDD include specific skill deficits, noncompliance, and sensory sensitivity. To help overcome these barriers to grooming independence, there are a number of interventions reviewed in the literature, including instruction, behavioral skills training, video modeling, self-monitoring, pictorial cues, general case instruction, and sensory adaptation. Implementation of effective interventions to increase grooming skills promotes behavioral health in multiple ways. For example, increased and appropriate hand washing leads to lower rates of respiratory illnesses as well as diarrheal diseases in child care and school settings (Master et al. 1997; Niffenegger 1997; World Health Organization 2001).

Menstrual care is a highly important self-care skill for females that is often overlooked and research on improving menstrual care in females with IDD is lacking (Ersoy et al. 2009). Females with developmental disabilities are capable of learning to care for their menstruation when provided with behavioral skills training. Such intervention can lead to a significant improvement in the lives and families of females with developmental disabilities, and by extension, females with IDD who otherwise have to rely on parental or caregiver support to manage the private issue of menstruation.

Toothbrushing, flossing, and participating in dental exams are all important oral hygiene skills that yield improved oral health. Starting at the first showing of a tooth and at least by the age of 1 year old, it is recommended that children establish a dental "home" and participate in a dental examination and cleaning (Norwood and Slayton 2013). Poor oral health negatively impacts a person's ability to eat, sleep and function without pain. Chronic oral health problems contribute to increased rates of systemic illness (e.g., pneumonia). The two most common diseases of the mouth that can be lessened or prevented by adequate oral hygiene are dental caries (cavities) of the teeth, and gingivitis and periodontal disease, which affect the gums or gingiva and supporting structures of the teeth, respectively (Norwood and Slayton 2013). However, establishment and maintenance of adequate oral hygiene is problematic for many individuals with IDD. One of the most prevalent barriers to accessing dental care for children with IDD is problem behavior in the dental setting (Brickhouse et al. 2009; Lai et al. 2012). Another challenge to overcome is that for many individuals with IDD, learning how to independently brush teeth and floss daily requires significantly more resources than for children without IDD. Addressing each of these barriers is critical for improving the physical health of individuals with IDD across the lifespan in addition to increasing independence in self-care skills required for independent living.

This chapter describes the personal hygiene concerns of grooming, oral hygiene and menstrual care that are of priority for individuals with IDD and other neurodevelopmental disorders. A review of current research literature on effective interventions for each of these areas is provided. Given the available research, we describe practice recommendations that the clinician to consider when improving a client's personal hygiene is a priority.

Priority Concerns

Grooming

Grooming behaviors, such as hand washing, showering, shaving, hair care, and using health care products come with a number of health and social benefits. For instance, grooming can lead to the avoidance of disease and sickness (Walmsley et al. 2013). In addition, grooming has been found to have a positive effect on an individual's self-esteem as it often leads to increased social acceptance and relationships (Garff and Storrey 1998; Stokes et al. 2004). Being well groomed also influences other's perception of physical attractiveness (Barry et al. 1977). Our family, friends, and co-workers expect us to be well groomed. As an example, as children begin to transition into puberty, they are expected to independently shower on a daily basis and wear deodorant to hide potential body odor. Given these expectations from others, it is not surprising that the consequences of poor grooming often include social isolation and even termination from employment.

Unfortunately, a number of studies have found that individuals with developmental disabilities have difficulty with grooming across all levels of functioning and ages. Overall, grooming problems has been identified as a barrier to integration into mainstream environments for individuals with developmental disabilities (Bolte and Poustka 2002; Carter et al. 1998; Garff and Storrey 1998; Matson et al. 2012; Palmen et al. 2012). For instance, Ellis et al. (2006) noted that the difficulty that some children have with applying sunscreen might prevent them from joining outdoor activities with their same aged peers. Additionally, poor grooming has been found to be primary reason that individuals with developmental disabilities are removed from supported employment settings (Garff and Storrey 1998; Reisman and Reisman 1993).

Difficulty with grooming is related to a number of factors. For one, the severity of a client's symptoms and motor and language impairments, contribute to poor grooming skills (Matson et al. 2012). Additionally, compliance is a major concern during grooming tasks, as clients are often avoidant or demonstrate significant problem behavior (DeLeon et al. 2008; Matson et al. 2012). One potential reason that clients may avoid grooming is due to sensitivity to sensory stimuli (e.g., tactile stimulation; Ellis et al. 2006). An issue cited in the literature is a concern of prompt dependency, specifically, that caregivers often are completing or prompting clients to complete many personal hygiene tasks (Cridland et al. 2014;

Palmen et al. 2012). Unfortunately, when individuals become prompt dependent, any change in that environment, such as variations in schedule or staff turnaround, may lead to a disruption of that grooming behavior.

Oral Hygiene

Establishing oral hygiene skills begins at the time a baby's first tooth appears and extends throughout one's lifespan. Maintaining oral hygiene leads to similar social consequences outlined in the grooming section. Additionally, failure to maintain adequate oral hygiene often leads to numerous oral health problems including gingivitis, plaque build-up, and dental caries (Fickert and Ross 2012; Norwood and Slayton 2013). To establish good oral hygiene one needs to engage in daily tooth brushing and flossing (ideally twice per day) as well as dental check-ups every six months. Learning to brush one's teeth is one of the first important personal hygiene skills we learn. Unfortunately, many parents report that their children require some assistance in oral hygiene skills of tooth brushing and flossing (Bishop et al. 2013). In addition, a substantial percentage of adults (47 %) with ASD do not independently and regularly brush their teeth (Orellana et al. 2012). Some of the reported reasons for this deficiency include a client's level of communication skills, listening repertoire, and motor skills. Parents report that a major barrier in completing toothbrushing with their child is due to problem behavior (Bishop et al. 2013). Due to some of the difficulties in establishing independent toothbrushing and other oral care activities for clients over the age of 5,[1] it is important to consider teaching parents or other caregivers, including clinicians, in how to provide oral care (Bishop et al. 2013).

Certainly good toothbrushing and flossing skills are helpful in maintaining oral hygiene. Another important skill is participation in routine (i.e., semi-annual) dental examinations. In ideal circumstances this includes establishing a consistent dental home (i.e., dental office) for the client. This goal is not always easy as some families report difficulty finding a dentist who is willing to care for their child or adolescent (Norwood and Slayton 2013). Unfortunately, there are simply not enough pediatric dentists who have training in providing care to children with developmental needs (Norwood and Slayton 2013). Finding and establishing a dental home for individuals can be challenging for several client-related reasons (Graudins et al. 2012). These include but are not limited to, disruptive or problematic behavior, level of receptive and expressive language, ability to follow multistep directions, anxiety or fear of dental exams and the cost of dental care to parents (Loo et al. 2008; Lai et al. 2012; Marshall et al. 2007; Norwood and

[1]The Centers for Disease control and Prevention recommend that parents brush their child's teeth until the child can use the toothbrush which is usually around age 4 or 5 years old (http://www.cdc.gov/oralhealth/pdfs/brushupquiz.pdf).

Slayotn 2013; Stein et al. 2014). In many instances, children with IDD consistently require more restraint during dental cleaning compared to same age peers without IDD (Stein et al. 2014). It is easy to imagine how difficulty in attending regular dental appointments might lead families to make these types of appointments for their child less regularly, which might negatively impact oral health. Identifying ways to improve behavior within the dental care setting would improve maintenance of proper oral hygiene for many individuals with IDD.

Menstrual Care

For females, menstrual care can easily be described as the most critical personal hygiene skill (Ersoy et al. 2009). Appropriate menstrual care can affect a wide range of quality of life indices for individuals with developmental disabilities. For example, outings in the community may be limited during menarche due to the possibility of soiling and odor (Kreutner 1981). Specific activities, such as swimming may also be restricted (Grover 2011). In some cases, individuals with developmental disabilities may even miss work or school if there is significant concern that she may not be able to manage menstruation on her own (Yaacob et al. 2012). The lack of independent menstrual care skills may also adversely affect interpersonal relationships for individuals with developmental disabilities. If familial or paid caregivers are left with the responsibility of menstrual care management, the potential for negative interactions increases. Indeed, caregivers frequently report menstrual care to be a highly distressing aspect of caring for their child with a developmental disability (Atkinson et al. 2003; Carlson and Wilson 1996; Mason and Cunningham 2008; Saltonstall 2007). Such assistance may also be distressing from the perspective of individuals with a developmental disability if they are able to recognize the societal norms around menstruation and thus demonstrate understanding of the private nature of this self-care skill. Thus, it may be particularly embarrassing for individuals with developmental disabilities to seek assistance from caregivers in managing their menstrual care (Rodgers 2001; Rodgers and Lipscombe 2005). Finally, relying on others to manage menstrual care potentially increases the risk for sexual abuse in this already vulnerable population.

Unfortunately, menstrual care instruction for individuals with developmental disabilities has received relatively little empirical attention within the self-care literature (Ersoy et al. 2009). Moreover, teaching independent menstrual care skills to individuals with developmental disabilities poses significant difficulty given the potential for an invasion to the individual's privacy (Ersoy et al.). Historically, the primary approach for managing menstruation in women with developmental disabilities focused on sterilization by either endometrial ablation or hysterectomy (Backeljauw et al. 2004; Grover 2011). Fortunately, legal and ethical advances in the last several decades have significantly curbed the use of sterilization practices (American Academy of Pediatrics Committee on Bioethics 1999). Although hysterectomies are much less common, a large proportion of females with developmental disabilities are prescribed a continuous oral contraceptive pill regimen in order to eliminate periods (Hamilton et al. 2011; Lennox et al. 2005). Although much less invasive, the long-term effects of manipulating the natural menstrual cycle is unclear (Backeljauw et al. 2004). Moreover, the lack of regular menstruation may increase the risk of sexual abuse since the risk of pregnancy is no longer a deterrent for potential abusers (Brady and Grover 1997). As an alternative to medically inducing amenorrhea, behavioral interventions were developed to teach independent menstrual care skills to females with developmental disabilities.

Research Findings on Effectiveness and Efficacy of Methods and Procedures

Research on effectiveness of interventions for the development and teaching of personal hygiene skills includes different methods and procedures that have been evaluated for each of the personal hygiene skills described in this chapter. To aid in assisting the reader with identifying relevant interventions, a sample of articles for each personal hygiene area (i.e., grooming, oral hygiene, and menstrual care) is provided in Table 3.1. For each study, we present information about the participants, intervention, the study's certainty of evidence, and the strength of the study's findings. A study's certainty of evidence was judged based on how well it followed the standards of single case research. Studies were placed in one of three categories: suggestive, preponderant, or conclusive. Studies were placed in the lowest category, suggestive, if weaknesses in the study interfered with conclusions about the intervention, for instance, using a nonexperimental A-B design, no or poor treatment fidelity and/or interobserver agreement, and insufficient information for replication of the study. Studies were placed in the middle category, preponderant, if there were noticeable weaknesses with the study's baseline measurement that reduced confidence that the intervention led to a change in behavior. The final level, conclusive, suggests the highest confidence in the findings and did not exhibit any of the flaws mentioned.

Grooming

Fortunately, there have been several studies examining the effectiveness of behavioral procedures targeting grooming skills for learners with developmental disabilities (Saloviita and Tuulkari 2000). Typically, these procedures are presented as part of a larger intervention package, which include a number of different components (Stokes et al. 2004). As such, the behavioral procedures discussed below were often combined with other procedures, rather than in isolation.

Table 3.1 Review of a Sample of Personal Hygiene Research Studies

Group Design Studies

Type of skill targeted	Authors	Title	Year	Population	Intervention	A comparison or control group in addition to intervention group?	Intervention group differences statistically significant?	Moderate power?	Intervention manual or equivalent used?	Reliable and valid treatment outcome measures included?	Overall rating: (suggestive, prepon-derant, conclusive)
Handwashing; Showering; Menstruation	Fabish & Thompson	The use of Filmstrips in Teaching Personal Hygiene to Moderately Retarded Adults	1970	Intellectual disability (mod-erate) (no ages provided)	Modeling; Filmstrips	Yes	Yes	No	Yes	No	Preponderant (no power analysis; unreliable outcome measures)
Showering	Matson, DiLorenzo, & Esveldt-Dawson	Independence Training as a Method of Enhancing Self-Help Skills Acquisition of the Mentally Retarded	1981	Moderate to Severe Intellectual Disability (21 to 55)	Psychoeducation, Modeling, Feedback, Self- and Other-Evaluation, Social Reinforcement	Yes	Yes	No	Yes	Yes	Preponderant (power not reported)
Showing	Matson, Marcheti, & Adkins	Comparison of Operant and Independence Training Procedures for Mentally Retarded Adults	1980	Intellectual Disability (moderate to profound; 22 to 57 years old)	Verbal prompts; modeling; manual guidance; social reinforcement; shaping; fading; chaining; tangible reinforcement; self-monitoring	Yes	Yes	No	Yes	Yes	Preponderant (power not reported)

(continued)

Table 3.1 (continued)

Single Subject Design Studies

Type of skill targeted	Authors	Title	Year	Population	Intervention	Experimental design	Adequate Treatment or Procedural Fidelity?	Adequate Interobserver Agreement?	Sufficient information for replication?	Overall rating (suggestive, preponderant, conclusive)
Eye Care - Wearing Glasses	DeLeon, Hagopian, Rodriguez-Catter, Bowman, Long, & Boelter	Increasing Wearing of Prescription Glasses in Individuals with Mental Retardation	2008	Intellectual Disability (moderate to severe) (4 to 19 years old)	Component Analysis: NCR; Response Blocking; Response Cost	Reversal; Multielement	No	Yes	Yes	Suggestive; no fidelity
Handwashing	Rosenberg, Schwartz, & Davis	Evaluation the Utility of Commercial Videotapes for Teaching Handwashing to Children with Autism	2010	Autism (3 to 5 year olds)	Commerical Video Modeling; Custom Video Modeling	Multiple Baseline Across Participants	Yes	Yes	Yes	Conclusive
Handwashing	Walmsley, Mahoney, Durgin, & Poling, 2013	Fostering Hand Washing Before Lunch By Students Attending a Special Neeeds Young Adult Program	2013	Developmental Disabilities (20 to 25 years)	Psychoeducation, least-to-most prompting, lottery system, immediate feedback	Multiple Baseline Across Groups	No	Yes	Yes	Suggestive; no fidelity

(continued)

Table 3.1 (continued)

Handwashing and Facewashing	Treffry, Martin, Samels, & Watson, 1970	Operant Conditioning of Grooming Behavior of Severely Retarded Girls	1970	Intellectual Disability	Positive reinforcement, time-out from positive reinforcement, punishment, fading, and task analysis	A-B Design	No	No	No	Suggestive; no fidelity, no IOA, no baseline, not enough for replication
Skincare	Ellis, Ala'i-Rosales, Glenn, Rosales-Ruiz, Greenspoon	The Effects of Graduate Exposure, Modeling, and Contingent Social Attention on Tolerance to Skin Care Products with Two Children with Autism	2006	Autism (4 years old)	Graduated exposure, modeling, contingent attention, task analysis	Changing Criterion with Multiple Baseline Across Prodcuts	No (inadequate sessions)	Yes	Yes	Suggestive; no fidelity
Grooming (washing hands, face, and armpits)/ Toothbrushing	Saloviita & Tuulkari	Cognitive-Behavoural Treatment Package for Teaching Grooming Skills to a Man with an Intellectual Disability	2000	Moderate Intellectual Dsiability (41 years old)	Self-management, pictorial prompts, psychoeducation, social attention	Multiple Baseline Across Behaviors	Yes	No	Yes	Suggestive; inadequate fidelity (16%)
Grooming (showering, dressing)/ Toothbrushing/ Toileting/ Cleaning	Jarman, Iwata, & Lorentzson	Development of Morning Self-Care Routines In Multiply Handicapped Persons	1983	Moderate to Severe Intelectual Disability (14 to 57 years old)	Token economy for single behaviors; token economy for behavioral chain	Group Multiple Baseline Across Behaviors	No	No (inadequate sessions)	Yes	Suggestive (no fidelity; inadequate IOA; intervening on increasing baseline)

(continued)

Table 3.1 (continued)

Grooming - Facewashing; Shaving; Toothbrushing; Hair Combing; Glasses Cleaning	Thinesen & Bryan	The Use of Sequential Pictorial Cues in the Initiation and Maintenance of Grooming Behaviors with Mentally Retarded Adults	1981	Intellectual Disability (mild to moderate; 28-42 years)	Psychoeducation; Modeling; Pictorial cues; tangible reinforcement	Group Multiple Baseline Across Behaviors	No	Yes	Yes	Suggestive; no fidelity
Shaving; Toothbrushing; Cleaning Face	Garff & Storey	The Use of Self-Management Strategies for Increasing Appropriate Hygiene of Persons with Disabilities in Supported Employment Settings	1998	Intellectual Disability (26 to 56 year old)	Preference assessment; task analysis; modeling; self-management; reinforcement	A-B	No	Yes	Yes	Suggestive; AB design; no fidelity
Clean/combed hair; toothbrushing; showering, shaving, handwashing, fingernail care, clean shirt/pants	Barry, Apolloni, & Cooke	Improving the Personal Hygiene of Mildly Retarded Men in a Community-Based Residential Training Program	1977	Intellectual Disability (20 to 25 years)	Psychoeducation; pictorial prompts; behavior contracting	Multiple Baseline Across Participants	No	Yes	No	Suggestive; no fidelity; insufficient information for replication

(continued)

Table 3.1 (continued)

Menstraul Care	Richman, Reiss, Bauman, & Bailey	Teaching Menstrual Care to Mentally Retarded Women: Acquisition, Generalization, and Maintenance	1984	Mild to Severe Intellectual Disability (28 to 44 years)	Verbal prompts; physical guidance; forward chaining; token economy; social reinforcement; tangible reinforcement	Multiple Baseline Across Participants	No	Yes	Yes	Conclusive
Menstraul Care	Richman, Ponticas, Page, & Epps	Simulation Procedures for TeachingIndependent Menstrual Care toMentally Retarded Persons	1986	Moderate to Severe Intellectual Disability (17 to 21 years)	Modeling with a Doll; forward chaining; verbal prompts; physical guidance; social reinforcement; tangible reinforcement	Multiple Baseline Across Participants and Behaviors	No	Yes	Yes	Conclusive
Menstraul Care	Epps, Stern, & Horner	Comparison of Simulation Training on Self and Using a Doll for Teaching Generalized Menstrual Care to Women with Severe Mental Retardation	1990	Severe to Profound Intellectual Disability (15 to 37 years)	On-self modeling; modeling with a doll; forward chaining; verbal prompts; physical guidance; social reinforcement; tangible reinforcement	Split Multiple Baseline Across Subjects	No	No	Yes	Conclusive for on-self modeling only; doll modeling found to be ineffective for generalization of menstraul care skills

(continued)

Table 3.1 (continued)

Menstraul Care	Klett & Turan	Generalized Effects of Social Stories with Task Analysis for Teaching Menstrual Care to Three Young Girls with Autism	2011	Autism (9 to 12 years)	Social Story; social reinforcement	Multiple Baseline Across Participants and Behaviors	No	No	Yes	Preponderant
Menstraul Care	Ersoy, Tekin-Iftar, & Kircaali-Iftar	Effects of Antecedent Prompt and Test Procedure on Teaching Simulated Menstrual Care Skills to Females with Developmental Disabilities	2009	Mild to Moderate Developmental Disability (12 to 14 years)	Antecedent Prompts and Test Procedure (APTP); modeling, tangible reinforcement	Multiple Probe Design Across Participants	Yes	Yes	Yes	Conclusive
Compliance in toothbrushing	Bishop, Kenzer, Coffman, Tarbox, Tarbox, & Lanagan	Using stimulus fading without escape extinction to increase compliance with toothbrushing in children with autism	2013	Three children with ASD (4-5 years old)	Stimulus fading hierarchy, reinforcement.	Multiple Baseline Across Participants	No	Yes	Yes	Suggestive; no fidelity

(continued)

Table 3.1 (continued)

Compliance in dental exam	Cuvo, Godard, Huckfeldt, & DeMattei	Training children with autism spectrum disorders to be compliant with an oral assessment	2010	Five children with ASD (3 to 5 years old)	Behavioral treatment package: Video modeling, stimulus fading hierarchy, prompintg, distraction, differential reinforcement, escape extinction and preference assessment	Multiple Probe Across Responses	Yes	Yes	Yes	Conclusive
Compliance in dental exam	Luscre & Center	Procedures for reducing dental fear in children with autism	1996	Three children with ASD (6-9 years old)	Behavioral treatment package: Video modeling, systematic desensitization with guided mastery, reinforcement	Multiple Baseline Across Participants	No	Yes	Yes	Suggestive; no fidelity
Dental staff training	Graudins, Rehfeldt, DeMattei, Baker, & Scaglia	Exploring the efficacy of behavioral skills training to teach basic behavior analytic techniques to oral care providers	2012	Three oral care providers	Behavioral skills training in management of child behavior during dental exam.	Multiple Baseline Across Participants	Yes	Yes	Yes	Preponderant

Task analysis. Grooming does not consist of one behavior, but is instead made up a number of steps, which is commonly known as a behavior chain. For instance, shaving involves (a) turning sink on; (b) wetting face; (c) rubbing the shaving cream on hands to face; (d) lightly putting razor to cheek and pulling razor down, and so on. To teach grooming skills, the behavior chain is often broken down into a *task analysis*, or breaking the skill into smaller, teachable units in sequential order (Klett and Turan 2012). Teaching each individual part of chain is a successful way to promote grooming independence (Jarman et al. 1983).

Prompting. One of the simpler procedures for teaching grooming skills is *prompting*, which may include a verbal statement, gesturing, hand-over-hand teaching, and physical guidance through the behavior. Clinicians can prompt either using a *most-to-least* (most intrusive prompts used at first) procedure or a *least-to-most* (slowly increasing the intrusiveness of the prompt) procedure. Prompting has been found to work in teaching grooming skills to both children and adults with developmental disabilities. For instance, in an early study, Treffry et al. (1970) taught 11 girls with severe intellectual disability to wash their hands using least-to-most prompting (verbal prompting then physical guidance) while Matson et al. (1980) used least-to-most prompting (verbal then physical prompting) with modeling to teach adults with intellectual disability living in an institution a number of self-care skills in a group format. Finally, Walmsley et al. (2013) used least-to-most prompting (gesturing, partial physical guidance, and full guidance) and modeling to teach hand washing skills to young adults with developmental disabilities.

Video modeling. Recently, the increased availability of affordable technology had made *video modeling*, or demonstrating how to complete a behavior using video, an appealing way to teach grooming skills. Video modeling allows for consistency of the model and accessibility, as the model can be shown on a smart phone or tablet, in a modality that a learner may prefer. In one study using video modeling to teach hand washing skills to three preschool age boys with ASD (Rosenberg et al. 2010), a commercially purchased video modeling program was compared to custom made videos that used a favorite peer or sibling as the model. Videos were shown to the children twice followed by a verbal prompt to "wash your hands just like on the tape." Two out of the three students improved using the custom made video modeling and one child learned most of the skill from the commercial video tape.

Pictorial cues. In the case where learners have already acquired the skill but are not engaging in it independently, the use of pictorial cues, or showing the sequence of the skill in pictures, has been found to be effective. For instance, in one study that taught morning routine behaviors of face washing, shaving, combing hair, and other tasks to three adults with mild intellectual disability (Thinesen and Bryant 1981), pictorial cues were set up so that three pictures associated with each task were shown in a book that was followed by a picture of a reinforcer. Interestingly, as the learners began to engage in the behavior, they eventually only looked at the first picture, indicating that the one picture may have cued the entire routine sequence. In another investigation of pictorial cues (Saloviita and Tuulkari 2000), one adult with moderate intellectual disability learned tooth brushing, showering and face, hands and armpit washing using four pictures associated with each behavior in conjunction with instruction and least-to-most prompting. In addition to pictorial cues, film strips, which include more steps showing the sequence of a target behavior, have also been used effectively to promote grooming independence (Faibish and Thompson 1970).

Contingency contracts and token economies. The use of *contingency contracts* and *token economies* (arrangements that specify the behaviors that lead to reinforcement) is another way to promote independent grooming after the learner has already been taught the skills or if the learner is noncompliant. For instance, Jarman et al. (1983) used a token economy with a group of adults with moderate to severe intellectual disability on six self-care behaviors they had be trained on previously. The adults initially received reinforcement for performing three behaviors independently, which was eventually expanded to completing all six behaviors to receive tokens. In another study that examined the use of a contingency contract with three adults with mild intellectual disability for promoting independence of ten grooming behaviors, adults were initially reinforced for performing five out of the ten behaviors, which was increased by one behavior until all ten behaviors were performed (Barry et al. 1977).

Self-monitoring. Self-monitoring, where the learner themselves record instances of behavior to receive reinforcement, has also been found to be effective as a way to promote grooming independence, without adding an increased workload for caregivers. For instance, in an early study, Matson et al. (1980) used self-monitoring to teach a group of adults with moderate to profound intellectual disability showering and other behaviors by placing a poster board in a public place. When the learners engaged in a grooming task, they put a star next to their name. Compared to two other groups, the self-monitoring group was the only group that showed marked improvement in skills. Plus, the staff had favorable opinions, as it did not lead to an increased workload. In another study Garff and Storey (1998) used self-monitoring to teach three adults with mild intellectual disability shaving, tooth brushing, and cleaning their face and clothes using checklists made directly from a task analysis. Clients were told they would receive reinforcement if they met a particular criterion (e.g., shaving for four days in a week). Learners had an increase of "appropriate hygiene days" and their peers rated them as being more acceptable.

Sensory adaptation. When clients are avoiding grooming due to sensory sensitivity, helping them habituate to the sensitivity, or *sensory adaptation*, is warranted. In one study, DeLeon et al. (2008) targeted wearing prescription eyeglasses in four learners with moderate to severe intellectual disability. The intervention package included noncontingent reinforcement of preferred items (items presented independent of their behavior), continuous attention, blocking the removal of glasses, and removal of preferred items and attention for 30 s for the removal of glasses. Intervention was effective for three of the learners; one individual only needed non-contingent reinforcement and never received the full treatment package. In another study, Ellis et al. (2006) examined ways to increase tolerance to putting on lotion in in two preschool aged children with ASD.,

Intervention features a graduated exposure procedure by slowly introducing the product through looking, smelling, touching, and dabbing, along with modeling and a token economy. Both children were able to successfully complete the program with increased acceptance of the lotion.

Oral Hygiene

Similar to grooming, interventions for improving tooth-brushing skills are established in the behavioral literature. Notably, independent tooth brushing is sometimes considered a grooming skill. Less interest has been on teaching others to assist in tooth brushing skills and on how to improve skills required for routine dental examinations. The oral hygiene section covers training of oral health care providers, training of caregivers in oral care as well as compliance training for participating in dental exams.

Psychoeducation and training of caregivers in toothbrushing. One step in improving oral hygiene is providing education to parents, caregivers, and dental care staff (Faulks and Hennequin 2000). Fickert and Ross (2012) examined the effects of a caregiver education program in providing oral care to individuals with developmental disabilities. The participants in the study were caregivers who worked in community living residence and were responsible for providing oral hygiene to the individuals living there. A four-hour long educational component including modeling of appropriate tooth brushing and flossing techniques was conducted. Based on post-test scores and a 3-month follow up, the program was successful in increasing caregiver knowledge and compliance in providing adequate oral care to individuals in the residential setting. Interestingly, flossing was reportedly the most difficult to complete for most caregivers.

A recent study by Bishop et al. (2013) implemented a behavioral intervention package consisting of contingent reinforcement for compliance and stimulus fading hierarchy to increase compliance young children with ASD during toothbrushing by clinicians. The intervention was successful for all participants and generalized to parents. This study used a 30-step stimulus fading hierarchy that began with flashing the toothbrush from a distance to brushing teeth for 60s. Stimulus fading probes were conducted after mastery of every third step and at pre-determined steps which allowed participants to move through the hierarchy more quickly and eliminated on average 50 % of the steps.

Behavioral skills training for dental care staff. Lai et al. (2012) suggest increased education of dentists and dental hygienists behavioral management strategies in the dental setting. In addition, they recommend the use of strategies to help prepare child patients for a dental exam such as scheduling the appointment during an optimal time for the individual and preparing parents and the child more generally.

Graudins et al. (2012) examined a behavioral skills training package to teach dental staff behavior analytic techniques to decrease problem behavior in children with ASD during dental examinations. The study was implemented with three oral care providers in a dental setting. Participants watched a video model describing and showing how to conduct a dental exam and manage challenging behaviors by using differential reinforcement and escape extinction. Participants' role played critical interactions and were provided feedback. When participants mastered the skills, they practiced their skills in the in vivo setting with the child patients.. The training package took approximately 4 h to complete, was successful for all three participants, and generalized as well. Importantly, all participants demonstrated competence post-training and reported high levels of social validity of the training.

Compliance training packages. Luscre and Center (1996) implemented an intervention package that consisted of systematic desensitization, video peer modeling and contingent reinforcement. A stimulus hierarchy was developed consisting of 13 steps for completion of the dental exam. Systematic desensitization was utilized given that it is an empirically-supported treatment for specific phobia and noncompliance was conceptualized as fear or phobic avoidance (Jennett and Hagopian 2008). In systematic desensitization, anti-anxiety stimuli (e.g., music, play-doh, and other stimuli that elicit a positive response) were incorporated in sessions as a method of counter-conditioning. The intervention was conducted in an analog setting and then generalized to an in vivo setting. The intervention was partially successful in that some variability in compliance was observed in the dental setting.

Cuvo et al. (2010) implemented a similar behavioral training package for young children with ASD. A video of a peer model was part of the behavioral intervention package. Still photos from the video and photos of reinforcers were included as photo prompts to be used at the beginning of each session to assist in preparing the participant for the exam. Differential reinforcement in the form of praise was provided for every 10 s of compliance during the session. An escape extinction procedure was in place for noncompliant behavior. The dental exam was divided into 8 components and training on components where noncompliance occurred was provided in the study. A stimulus fading hierarchy was developed for each of the eight components. This hierarchy was similar to the hierarchy used in systematic desensitization procedures. The behavioral intervention package was successful for each child and generalization to the dental care setting and with a dental care provider was demonstrated.

Menstrual Care

Richman et al. (1984, 1986) can be credited with the two pioneering empirical studies of teaching independent menstrual care skills to women with intellectual disabilities. The authors developed a highly comprehensive task analysis of menstrual care skills that included three sub-skills: (a) menstrual stain on underwear, (b) menstrual stain on a sanitary pad, and (c) menstrual stain on both underwear and sanitary pad. Each sub-skill was comprised of approximately 20 steps such as "Identify stained under-wear; Obtain clean pad; Obtain clean underwear….."

Additionally, Richman et al. (1984) identified several prerequisite skills required for independent menstrual care. Given the skills required for adequate menstrual care, participants were only selected for participation in the study if they were ambulatory, proficient in toilet training skills, and able to respond to simple instructions.

Self-simulation behavior skills training package. The treatment package developed by Richman et al. (1984, 1986) combined several behavioral techniques including prompting, modeling, physical guidance, and reinforcement. Participants were prompted with the instruction "Check your pants," and a *forward chaining* procedure was implemented. Forward chaining describes a technique in which participants are taught a complex behavior skill, such as menstrual care, in a chain or series of steps. In this procedure, the first step in the task analysis is taught until participants demonstrate mastery, at which point the second step in the chain is introduced. This procedure was also combined with prompting, social reinforcement, and a token economy reinforcement system to teach menstrual care skills. If participants were unable to complete a task in the menstrual care chain, they were provided with verbal prompts and when needed, modeling and/or physical prompts. Social praise was provided once the task was completed correctly. Moreover, upon completing the chain, participants received points as part of a token economy package. The training package was highly effective in teaching independent menstrual care skills and was found to generalize to independent care of menstruation for all participants.

A key component in the training package developed by Richman et al. (1984) is the use of "simulated" or "practice" periods which likely account for generalization of menstrual care skills to the presence of in vivo menstruation. Practice periods are an important component of any training package designed to teach menstrual care skills because relying on natural menstruation to occur restricts the potential schedule for training sessions and inhibits prepubescent females from participation. Also, practice periods ensure that participants receive training in appropriately responding to discriminative stimuli (Richman et al. 1984). In this manner, the participant learns the appropriate cue (a red stain on the underwear), which initiates a self-care chain.

Doll-simulation behavioral skills training. An alternative to practice periods and self-instruction is the use of dolls to teach menstrual care skills. Richman et al. (1986) first demonstrated that behavioral skills training for menstrual care could be taught using a doll rather than the individual herself. This method of teaching menstrual care was found to be effective for females with profound to moderate developmental disabilities. Using a doll also has several advantages as compared to self-instruction. For example, doll training allows for sessions to occur in a classroom or home setting, rather than a private setting such as the bathroom and avoids exposing the individual to embarrassing and uncomfortable situations. In support of evidence for this claim, Epps et al. (1990a) demonstrated that females who did not work professionally with individuals with developmental disabilities rated doll training methods as more acceptable than self-training for teaching menstrual care skills, due to the less invasive nature of this procedure.

Epps et al. (1990b) compared self-simulation and doll simulation and found that although doll-simulation is considered less intrusive and socially acceptable, self-simulation may be more effective in teaching menstrual care skills to females with moderate to severe developmental disabilities. However, for females with mild to moderate developmental disabilities, doll training may be sufficient (Ersoy et al. 2009).

Antecedent prompt and test procedure. In a more recent investigation on the use of dolls to teach menstrual care skills, Ersoy et al. (2009) examined the use of an *errorless learning procedure*. Errorless learning procedures are distinct from trial and error learning in that they attempt to minimize the possibility that the learner will make errors as she is learning a new skill. Ersoy et al. specifically examined the *antecedent prompt and test procedure* (*APTP*) for menstrual care skills. Intervention sessions in this procedure included a teacher who modeled how to change the sanitary napkin on a doll for the subject. Following the modeling, the teacher provided a *task direction prompt* ("Please change the sanitary napkin on the doll"). Immediately following this direction, the teacher provided a *controlling prompt* ("Take your doll to the bathroom") and further modeling (the teacher would then take the doll to the bathroom *without waiting for a response from the subject*). Using a multiple probe design across participants, the authors demonstrated effectiveness of the APTP procedure in teaching participants how to change sanitary napkins on a doll. Unfortunately, the authors did not assess for generalization to in vivo menstrual care skills, a significant limitation in this study. Nevertheless, parental report from two of three participants indicated generalization of the APTP procedure to menstrual care in thc home.

Social Stories. In addition to behavioral skills training packages, Social Stories may also be used to teach menstruation skills to individuals with developmental disabilities. Social Stories are visual and/or written guides that are often used to describe or teach a concept or skill (Gray and Garand 1993). Klett and Turan (2012) examined the effectiveness of a social story developed to teach menstruation skills to three pre-pubescent females on the autism spectrum. The social story was individualized for each female and included written and pictorial information designed to teach participants to identify when to change a dirty pad and how to fasten a clean pad onto their underwear. Notably, the researchers taught participant's mothers how to implement the intervention and how to conduct "practice period" probes to assess generalization of skills. All three participants showed improvement in their menstrual care skills post intervention. Unfortunately, generalization to in vivo periods was only possible for one participant as the other two participants did not menstruate until after the completion of the study. Thus, evidence for generalization of Social Stories for menstrual care skills in limited.

Social stories may be particularly appealing for parents who often struggle with discussing the difficult topic of menstruation with their daughters. An individualized script for introducing and teaching menstruation skills may reduce parental anxiety and simultaneously avoid the need to delegate the teaching of menstruation skills to educational personnel and treatment providers outside of the family Although Social Stories are easy to implement and appealing for parents, it is important to note that this intervention approach may only be appropriate for higher functioning individuals. For example, participants in this study possessed reading decoding and reading comprehension skills required for Social Stories. Thus, for individuals without reading skills, Social Stories may need to be supplemented with prompting, modeling, and reinforcement.

Practice Recommendations

There are several practice recommendations that apply to each of the areas of personal hygiene reviewed in this chapter. Therefore, each practice recommendation will be described using an example from grooming, oral hygiene, or menstrual care. The practice recommendations include identification of pre-requisite skills as well as the importance of assessment of certain client variables, preparation of clients, caregivers, and others prior to implementation of an intervention, developing a task analysis, considerations for skill acquisition, promoting independence, addressing sensory or anxiety issues (avoidance behavior), and promoting generalization and maintenance.

Pre-requisite Skills and Assessment of Client Variables

According to Anderson et al. (2007), a number of pre-requisite skills are necessary for clients prior to beginning hygiene-related interventions. These skills include attending to the hygiene activity (e.g., washing hands) for a minimum of 5–10 min (depending on the duration of the activity), responding to one's name, developing discrimination skills, following directions, imitating others' behaviors, and making choices. When teaching different personal hygiene skills, consider other pre-requisite skills specific to the target skill or behavior. As an example, prior to teaching menstrual care skills, females should possess toilet training skills.

Understanding of a client's learning characteristics and functioning level in the domains of communication, social skills, and motor skills is helpful in the planning stage and for selecting appropriate interventions. An assessment of the client's functioning should also precede intervention. There are several areas to consider in an assessment, such as whether the client (a) has been taught the skill in the past; (b) has been taught the skill but is not engaging in the behavior independently; (c) is prompt dependent; and (d) has sensory sensitivities interfering with a personal hygiene activity. Furthermore, there may be other variables that may be leading to avoidance of hygiene. The assessment should be conducted using interviews with parents, caregivers, and the clients themselves if they have communicative ability. Additionally, direct observations of the clients in the naturalistic settings should be conducted to evaluate baseline skills (i.e., how many steps on the task analysis can they complete independently). For example, when teaching menstrual care skills, assessment of intellectual or cognitive abilities might be helpful in selecting an intervention. Specifically, females with severe levels of intellectual impairment may benefit most from in vivo behavioral skills training and self-training; whereas, for females with milder forms of intellectual impairment, doll-simulation and Social Stories may be preferred. For interventions that will include the caregiver, such as assisting with tooth brushing, simple discrimination skills might be an important consideration as a pre-requisite skill. Identifying pre-requisite skills and an understanding of a client's functioning level across different developmental domains assists the clinician in selecting appropriate interventions, as well as in identifying how best to prepare the client and his or her caregivers or other clinicians for personal hygiene interventions.

Preparation of Clients, Caregivers and Others

Providing caregivers, other family members, and professional staff with information about IDD and other neurodevelopmental disorders can be helpful. However, client-specific information alone is not enough to guarantee intervention success. Describing the rationale for the intervention, the role of those involved in the intervention, and the short-term and long-term benefits of improving personal hygiene skills would likely be helpful as well. In order to provide the most benefit to the client, it is also important to emphasize the relative time table required for the intervention, the need for commitment from all involved in the intervention, and consistency of the implementation intervention. To illustrate this, we provide readers with an example of preparing caregivers and family members in improving menstrual care skills. Despite the availability of training methods, a large proportion of females with developmental disabilities are deprived of the opportunity to learn how to manage their own menstrual care (Rodgers and Lipscombe 2005). Given the availability of methods, Gomez et al. (2012) suggested that myths related to menstruation for individuals with developmental disabilities may be adversely impacting caregiver decisions related to menstrual management. For example, discomfort related to sexuality in females with developmental disabilities is a common experience for parents or caregivers and it may dissuade caregivers from engaging in conversations related to menstruation. For this reason, significant preparation may be required prior to implementing a training procedure to teach menstrual care.

It is essential that caregivers introduce the concept of menstruation to clients in a positive manner, as they are likely to model their caregiver's perceptions of menstruation. Ideally, the topic of menstruation should be broached *before* a female experiences menarche in order to adequately prepare the client for the changes her body will undergo through puberty (Gomez et al. 2012). Education should be provided in a developmentally appropriate manner using simple words and visual cues. Furthermore, it is essential that caregivers avoid negative reactions and respond calmly to the presence of menstrual stains. This positive approach should be consistent across all caregivers and individuals who may assist the client in management of her menstrual care (Gomez et al. 2012).

As a way to prepare both the client and her caregivers, we recommend practice periods prior to the onset of menarche (Gomez et al. 2012). The individual may be involved in the selection and purchase of menstrual care products and her preferences related to comfort should be considered. Involvement in decisions related to menses may improve the individual's perception of her menstrual cycle and the onset of puberty. Following the onset of menses, caregivers should assist the individual in preparing for each upcoming menstrual cycle. Females may be taught to independently chart their menstrual cycle so as to anticipate its onset. In cases where this is not possible, caregivers should include clients with the charting process as much as possible (Gomez et al. 2012).

Involvement of caregivers sometimes warrants additional consultation from the clinician. In the event that caregivers demonstrate anxiety or reluctance to teach personal hygiene skills, professionals should provide education and counsel caregivers towards selecting the least invasive procedure to manage personal hygiene. Using techniques such as motivational interviewing might be a consideration to help develop agreement on intervention goals and commitment (Siller et al. 2014).

Develop a Task Analysis

A task analysis can be developed for most personal hygiene skills and should be considered prior to developing a personal hygiene skill intervention. A task analysis of the target behavior should be completed, with the client's age and skill level (e.g., motor skills) taken into consideration. Some options for completing a task analysis are (a) watching another person perform the skill and recording the steps, (b) consulting with experts about the skill, or (c) performing the behavior yourself and recording the task. It is common for a task analysis to go through different versions before it is finalized. Examples of task analyses for the personal hygiene skills discussed in this chapter are presented in Tables 3.2, 3.3 and 3.4.

Skill Acquisition

For clients that have adequate verbal ability, providing education or instruction can be an effective component for teaching personal hygiene skills (Barry et al. 1977; Matson et al. 1980; Thinesen and Bryan 1981; Walmsley et al. 2013). In addition, if the client has stated a goal of increasing their social contacts or obtaining employment, instruction on the rationale of the target skill may help to motivate them during intervention. So too, having the client make a verbal response prior to the behavior can help increase the probability that they will engage in independent grooming. For instance, Stokes et al. (2004) used *correspondence training*,

Table 3.2 Sample task analysis of toothbrushing

Step	Description
1	Pick up the toothbrush
2	Wet the brush
3	Take the cap off toothpaste tube
4	Squeeze toothpaste tube to put paste on the brush
5	Brush the outside of the bottom row of teeth
6	Brush the outside of the top row of teeth
7	Brush the biting surface of the top row of teeth
8	Brush the biting surface of the bottom row of teeth
9	Brush the inside surface of the bottom row of teeth
10	Brush the inside surface of the top row of teeth
11	Spit into the sink
12	Pick up the cup
13	Fill cup with water
14	Rinse teeth with water
15	Spit out water
16	Rinse the brush
17	Place the brush in the holder
18	Pick up the hand towel
19	Wipe mouth
20	Screw cap back on toothpaste tube

Table 3.3 Sample task analysis of face washing

Step	Description
1	Turn on water
2	Adjust water until it is warm
3	Put hands together under the water
4	Bring hands to face to wet face
5	Put face wash (soap) on hands or washcloth
6	Rub face wash (soap) onto whole face
7	Put hands together under water
8	Bring hands to face to rinse face wash off
9	Rinse face until all face wash is gone
10	Turn off water
11	Pat face dry with towel
12	Dry hands

or having the clients "say, do, and report" as part of the intervention. This type of mediating response may help the client when the instructor cannot be present, such as when showering or cleaning after toileting is being taught.

Modeling and prompting can be used in conjunction with instruction in a *behavioral skills training* approach (Matson et al. 1980; Treffry et al. 1970). When using prompting, clinicians should decide on whether a most-to-least or

Table 3.4 Task analysis for menstrual skills (Richman et al. 1984)

Step	Description
1	Client walks into bathroom and doses the door
2	Pulls down underwear below knees and sits on toilet
3	Pulls up underwear and other clothes
4	Walks out of bathroom
5	Obtains box containing underwear, sanitary napkin, plastic bag, and paper bag
6	Walks into bathroom and doses door
7	Washes complete surface of hands and fingers with soap and water so no dirt or residue remains visible on area, dries, throws paper towel in trash
8	Brings box to stall, pulls down underwear below knees and sits on toilet
9	Removes soiled underwear
10	Places soiled underwear in plastic bag
11	Wipes vaginal area at least once to remove residual blood and drops paper in toilet
12	Puts on dean pair of underwear
13	Pulls tab off dean sanitary napkin
14	Disposes of strip in trashcan
15	Fastens sticky side of sanitary napkin lengthwise in underwear and presses into place
16	Pulls up underwear and other clothes
17	Flushes toilet
18	Washes hands as in step 7
19	Exits bathroom putting soiled underwear in laundry bag and plastic bag in trash
20	Places box in bedroom cabinet for storage

least-to-most prompting procedure is most appropriate. It will be important that immediate corrective feedback be used if the client engages in an error. It may also be helpful for clients if a permanent product was left after they engaged in the grooming behavior—for example, Walmsley et al. (2013) used a lotion that under black light showed how much of the clients' hands were covered by soap during washing. Other examples of such permanent products could include the residue left behind by deodorant or hand sanitizer and lotion than emits a smell when rubbed in for the appropriate amount of time.

If video modeling is determined to be an appropriate tool to teach a specific skill, it appears that using a familiar model in the video, such as an adult or peer, would be beneficial (Rayner et al. 2009). Additionally, it appears that having narration over the video model performing the skill, as well as showing the modeling receiving reinforcement, may be important components to promote acquisition (Rosenberg et al. 2010). Finally, if the model is shown receiving reinforcement in the video, then the client should receive similar reinforcement. Thus, conducting a preference assessment to determine appropriate reinforcers should be completed prior to making the video.

Promoting Independence

If assessment indicates that the client has already been taught the skill but does not behave independently, then token economies or contingency contracts may be effective (Jarman et al. 1983). Self-monitoring can also reduce caregiver response effort (Garff and Storey 1998; Saloviita and Tuulkair 2000). Ways to self-monitor include memory aides, checklists, or reminders on smart phones or tablets. For example, reminders can be programmed on a smart phone calendar or through an app to prompt a morning routine. It will be important to explain the contingencies, or what the client needs to do to receive reinforcement, prior to implement of the program.

Pictorial cues can also be used to prompt behaviors that may already be in the client's repertoire. Various stimuli can be used by creating picture books of the different steps of a task analysis or putting these pictures in a smart phone or tablet that the individual can flip through after an alarm goes off. Although the task analysis can be presented within in a book, there is some evidence that just one picture of the person initiating the behavior may be enough to start the behavior (Thinesen and Bryan 1981).

Considerations for Sensory Issues or Anxiety (Avoidance)

If clients avoid personal hygiene products due to sensory sensitivity or anxiety, a graduated approach can be considered (DeLeon et al. 2008) through systematically introducing the products to the client (e.g., increasing the amount of lotion to put on the skin), commonly referred to as s*ensory adaptation* for sensory sensitivity, and *stimulus fading with contingent reinforcement* for avoidance (Luscre and Center 1996; Cuvo et al. 2010). DeLeon et al. (2008) also suggest providing continuous access to preferred stimuli during training, which might serve as a counter conditioning process similar to systematic desensitization. Applying escape extinction might also be warranted given the situation and individual (Cuvo et al. 2010). Instructors and caregivers should anticipate a slow process when addressing sensory adaptation or avoidance (DeLeon et al. 2008). For example, the application of deodorant can be completed using small steps in a sequence of smelling deodorant, touching it with finger, applying it to arm, apply one swipe to underarm, apply two swipes to underarm, and so on.

Generalization and Maintenance

When developing an intervention to improve personal hygiene, it is important to consider maintenance and generalization. One way to address maintenance is planning on how to fade out reinforcement. For example, when using self-monitoring or a contingency contract for a morning routine of three behaviors, clients may initially receive dense reinforcement, such as reinforcement for completing each behavior, which can be faded to receiving reinforcement for every two behaviors, then every three behaviors, to completing three behaviors daily for a week, to fading out reinforcement entirely. Generalization can be targeted by using the intervention across a range of different situations relevant to the client, and with caregivers who will often be working with the client. For instance, if using video modeling to teach hand washing skills to children, the video can be shown on a smart phone in the home bathroom, school bathroom, or public bathroom prior to the client engaging in the behavior. It is recommended that generalization be targeted once the client exhibits the steps on the task analysis independently (Martin et al. 1982). Another strategy for generalization is *general case instruction,* or presenting the client with many examples of what they will encounter in their natural environment (Stokes et al. 2004). Specifically, when teaching hand washing, different types of faucets and soaps can be presented; when teaching hair combing, different types of hairbrushes and combs can be presented; or, when teaching shaving, manual and electric razors can be presented.

Conclusion

Grooming, menstrual care and oral hygiene are important for individuals with IDD for health promotion and ensuring opportunities for increased socialization, participation in inclusion environments, and access to vocational opportunities. There are many effective interventions and treatment packages to guide the practitioner in teaching and maintaining personal hygiene across the lifespan. Involvement of the client, family, and others, such as dental care staff, can all play a role in improving personal hygiene. Future research in these areas, especially with respect to menstrual care and other areas within personal hygiene that have not received as much attention is needed.

Across all the personal hygiene skills described in this chapter it is imperative to involve clients and parents/caregivers in all aspects of assessment, intervention, and maintenance/generalization. A critical step is providing factual information to parents or caregivers about the importance of personal hygiene and addressing any misconceptions they might have in considering skill development in this area. The client and family should be included in the development of behavior plans, for example, identifying contingencies for reinforcement and the specific reinforcement that will be used in a contingency contract. The client and family members can also assist in identifying preferred products (e.g., toothbrushes, deodorant scents, soap vs. body wash, etc.) to use for different hygiene tasks. Improving client and family involvement in the development and implementation of behavioral interventions will likely increase the success for the client.

References

American Academy of Pediatrics, Committee on Bioethics. (1999). Sterilization of minors with developmental disabilities. *Pediatrics, 104*, 337.

Anderson, S. R., Jablonski, A. L., Thomeer, M. L., & Knapp, V. M. (2007). *Self-help skills for people with autism: A systematic teaching approach*. Bethesda: Woodbine House.

Atkinson, E., Bennett, M. J., Dudley, J., Grover, S., Matthews, K., Moore, P., et al. (2003). Consensus statement: Menstrual and contraceptive management in women with an intellectual disability. *The Australian and New Zealand Journal of Obstetrics and Gynaecology, 43*(2), 109–110.

Backeljauw, P. F., Rose, S. R., & Lawson, M. (2004). Clinical management of menstruation in adolescent females with developmental delay. *The Endocrinologist, 14*(2), 87–92.

Barry, K., Apolloni, T., & Cooke, T. P. (1977). Improving the personal hygiene of mildly retarded men in a community-based residential training program. *Corrective & Social Psychiatry & Journal of Behavior Technology, Methods & Therapy, 23*(3), 65–68.

Bishop, M. R., Kenzer, A. L., Coffman, C. M., Tarbox, C. M., Tarbox, J., & Lanagan, T. M. (2013). Using stimulus fading without escape extinction to increase compliance with toothbrushing in children with autism. *Research in Autism Spectrum Disorders, 7*(6), 680–686.

Bölte, S., & Poustka, F. (2002). The relation between general cognitive level and adaptive behavior domains in individuals with autism with and without co-morbid mental retardation. *Child Psychiatry and Human Development, 33*(2), 165–172. doi:10.1023/A:1020734325815

Brady, S., & Grover, S. (1997). *The sterilization of girls and young women in Australia: A legal, medical and social context*. Sydney, Australia: Human Rights and Equal Opportunity Commission.

Brickhouse, T. H., Farrington, F. H., Best, A. M., & Ellsworth, C. W. (2009). Barriers to dental care for children in Virginia with autism spectrum disorders. *Journal of Dentistry for Children, 76*(3), 188–193.

Carlson, G., & Wilson, J. (1996). Menstrual management and women who have intellectual disabilities: Service providers and decision-making. *Journal of Intellectual and Developmental Disability, 21*(1), 39–57.

Carter, A. S., Volkmar, F. R., Sparrow, S. S., Wang, J. J., Lord, C., Dawson, G., et al. (1998). The Vineland adaptive behavior scales: Supplementary norms for individuals with autism. *Journal of Autism and Developmental Disorders, 28*(4), 287–302.

Cridland, E. K., Jones, S. C., Caputi, P., & Magee, C. A. (2014). Understanding high-functioning autism during adolescence: A personal construct theory approach. *Journal of Intellectual and Developmental Disability, 39*(1), 108–118. doi:10.3109/13668250.2013.870331

Cuvo, A. J., Godard, A., Huckfeldt, R., & DeMattei, R. (2010). Training children with autism spectrum disorders to be compliant with an oral assessment. *Research in Autism Spectrum Disorders, 4*(4), 681–696.

DeLeon, I. G., Hagopian, L. P., Rodriguez-Catter, V., Bowman, L. G., Long, E. S., & Boelter, E. W. (2008). Increasing wearing of prescription glasses in individuals with mental retardation. *Journal of Applied Behavior Analysis, 41*(1), 137–142. doi:10.1901/jaba.2008.41-137

Ellis, E. M., Ala'i-Rosales, S. S., Glenn, S. S., Rosales-Ruiz, J., & Greenspoon, J. (2006). The effects of graduated exposure, modeling, and contingent social attention on tolerance to skin care products with two children with autism. *Research in Developmental Disabilities, 27*(6), 585–598. doi:10.1016/j.ridd.2005.05.009

Epps, S., Prescott, A. L., & Horner, R. H. (1990a). Social acceptability of menstrual-care training methods for young women with developmental disabilities. *Education & Training in Mental Retardation*.

Epps, S., Stern, R. J., & Horner, R. H. (1990b). Comparison of simulation training on self and using a doll for teaching generalized menstrual care to women with severe mental retardation. *Research in Developmental Disabilities, 11*(1), 37–66.

Ersoy, G., Tekin-Iftar, E., & Kircaali-Iftar, G. (2009). Effects of antecedent prompt and test procedure on teaching simulated menstrual care skills to females with developmental disabilities. *Education and Training in Developmental Disabilities, 44*(1), 54–66.

Faibish, G. M., & Thompson, M. M. (1970). The use of filmstrips in teaching personal hygiene to the moderately retarded adolescent. *Education and Training of the Mentally Retarded, 5*(3), 113–118.

Faulks, D., & Hennequin, M. (2000). Evaluation of a long-term oral health program by carers of children and adults with intellectual disabilities. *Special Care Dentistry, 20*, 199–208.

Fickert, N. A., & Ross, D. (2012). Effectiveness of a caregiver education program on providing oral care to individuals with intellectual and developmental disabilities. *Intellectual and Developmental Disabilities, 50*(3), 219–232.

Garff, J. T., & Storey, K. (1998). The use of self-management strategies for increasing the appropriate hygiene of persons with disabilities in supported employment settings. *Education and Training in Mental Retardation and Developmental Disabilities, 33*(2), 179–188.

Gomez, M. T., Carlson, G. M., & Van Dooren, K. (2012). Practical approaches to supporting young women with intellectual disabilities and high support needs with their menstruation. *Health Care for Women International, 33*(8), 678–694.

Gray, C. A., & Garand, J. D. (1993). Social stories: Improving responses of students with autism with accurate social information. *Focus on Autistic Behavior.*

Graudins, M. M., Rehfeldt, R. A., DeMattei, R., Baker, J. C., & Scaglia, F. (2012). Exploring the efficacy of behavioral skills training to teach basic behavior analytic techniques to oral care providers. *Research in Autism Spectrum Disorders, 6*(3), 978–987.

Grover, S. R. (2011). Gynaecological issues in adolescents with disability. *Journal of pediatrics and child health, 47*(9), 610–613.

Hamilton, A., Marshal, M. P., & Murray, P. J. (2011). Autism spectrum disorders and menstruation. *Journal of Adolescent Health, 49*(4), 443–445.

Jarman, P. H., Iwata, B. A., & Lorentzson, A. M. (1983). Development of morning self-care routines in multiply handicapped persons. *Applied Research in Mental Retardation, 4*(2), 113–122.

Jennett, H. K., & Hagopian, L. P. (2008). Identifying empirically supported treatments for phobic avoidance in individuals with intellectual disabilities. *Behavior Therapy, 39*(2), 151–161.

Klett, L. S., & Turan, Y. (2012). Generalized effects of social stories with task analysis for teaching menstrual care to three young girls with autism. *Sexuality and Disability, 30*(3), 319–336.

Kreutner, A. K. (1981). Sexuality, fertility, and the problems of menstruation in mentally retarded adolescents. *Pediatric Clinics of North America, 28*(2), 475–480.

Lai, B., Milano, M., Roberts, M. W., & Hooper, S. R. (2012). Unment dental needs and barriers to dental care among children with autism spectrum disorders. *Journal of Autism and Developmental Disorders, 42*, 1294–1303. doi:10.1007/s10803-011-1362-2

Lennox, N., Beange, H., Davis, R., Durvasula, S., Edwards, N., et al. (2005). *Management Guidelines: Developmental Disability*. Melbourne: Therapeutic Guidelines Limited.

Loo, C. Y., Graham, R. M., & Hughes, C. V. (2008). The caries experience and behavior of dental patients with autism spectrum disorder. *Journal of the American Dental Association, 139*, 1518–1524.

Luscre, D. M., & Center, D. B. (1996). Procedures for reducing dental fear in children with autism. *Journal of Autism and Developmental Disorders, 26*(5), 547–556.

Marshall, J., Sheller, B., Williams, B. J., Mancl, L., & Cowan, C. (2007). Cooperation predictors for dental patients with autism. *Pediatric Dentistry, 29*, 369–376.

Martin, J. E., Rush, F. R., & Heal, L. W. (1982). Teaching community survival skills to mentally retarded adults: A review and analysis. *Journal of Special Education, 16*(3), 243–267.

Mason, L., & Cunningham, C. (2008). An exploration of issues around menstruation for women with down syndrome and their carers. *Journal of Applied Research in Intellectual Disabilities, 21*(3), 257–267.

Master, D., Hess Longe, S. H., & Dickson, H. (1997). Scheduled hand washing in an elementary school population. *Family Medicine, 29*, 336–339.

Matson, J. L., Hattier, M. A., & Belva, B. (2012). Treating adaptive living skills of persons with autism using applied behavior analysis: A review. *Research in Autism Spectrum Disorders, 6*(1), 271–276. doi:10.1016/j.rasd.2011.05.008

Matson, J. L., Marchetti, A., & Adkins, J. A. (1980). Comparison of operant- and independence-training procedures for mentally retarded adults. *American Journal of Mental Deficiency, 84*(5), 487–494.

Myles, B. S. (Ed.). (2005). *Children and youth with Asperger syndrome: Strategies for success in inclusive settings*. Beverly Hills: Sage.

Niffenegger, J. P. (1997). Proper handwashing promotes wellness in childcare. *Journal of Pediatric Health Care, 11*, 26–31.

Norwood, K. W. Jr., Slayton, R. L., & Council on Children with Disabilities and Section on Oral Health. (2013). Oral health care for children with developmental disabilities. *Pediatrics, 131*, 614–619. doi:10.1542/peds.2012-3650

Orellana, L. M., Silvestre, F. J., Martinez-Sanchis, S., Martinez-Mihi, V., & Bautista, D. (2012). Oral manisfestations in a group of adults with autism spectrum disorder. *Medicina Oral, Patoligia Oral y Circugia Bucal, 17*(3), 415–419. doi:10.4317/medoral.17573

Palmen, A., Didden, R., & Lang, R. (2012). A systematic review of behavioral intervention research on adaptive skill building in high-functioning young adults with autism spectrum disorder. *Research in Autism Spectrum Disorders, 6*(2), 602–617. doi:10.1016/j.rasd.2011.10.001

Rayner, C., Denholm, C., & Sigafoos, J. (2009). Video-based intervention for individuals with autism: Key questions that remain unanswered. *Research in Autism Spectrum Disorders, 3*(2), 291–303. doi:10.1016/j.rasd.2008.09.001

Reisman, E. S., & Reisman, J. I. (1993). Supervision of employees with moderate special needs. *Journal of Learning Disabilities, 26*(3), 199–206. doi:10.1177/002221949302600307

Richman, G. S., Ponticas, Y., Page, T. J., & Epps, S. (1986). Simulation procedures for teaching independent menstrual care to mentally retarded persons. *Applied Research in Mental Retardation, 7*(1), 21–35.

Richman, G. S., Reiss, M. L., Bauman, K. E., & Bailey, J. S. (1984). Teaching menstrual care to mentally retarded women: Acquisition, generalization, and maintenance. *Journal of Applied Behavior Analysis, 17*(4), 441–451.

Rodgers, J. (2001). Pain, shame, blood, and doctors: How women with learning difficulties experience menstruation. In *Women's Studies International Forum* (Vol. 24, No. 5, pp. 523–539). Pergamon.

Rodgers, J., & Lipscombe, J. (2005). The nature and extent of help given to women with intellectual disabilities to manage menstruation. *Journal of Intellectual and Developmental Disability, 30*(1), 45–52.

Rosenberg, N. E., Schwartz, I. S., & Davis, C. A. (2010). Evaluating the utility of commercial videotapes for teaching hand washing to children with autism. *Education and Treatment of Children, 33*(3), 443–455. doi:10.1353/etc.0.0098

Saloviita, T. J., & Tuulkari, M. (2000). Cognitive-behavioural treatment package for teaching grooming skills to a man with an intellectual disability. *Scandinavian Journal of Behaviour Therapy, 29*(3–4), 140–147. doi:10.1080/028457100300049773

Saltonstall, B. (2007). *Mothers raising daughters with cognitive delay: Reflections on menarche & menstruation*. Burleigh: Pristine Publisher.

Sheppard, L. (2006). Growing pains: A personal development program for students with intellectual and developmental disabilities in a specialist school. *Journal of Intellectual Disabilities, 10*, 121–142.

Siller, M., Morgan, L., Turner-Brown, L., Baggett, K. M., Baranek, G. T., Brian, J., et al. (2014). Designing studies to evaluate parent-mediated interventions for toddlers with autism spectrum disorder. *Journal of Early Intervention*. Online January 17, 2015. doi:10.1177/1053815114542507

Stein, L. I., Lane, C. J., Williams, M. E., Dawson, M. E., Polido, J. C., & Cermak, S. A. (2014). Physiological and behavioral stress and anxiety in children with autism spectrum disorders during routine oral care. *BioMed Research International*.

Stokes, J. V., Cameron, M. J., Dorsey, M. F., & Fleming, E. (2004). Task analysis, correspondence training, and general case instruction for teaching personal hygiene skills. *Behavioral Interventions, 19*(2), 121–135. doi:10.1002/bin.153

Thinesen, P. J., & Bryan, A. J. (1981). The use of sequential pictorial cues in the initiation and maintenance of grooming behaviors with mentally retarded adults. *Mental Retardation, 19*(5), 246–250.

Treffry, D., Martin, G., Samels, J., & Watson, C. (1970). Operant conditioning of grooming behavior of severely retarded girls. *Mental Retardation, 8*(4), 29–33.

Walmsley, C., Mahoney, A., Durgin, A., & Poling, A. (2013). Fostering hand washing before lunch by students attending a special needs young adult program. *Research in Developmental Disabilities, 34*(1), 95–101. doi:10.1016/j.ridd.2012.08.002

World Health Organization. (2001). *Water for health: Taking charge*. Available at http://www.who.int/water_sanitation_health/wwdreportchap4.pdf

Yaacob, N., Nasir, N. M., Jalil, S. N., Ahmad, R., Rahim, N. A. R. A., Yusof, A. N. M., et al. (2012). Parents or caregiver's perception on menstrual care in individuals with down syndrome. *Procedia-Social and Behavioral Sciences, 36*, 128–136.

Chapter 4
Increasing and Maintaining Exercise-Physical Activity

James K. Luiselli

Inadequate exercise-physical activity in children and adults can lead to obesity, diabetes, and cardiovascular disease, among other health-threatening conditions (Dowda et al. 2004; Reilly and Kelly 2011; Yamaki et al. 2011). Conversely, serious medical problems can be reduced and possibly prevented by exercising and being physically active (Ekelund et al. 2012; Ross et al. 2000). For children, the Centers for Disease Control recommended 60 min of moderate-to-vigorous physical activity (MVPA) every day (Centers for Disease Control 2008). Physical activity guidelines for adults specify 150 min of MVPA per week by exercising 30 min daily, five days per week, in bouts lasting a minimum of 10 min (Centers for Disease Control 2008; Haskell et al. 2007). Unfortunately the majority of children and adults do not regularly achieve these performance criteria (Troiano et al. 2008).

Similar to the population at large, many people with intellectual and developmental disabilities (IDD) have sedentary lifestyles, do not exercise, and lack health-promoting physical outlets (Heath and Fentem 1997; Luiselli (2014); Rimmer 1999). A survey by Rimmer et al. (2004) revealed that 56 % of "people with disabilities" reported having no leisure-time physical activities. Tracking a large group of adults (18–64 years old) who had hearing, vision, cognitive, and motor disabilities, Carroll et al. (2015) found that 47.1 % were physically inactive compared to 26.1 % of adults without disabilities. By not achieving sufficient levels of exercise and cardiovascular exertion, positive health status in people with IDD is seriously compromised (Mann et al. 2006; Peterson et al. 2008; Seekins et al. 2005).

J.K. Luiselli (✉)
North East Educational and Developmental Support Center, 1120 Main Street, Tewksbury, MA 018776, USA
e-mail: jluiselli@needsctr.org

J.K. Luiselli
Clinical Solutions, Inc., Beverly, MA, USA

J.K. Luiselli (ed.), *Behavioral Health Promotion and Intervention in Intellectual and Developmental Disabilities*, Evidence-Based Practices in Behavioral Health,
DOI 10.1007/978-3-319-27297-9_4

There are several factors that impede and curtail exercise-physical activity among people with IDD. These limitations and barriers include persistent medical problems, social isolation, limited financial resources, and exposure to unhealthy living conditions (Emerson 2007; Scepters et al. 2005). As well, many people with IDD and their families do not have access to information about health promotion and preventive services emphasizing exercise-physical activity (Krahn et al. 2006). It behooves behavioral healthcare professionals to identify the person-specific, family, systems-level, and societal influences that make it difficult for people with IDD to be physically fit and maintain sound health status across the lifespan (Luiselli 2015a, b; U.S. Public Health Service (USPHS) 2002; U.S. Department of Health and Human Services 2005).

Beyond health benefits, routine exercise-physical activity has a positive effect on mood, reduces stress, and lessens anxiety sensitivity (Otto and Smites 2011). Research further supports that by engaging in MVPA, people with IDD and other neurodevelopmental disorders have improved self-concept, enhanced intellectual functioning, and better adjustment within educational and habilitation settings (Gabler-Halle et al. 1993a, b; Oriel et al. 2011; Rosenthal-Malek and Mitchell 1997). There is also evidence that strategically planned antecedent exercise-physical activity is associated with fewer problem behaviors and more sustained attention during instructional opportunities (Cannella-Malone et al. 2011; Morrison et al. 2011).

One additional consideration is that most care-providers for people with IDD endorse the need for and salutary effects from exercise-physical activity. For example, Glidden et al. (2011) found that parents reported positive family impact, high degree of happiness, and fulfilling expectations by having their children (12–49 years old) participate in Special Olympics. In a related social validity study by Luiselli et al. (2013b), education service providers consistently endorsed exercise and athletic pursuits for improving learning, mood, sleep, and personal happiness of children and youth with autism and other neurodevelopmental disorders.

This chapter reviews exercise-physical activity in IDD by focusing on practice and research applications with children and adults. In the first section of the Chap. 1 address measurement methods in order to properly monitor indices such as exercise frequency and duration, patterns of physical activity, energy expenditure, and adherence. This section also discusses how functional analysis methodologies can be used to isolate contextual variables affecting exercise-physical activity and to inform intervention decision making. Next, the chapter considers effective performance improvement strategies with typically developing children and adults. This information provides a background for presentation of intervention objectives, procedures, and results with people who have IDD. In the concluding section "Measurement" present several practice recommendations.

Measurement

Measurement of exercise-physical activity is needed to properly evaluate the results of intervention plans, revise procedures through data-based decision making, and monitor post-intervention maintenance. Measurement also extends to exercise-physical activity adherence and compliance. Additionally, measurement data are often incorporated as graphic performance feedback, particularly when goal setting is a component of intervention (Luiselli and Reed 2011; Luiselli et al. 2011).).

Typically, exercise-physical activity is measured by mechanical instrumentation, direct observational coding, or both (Van Camp and Hayes 2012).

Mechanical Instrumentation

Actigraphy is the ambulatory measurement of physical activity (Tryon 2011). Pedometers and digital step counters represent a common type of instrumentation by which a wrist-worn device tallies the number of steps a person takes. Contemporary pedometers digitally convert steps into distance, are relatively inexpensive, and do not have a conspicuous appearance. They also allow for measurement when direct observation of exercise-physical activity is not possible. However, pedometers and digital step counters are limited because they do not control for the effects of a person's height on stride-length. These devices may also underestimate MVPA and their reliability and validity have been questioned (Butte et al. 2012). Beets and Pitetti (2011) have shown that one strategy for calculating MVPA from pedometer-generated data is to correlate step frequency (steps per minute) with a person's height and weight.

Another type of actigraphy incorporates computerized, accelerometer-based devices worn on the wrist, waist, and ankle. These devices "rapidly and simultaneously digitize movement in one, two, or three dimensions every 15, 30, or 60 s continuously 24 h a day for as many days as memory allows" (Tryon 2011, p. 29). There are many versions of accelerometers and widespread utilization in exercise-physical activity research (Van Camp and Hayes 2012). A strong feature of such instrumentation is the wireless uploading to websites that have the capacity to store, aggregate, and graph data.

Heart-rate monitors (HRMs), a third type of instrumentation, provide an indirect measure of physical exertion by recording electrical activity of the heart through a skin-contact monitor attached to a person's chest. Larson et al. (2011) found that HRM data in children matched more precisely with the intensity of physical activities than measurement from pedometers. Of course, other factors unrelated to exercise-physical activity can increase heart rate—therefore, it is necessary to correlate the data from HRMs with specific activity patterns and levels of physical exertion.

Despite their respective shortcomings, the different types of mechanical instrumentation are valuable for unobtrusive monitoring and recording of exercise-physical activity. Each instrumentation device should be tailored to specific dependent measures. Keep in mind, however, that pedometers, accelerometers, and HRMs can be applied simultaneously as a means of measuring co-variation among motor and physiological responses. Actigraphy combined with direct observation and possibly self-recording via rating scales and checklists would appear to be the most robust measurement methodology available to practitioners and researchers alike.

Direct Observational Coding

Several formal observation protocols have been designed for measuring children's physical activity. McKenzie et al. (1991) developed the *Behaviors of Eating and Activity for Children's Health Evaluation System* (*BEACHES*) as a method for documenting five defined activity levels when children are laying down, sitting, standing, walking, or being very active. The *BEACHES* uses an interval-based recording format to yield percentage measures of activity level. A similar protocol, the *System for Observing Play and Leisure Activity in Youth* (*SOPLAY*: McKenzie et al. 2000), codes intensity of physical activity within indoor and outdoor setting locations.

McIver et al. (2009) commented that despite the utility of *BEACHES* and *SOPLAY,* "they do not isolate the moment-to-moment social and environmental circumstances researchers might want to identify" (p. 2). The *Observation System for Recording Physical Activity in Children-Preschool* (*OSR-AC-P*), reported by Brown et al. (2006), advanced the previous observation protocols by further correlating intensity of physical activity with social context and other environmental conditions. An additional instrument, the *Observational System for Recording Physical Activity in Children-Home* (*OSRAC-H*: McIver et al. 2009), focuses exclusively on children's in-home physical activity according to the following dimensions: (a) physical activity levels, (b) physical activity types, (c) locations, (d) indoor activity contexts, (e) outdoor activity contexts, (f) activity initiation, (g) group compositions, (h) adult and peer prompts for physical activity, (i) parent and peer engagement, and (j) television viewing. Acquiring these data offers a broad and all-inclusive representation of children's physical activity within common home contexts and interactions.

With regard to research inquiry, Hustyi et al. (2011) conducted a study with two obese preschool children comparing the *Observation System for Recording Activity in Children* (*OSRAC*: McIver et al. 2009) with pedometer-recorded step counts. The children were observed during a 20-min outdoor recess period on a school playground. The *OSRAC* coded for five activity levels specified as stationary or motionless, stationary with limb or trunk movements, slow-easy movements, moderate rate movements, and fast movements. The number of steps both children took and their average *OSRAC* activity level co-varied during baseline phases and when they were exposed to an intervention plan that was intended to increase physical activity. Thus, this study demonstrated correspondence between actigraphy measured and direct observation activity data. Hustyi et al. (2011) concluded that "This correspondence suggests that either method of assessment can be used to evaluate interventions designed to increase physical activity in children" (p. 637).

Contextual and Functional Analysis

As noted previously, refined methods of direct observational coding not only quantify exercise-physical activity but also isolate the situations and conditions that occasion and maintain a person's behavior. In illustration, Hustyi et al. (2012) evaluated the effects of outdoor context on physical activity of four preschool children. Each child's activity level from the *OSRAC* (Brown et al. 2006) was recorded during outdoor playground sessions at a daycare center. These data were converted to a measure of MVPA according to the percentage of recording intervals that were scored at "level 4" (moderate rate movements) and "level 5" (fast movements). Within a multi-element experimental design, the children were exposed to sessions in the presence of *outdoor toys* (e.g., jump rope, bucket and shovel, soft baseballs), *access to fixed equipment* (e.g., slides, monkey bars, stairs), and an *open space* without the toys and equipment. These three conditions were further compared to a control phase in which the children sat at a table in a small area of the playground. All of the children had the highest levels of MVPA in the fixed-equipment condition and less physical activity with outdoor toys, in the open space, and under the control situation. This kind of assessment leads naturally to intervention options for increasing children's physical activity such as planned access to particular occasioning stimuli. Hustyi et al. (2012) acknowledged that interactive patterns with adults and peers as well as the social consequences of engaging in physical activity would also be expected to affect the results of this and similar contextual analysis.

Building on their earlier research, Larson et al. (2013) implemented a functional analysis of MVPA with two, 3-year old typically developing girls during outdoor play at their daycare center. The dependent measure was the percentage of recording intervals that were scored with "moderate" and "fast" movements on the *OSRAC-H* (McIver et al. 2009). In the functional analysis the MVAP of each child was measured within four conditions: (a) alone—no interaction or social consequences for MVPA, (b) attention contingent on MVPA, (c) adult interaction contingent on MVPA, and (d) escape from task demands contingent on MVPA. Results revealed that the children had the most MVPA when they received contingent attention and interactive play. These principal findings also had treatment implications because the MVPA in the attention and interaction conditions of the functional analysis was higher than levels recorded in a naturalistic baseline phase. That is, the findings suggest that children's MVPA might be easily promoted by having peers and adults interact with them during isolate or less vigorous play activities.

Larson et al. (2014b) reported another study showing the contribution of functional analysis in informing intervention decisions for increasing physical activity. The functional analysis included four, 4-year old preschool children during playground activities at their elementary schools. Similar to Larson et al. (2013), MVPA was measured from the percentage of recording intervals that were scored as "moderate" and "fast" movements from the *OSRAC-H* (McIver et al. 2009).

Following an initial naturalistic baseline phase the children participated in interactive play, attention, escape, alone, and control conditions, as described previously. All of the children had the highest MVPA during interactive play, followed by the contingent attention condition. Once again, these functional analysis findings "suggest that positive reinforcement in the form of both adult engagement and adult attention might play an important role in increasing activity levels of many children" (Larson et al. 2014a, b, p. 226).

Finally, Larson et al. (2014a) conducted a functional analysis of physical environments on activity levels of eight typically developing preschool children (3.4 years old) across different group compositions. Direct observation recording of MVPA occurred when the children were able to play with outdoor toys, on fixed equipment, and in a barren open space. These environments were manipulated further by having the children play alone, with one peer present, and in the company of 2–3 peers. This study found that six of the eight children were most active within the fixed equipment condition, while the remaining two children had similar levels in the open space. Compared to the alone condition, single or multiple peer presence accounted for the highest MVPA in all of the children. Therefore, physical activity was not only influenced by environmental context but was responsive to group composition. These findings offer further evidence about potential strategic interventions for fostering and maintaining desirable levels of physical activity among young children.

Exercise-Physical Activity Interventions with Typically Developing Populations

Most behaviorally-focused exercise-physical activity research has been conducted with typically developing children and adults. The themes of this research, described below, have been increasing exercise-physical activity to reap the associated health benefits but also to intervene with medical patients who had problems such as obesity, diabetes, and cardiovascular disease. These population-at-large studies identified several intervention procedures that have, to a small degree, been applied with and can likely be of value for people who have IDD. In presenting the following research, I have highlighted several specific procedures, noting that they are rarely applied in isolation but almost always combined in a multicomponent plan.

Positive Reinforcement-Contingency Contracting

In a study with undergraduate and graduate university students (20–33 years old), Wysocki et al. (1979) established a program to increase the number of aerobic points earned through planned exercise such as running, walking, cycling, swimming, tennis, and handball. The students contracted to acquire a criterion number of aerobic points each week. If successful, they "earned back" items of personal worth that had been deposited preceding the study. Items were also refunded when the students correctly submitted their aerobic points recording forms. In a multiple baseline design across students, contingency contracting increased substantially the number of aerobic points for seven of the eight participants. The method of positive reinforcement in this study was highly personalized and represents one strategy for dispensing exercise-contingent consequences.

More recently, Washington et al. (2014) illustrated another positive reinforcement procedure, a prize-based lottery, for increasing physical activity of 15 university students (18–26 years old). These participants wore an accelerometer device each day to record step counts that were wirelessly uploaded to a website. During intervention the students had to achieve a gradually accelerating number of daily steps in order to draw from a prize bowl stocked with raffle tickets. The tickets were assigned different values ranging from verbal praise to small ($5.00), medium ($15.00), large ($50.00), and jumbo ($120.00) prizes. The probability of obtaining a prize was inversely adjusted based on the respective increasing prize values. Eight of 10 students who completed the study had high to moderate increases in the number of steps taken daily. The increased activity in these cases was associated with decreasing pauses between episodes of activity exertion.

Monetary incentives have been employed in several studies to reinforce exercise engagement. Thus, Finkelstein et al. (2008) showed that adults who received financial rewards contingent on achieving daily walking goals were more active than non-reinforced control group participants. Petry et al. (2013) reported a similar finding with sedentary adults who earned monetary prizes upon achieving walking goals. And as described by Andrade et al. (2014), gradually thinning the schedule of activity-based monetary "rewards" with adults can be more effective in promoting walking than abruptly terminating reinforcement. In fact, fading reinforcement is a critical programing consideration for enhancing the therapeutic success and maintenance of incentive-focused intervention plans.

Goal Setting-Performance Feedback

Wack et al. (2014) included five women (18–28 years old) in a study to increase their weekly running distance through goal setting and performance feedback. Distance per running episode was recorded by a sport-sensor device, initially during a baseline phase and throughout intervention. Goal setting consisted of the women establishing daily, short-term distance goals and a long-term distance goal to be achieved by conclusion of the study. There were distance criteria for lowering, increasing, and maintaining the weekly goals. Each week a member of the research team showed the women a graphical display of their daily running distance and verbally commented about progress. Two of the five women increased running distance with this intervention; the other three women had similar results when short-term goals were changed from daily to weekly criteria. Commenting on these findings, Wack et al. (2014) suggested that, "Goal setting procedures in which criterion levels are set for an individual's behavior may function as an establishing operation that enhances the reinforcing value of goal achievement" (p. 184). The performance feedback may also have functioned as positive reinforcement.

Technology-Assisted Intervention

Van Wormer (2004) researched the effect of combining pedometers and brief E-counseling on physical activity of three adults (32–51 years old). In a baseline phase, the participants simply wore a pedometer to measure step counts. Next, they self-monitored activity by recording daily steps on a spreadsheet. With ongoing self-monitoring, an E-counseling component was added whereby a researcher reviewed each participant's step data, set performance goals, and delivered praise during a weekly, 10-min email conversation. The self-monitoring and self-monitoring plus E-counseling interventions were approximately equal in increasing daily step totals over baseline levels.

Targeting 12 sedentary adults who were 50 years of age and older, Kurti and Dallery (2013) incorporated accelerometer instrumentation to record steps taken, calories burned, and distance travelled. These activity data were automatically uploaded to a website that was accessible to the researchers. The participants could also login to a personal homepage that displayed a graph of their steps and related information. During one intervention phase, participants had to exceed prescribed step goals on at least three of five days each week before advancing to a higher goal. They were compensated with money for achieving and surpassing these goals. A second intervention phase only included the goal-setting component. Both of these internet-sourced programs dramatically increased the daily step total for 11 of the 12 participants, although results were slightly more robust with activity-contingent monetary consequences.

Exergaming

The format for exergaming is that "video games or various auditory and visual stimuli are paired with different types of exercise equipment and activities and the individual must engage in physical activity to play the game or produce the auditory or visual stimulation" (Fogel et al. 2010, p. 592). It has been shown that playing exergames can increase energy expenditure in typically developing children (Graf et al. 2009; Mhurchu et al. 2008), and that they enjoy exergaming more than a conventional form of exercise such as treadmill walking (Leiringer et al. 2010). One possible reason for the superiority of exergaming is that it heightens motivation to be active because the types of stimulation and games can be matched to a child's preferences. In research with elementary school students, Fogel et al. (2010) and Shayne et al. (2012) compared exergaming to traditional physical education classes. The students consistently had more physical activity and opportunity to engage in physical activity with exergaming.

Exercise-Physical Activity Intervention in IDD

In a survey of exercise-physical activity research among children and youth with autism spectrum disorder (ASD), Lang et al. (2010) found that 61 % of published studies had to do with jogging or running. Other less frequent types of exercise-physical activity were bike riding, weight training, roller skating, swimming, and water aerobics. Similarly, Sowa and Meulenbroek (2012) completed a meta-analysis of research with children and adults who had ASD, finding that jogging and swimming were the two most frequently studied physical activities, followed by horseback riding, weight training, and walking. Though informative, the reviews by Lang et al. (2010) and Sowa and Meulenbroek (2012) must be qualified by the specific ASD population they targeted and the diverse objectives of the exercise-physical activity plans in those studies. Promoting jogging and running, for example, was not selected solely to improve health or offer pleasurable exercise outlets but in some cases to decrease challenging behaviors through antecedent intervention (Celiberti et al. 1997; Elliot et al. 1994; Gordon et al. 1986).

Lancioni et al. (2009) focused on locomotor behavior in a review of research with children who had cerebral palsy, Down syndrome, Rett syndrome, and other developmental disabilities. Eighty-one percent (81 %) of these studies featured treadmills, while proportionately fewer programs utilized walkers with micro-switch activated sensory stimulation. To reiterate, these findings should be interpreted relative to the population characteristics and the inclusion of only treadmills and micro-switch technology as methods for facilitating exercise-physical activity.

The reviews by Lang et al. (2010), Sowa and Meulenbrock (2012), and Lancioni et al. (2009) consistently identified health and related benefits from exercise-physical activity, most notably improved physical fitness, functional ambulation, walking endurance, motor responsiveness, activity engagement, and social skills. Among the specific health outcomes from physical activity in adolescents with ASD, a systematic review of research by Sorensen and Zarrett (2014) revealed the strongest effects for cardiovascular and aerobic fitness, flexibility, endurance, and motor abilities.

There are several examples of early ABA research in the area of exercise-physical activity with people who have IDD and other neurodevelopmental disabilities. Luyben et al. (1986) took a team sports approach by teaching a side-of-the-foot soccer pass to three adults (24–52 years old) with IDD using a combination of verbal and manual prompting, prompt-fading, praise, and visual cues. A trainer followed a 9-step task analysis during individual sessions with each participant. The training program was successful but somewhat limited because the participants were not taught to pass the soccer ball to a peer or in the context of team play. Nonetheless, the study is notable for being one of the first to integrate behavioral training and athletic performance with an underserved population.

Dowa and Dove (1980) included four categories of "swimming behavior" within a rating checklist comprised of 35 responses. The participants were three children with spina bifida, although their level of intellectual functioning was not indicated in the published study. The dependent measure was the number of swimming responses from the checklist each child achieved during scheduled sessions at a summer camp. During intervention the children watched themselves swimming in brief segments of self-modelling videotapes which captured "performed behaviors superior to those previously observed on the checklist" (p. 53). Compared to their baseline performance, all of the children had moderate increases in the number of checklist behaviors achieved when they viewed the self-modelling videotapes. A noteworthy feature of this study is that it predated the development of video modelling technology which has become a popular instructional approach in IDD (Darden-Brunson et al. 2008; Nikopoulos et al. 2015) and more recently been applied to athletic performance enhancement (Boyer et al. 2009; Luiselli et al. 2011).

Rogers et al. (2010) further investigated methods for teaching swimming to three children (10–12 years old) with autism. The swimming responses were executing a flutter kick, stroking with a front-crawl motion, and turning head to the side. A trainer implemented constant time-delay prompting with each child, a procedure that was intended to minimize errors and produce fluent skill acquisition. This intervention was highly effective with all of the children in building these foundational swimming skills. The study also highlights a variant of "errorless" teaching in the context of exercise-physical activity intervention.

Cameron and colleagues (Cameron and Cappello 1993; Cameron et al. 2005) illustrated the positive effect of stimulus shaping and stimulus transfer procedures within programs to enhance exercise-physical activity. The participant in Cameron and Cappello (1993) was a 21-year old man with Down syndrome preparing for jumping hurdles at a Special Olympics track event. Before training he would not jump over a hurdle at any height. His program consisted of an 11-step protocol that initially had him step over four hurdles that were flat on the floor. The hurdles were gradually raised in fixed increments, reaching a terminal height of 12 inches. After 37 training sessions the man was able to clear hurdles consistently at this placement height. He also performed successfully in the Special Olympics event six months later.

Citing bike riding is a versatile form of exercise, Cameron et al. (2005) taught a 9-year-old boy diagnosed with Asperger syndrome to initially pedal for 5 min on a stationary kinetic trainer. The next series of steps increased his time pedaling to 15 min, then instructed him to brake, and finally dismount. At this stage of the intervention the bike was removed from the kinetic trainer and the boy was prompted to glide on his bike over a slightly declining grassy slope. With further shaping and stimulus transfer procedures, his bike riding was extended to a roadway in front of his house, which the boy successfully accomplished and was able to maintain many months later.

Several more recent studies have expanded exercise-physical activity interventions to include different combinations of procedures and contemporary technology devices. LaLonde et al. (2014) recruited five adults (21–26 years old) with ASD for a program to increase the number of steps they walked each day at a post-secondary educational facility. Four of the adults had BMIs in the "obese" range and the fifth adult was classified as being "overweight." They wore a small pedometer to record step frequency, synchronized with a laptop computer, and programmed to transmit data to a central source. Preceding intervention, tokens (stickers) were provided to the adults when they attached and removed their pedometers correctly at the start and conclusion of each day respectively. They were not able to see the step numbers on the pedometers, nor were procedures in effect to encourage walking. Intervention consisted of the adults setting daily step-frequency goals that were gradually increased as progress was achieved. The adults could earn valued "prizes" whenever they matched or exceeded their goals. Evaluated in a multiple baseline design, goal setting and positive reinforcement consistently increased the number of steps the adults took each day, with all of them surpassing 10,000 or more steps by conclusion of the study. The exercise-physical activity program was easily integrated within the setting and every adult rated it positively.

Luiselli et al. (2013a, b) implemented several methods of behavioral coaching for preparing two adults with IDD (20 and 21 years old) to participate in a Special Olympics 100 m sprint event. In a baseline phase lasting one day, they were timed during three sprints without specific training. Within five sequential intervention phases, each adult (a) set gradually increasing sprint-time goals, (b) received verbal performance feedback, (c) earned preferred objects upon exceeding their goals, and (d) watched video models of a coach demonstrating proper sprinting technique. Results showed that average sprint time for one of the adults was below his baseline average during each of the five intervention phases. For the other adult, average sprint time during intervention phases was also lower, albeit comparable to his baseline average. Both adults had their fastest sprint times in the intervention phase that combined goal-setting, performance feedback, and positive reinforcement. These times were also maintained when they ran at the Special Olympics event one week following the study.

Walking is a simple, inexpensive, and convenient form of exercise, but many people with IDD are not able to ambulate fluently because they have motor, sensory, and orthopedic impairments. Lancioni and colleagues (Lancioni et al. 2010; Lancioni et al. 2012; Lancioni et al. 2013) have published extensive research showing that assistive technology devices can be used to facilitate and maintain walking in otherwise inactive children and adults who have IDD and multiple disabilities. In Lancioni et al. (2014), the researchers designed optic micro-switches on the heels of shoes that when activated through walking, triggered sources of preferred sensory stimulation intended to function as positive reinforcement. One case involved a 23-year-old man with ID, blindness, and hearing loss. During daily ambulation sessions he had the opportunity to walk a defined travel distance under baseline conditions without micro-switch activation and during intervention in which his steps produced several seconds of preferred vibratory stimulation. The second participant was a 10-year-old girl who also had ID, vision impairment, and hearing loss. She was involved in a similar baseline-intervention evaluation except her preferred step-contingent stimulation was music and blinking lights. Intervention with both participants increased the percentage of their independent travel and reduced the average time traversing the travel route. Summarizing the results, Lancioni et al. (2014) commented that micro-switch-aided programs represent a vital technology for individuals who have IDD and motor disabilities, enabling them to exercise through planned and spontaneous ambulation.

Though preliminary, exergaming may be promising for health promotion and intervention in IDD. Lotan et al. (2009) implemented a virtual reality program of game-like exercises with 30 adults (*M* age = 52.3 years) who had moderate IDD and compared effects with 30 adults (*M* age = 54.3 years) in a matched-control group. The program consisted of two, 30-min sessions each week for a duration of 5–6 weeks. Intervention group participants had significant improvements in physical fitness as measured by a modified 12-min walk-run (Modified Cooper Test) and the Total Heart Beat Index (THBI). The control and intervention groups did not differ significantly on the Energy Expenditure Index (EEI).

Dickinson and Place (2014) designed a randomized control trial (RCT) with 100 children (10–11 years old) who had autism to evaluate the contribution of a computer-based activity program on cardiopulmonary fitness and BMI. All of the children participated in standardized physical education classes at school consisting of two, 30–40 min sessions per week of basketball, gymnastics, swimming, dance, and ball games. Half of the children (intervention group) were further exposed to computer game activities for a period of 15 min each day, three times per week. The activities were organized around Olympic events such as fencing, aquatics, rowing, archery, shooting, and gymnastics. After one year, the intervention group children had statistically significant improvement on all measures from a fitness test battery other than flexibility. These gains were also significantly better than the fitness outcomes among the children who did not have access to the computer-based activity program.

Finally, Knights et al. (2014) evaluated an internet exergame cycling program on cardiovascular fitness of eight youth with cerebral palsy. Several health measures were taken before and following a 6-weeks course of intervention. Significant post-intervention improvements were obtained on the Gross-Motor Functional Classification System (GMFCS)-Level III but on none of the other dependent measures. These limited findings should also be qualified by the absence of a comparative control group.

Summary

The research reviewed in this chapter supports several behavioral intervention procedures for increasing and maintaining exercise-physical activity among children and adults with IDD. Most commonly, studies have evaluated shaping, positive reinforcement, goal-setting, and stimulus control methods, albeit in different combinations and targeting diverse intervention objectives. Technology advancements, in particular, define more contemporary applications, as revealed with pedometer-accelerator activated measurement systems and interventions that incorporate video modeling and internet-sourced modalities.

Nevertheless, the exercise-physical activity research literature in IDD is not robust. Commenting about this matter in the case of adolescents with ASD, Sorensen and Zarrett (2014) wrote, "This lack of research is particularly surprising due to (1) the higher risk of chronic disease, (2) higher rates of overweight and obesity, (3) higher rates of sedentary behavior, (4) lower rates of physical activity among adolescents with ASD relative to non-affected peers, and (5) studies demonstrating similar benefits (e.g., health, cognitive, emotional, and behavioral) for typically developing individuals during adolescence and across the lifespan" (p. 350). These same factors apply to the state of research with people who have IDD. Thus, a critical objective going forward is overcoming the barriers to pursuing health promotion and intervention in IDD, thereby increasing research dissemination that translates to effective and "user friendly" clinical practices.

A second limitation is that much of the exercise-physical activity intervention research to date has not reported definitive health measures. Instead, studies have generally recorded direct observational and instrumentation-generated data such as steps taken (LaLonde et al. 2014), running speed (Luiselli et al. 2013a, b), and percentage of time demonstrating motor responses (Lancioni et al. 2014). Certainly, it can be assumed that properly planned and executed exercise-physical activity should confer health benefits. However, standardized measures of energy expenditure, heart rate, functional movement, BMI, cardio-respiratory output, and other similar indices should be the basis of health-focused research, notwithstanding the corollary changes that can be attained for cognitive functioning and challenging behaviors (Anderson-Hanley et al. 2011).

Practice Recommendations

Medical screening is a necessity before initiating an exercise-physical activity program with a child or adult who has IDD. A physical examination would be required to rule out health impairments or limitations that might contraindicate certain types of exercise or increasingly strenuous activities. Medical evaluation is particularly crucial when the exercise-physical activity program is part of a plan that addresses health-compromising conditions such as obesity and diabetes (Fleming 2011). Persons taking psychotropic medications must also be examined in order to prevent possible negative consequences from exercising and becoming more physically active. These concerns apply similarly throughout intervention.

Most people with IDD receive educational and habilitation services in schools, community settings, congregate living arrangements, and homes. Teachers, therapists, direct-care staff, and parents are usually responsible for implementing intervention procedures. Hence, these and other care-providers must be properly trained, supervised, and taught the skills necessary to promote exercise-physical activity in their respective settings.

Training care-providers is most effective when it is competency-based and conducted in vivo (Luiselli 2011, 2015a, b; Parson et al. 2013). The basis for this training is instructing a teacher, therapist, or parent to implement clearly defined and observable behaviors that improve performance of service recipients. The role of a care-provider in an exercise-physical activity intervention could be establishing relatively rudimentary actions with a child or adult such as walking and running (LaLonde et al. 2014; Lancioni et al. 2009), or gradually building more complex repertoires such as shooting a basketball (Lo et al. 2014). Accordingly, the methods for training care-providers must be geared to the learning objectives and requisite behaviors that constitute the type of exercise-physical activity. Some training may be possible in a didactic or simulated context but as noted, should ultimately be instituted in the natural environment in order to facilitate generalization and occasion performance during "real world" conditions.

Another facet of training is supervising care-providers to ensure they implement procedures with integrity (Hagermoser Sanetti and Kratochwill 2014). Intervention integrity is assessed by observing care-providers interacting with service recipients and recording whether they accurately followed a prescribed (usually written) intervention plan. A key element of such assessment is having the supervisor provide performance feedback by praising the care-provider for procedures applied properly and correcting procedures that were misapplied. These interactions with the supervisor include verbal reminders, demonstration, and additional practice (DiGennaro Reed and Codding 2011). Absent intervention integrity assessment, it is not possible to judge whether a seemingly ineffective plan is the result of inaccurate implementation or the intervention procedures themselves.

As an example of intervention integrity assessment, the study by LaLonde et al. (2014) to increase walking by young adults with ASD had a member of the research team present each morning to document that the participants wore their accelerometer devices, filled out data sheets, and correctly completed other steps in their self-managed plans. The overall integrity score was 98 %. The researchers also observed the participants during 30 % of their school days and verified that the accelerometer devices were worn 100 % of the time. Less impressive intervention integrity would trigger additional participant training until performance improves to an acceptable standard.

Beyond the direct measurement of outcome indicators, social validity is a critical determinant of intervention success (Kazdin 1977; Wolf 1978). One emphasis of social validity is verifying that intervention rationale, goals, and techniques are reasonable. As it applies to exercise-physical activity, a program for teaching swimming to children with IDD might begin by surveying swimming instructors to confirm a proposed task analysis of arm, head, and leg motions. Exemplifying this approach, Luiselli et al. (2013a, b) referenced the Special Olympics rules for running the 100 m sprint before creating an 8-step task analysis that guided their behavioral coaching intervention with two young adults.

A second purpose of social validity assessment is soliciting opinions about intervention satisfaction and acceptability. It is possible, for example, that a very effective intervention plan is not rated favorably by care-providers and service recipients because the procedures are perceived as being burdensome, stigmatizing, or complex. Referring to LaLonde et al. (2014) again, the researchers approached social validity assessment by asking the participants whether they did ("yes") or did not ("no") like wearing the accelerometer device each day and would they want to wear it and set walking goals in the coming year? Based on a 7-point Likert-type scale (1 = very, 7 = not at all), the instructor also responded to questions from the modified *Treatment Acceptability Rating Form Revised* (*TARF-R*) (Reimers et al. 1992): (a) how acceptable was the treatment, (b) how willing were you to carry-out the treatment, and (c) how effective was the treatment? When social validity is poor, the task is to revise the components of intervention plans that were rated less favorably. A related consideration is that positively regarded intervention plans by care-providers predicts stronger post-intervention maintenance (Kennedy 2002)—that is, individuals will continue to implement procedures that they like and approve.

Concerning maintenance, there are several strategies for sustaining the positive effects of exercise-physical activity programs. Kurti and Dallery (2013) correctly opined that people are more likely to remain active and adhere to prescribed regimens that require minimal equipment, can be performed conveniently, and are inexpensive. Adults, for example, prefer home-based activities and may engage more with web-presented routines (Brawley et al. 2003). Since most people with IDD will require close supervision, home-centered, easily accessed, and relatively simple physical activities such as exergaming (Fogel et al. 2010; Shane et al. 2012) and walking (LaLonde et al. 2014; Lancioni et al. 2014) can be maintenance-facilitating.

Motivation, of course, is another influence on sustaining exercise-physical activity. Therefore, it is imperative to assess a person's preferences, ideally using formal, choice-methods that have proven to be effective in identifying positively reinforcing stimuli (Tiger and Kliebert 2011). Gradually "thinning" the schedule of reinforcement and systematically varying preference options are other strategies for promoting maintenance. Self-monitoring with goal setting may also contribute to post-intervention maintenance subsequent to reinforcement fading.

Emphasizing a point made earlier in the chapter, multi-method measurement, whenever possible, is the optimal approach for evaluating exercise-physical activity interventions with people who have IDD. In the case of a walking program, these measures would include steps taken, distance, duration, and physiological outcomes such as respiration and heart rate. Again, other data (e.g., weight, BMI, blood markers) are further indicated when the priority of an exercise-physical activity intervention plan is health improvement.

In summary, behavioral intervention can facilitate, increase, and maintain exercise-physical activity in people with IDD. Despite the efficacy of past and recent research demonstration, additional inquiry is needed to replicate and expand previous findings across child and adult populations and encompassing new methodologies. Varied technological adaptations and innovations will further contribute to promoting exercise-physical activity with individuals who have IDD and complicated motor and sensory impairments (Lancioni et al. 2012). As research continues to inform practices, schools, community settings, and families will be expected to support and prompt access to exercise-physical activity in ways that are convenient and economical (Tyler et al. 2014). After-school programs, in-home consultation, community clubs, peer-buddy arrangements, and environmentally-adapted athletic training facilities are just some of the outlets that can encourage people with IDD and their families to become more active. An emphasis on multidisciplinary collaboration among physicians, rehabilitation specialists, nutritionists, and allied professionals is another worthwhile and necessary endeavor for delivering exemplary services.

References

Anderson-Hanley, C., Tureck, K., & Schneiderman, R. L. (2011). Autism and exergaming: Effects on repetitive behaviors and cognition. *Psychology Research and Behavior Management, 1*, 129–137.

Andrade, L. F., Barry, D., Litt, M. D., & Petry, N. M. (2014). Maintaining high activity levels in sedentary adults with a reinforcement-thinning schedule. *Journal of Applied Behavior Analysis, 47*, 523–536.

Beets, M. W., & Pitetti, K. H. (2011). Using pedometers to measure moderate-to-vigorous physical activity for youth with intellectual disability. *Disability and Health Journal, 4*, 46–51.

Boyer, E., Miltenberger, R. G., Batsche, C., & Fogel, V. (2009). Video modeling by experts with video feedback to enhance gymnastics skills. *Journal of Applied Behavior Analysis, 42*, 855–860.

Brawley, L. R., Rejeski, W. J., & King, A. C. (2003). Promoting physical activity for older adults: The challenges for changing behavior. *American Journal of Preventive Medicine, 25*, 172–183.

Brown, W. H., Pfeiffer, K., McIver, K. L., Dowda, M., Almeida, J., & Pate, R. (2006). Assessing preschool children's physical activity: An Observational System for Recording Physical Activity in Children—Preschool Version (OSRAC-P). *Research Quarterly for Exercise and Sport, 77*, 167–176.

Butte, N. F., Ekelund, U., & Westerterp, K. R. (2012). Assessing physical activity using wearable monitors: Measures of physical activity. *Medicine and Science in Sports and Exercise, 44*, S5–S12.

Cameron, M. J., & Cappello, M. J. (1993). "We'll cross that hurdle when we get to it": Teaching athletic performance within adaptive physical education. *Behavior Modification, 17*, 136–147.

Cameron, M. J., Shapiro, M. J., & Ainsleigh, S. A. (2005). Bicycle riding: Pedaling made possible through positive behavioral interventions. *Journal of Positive Behavioral Interventions, 7*, 153–158.

Cannelle-Malone, H. I., Tullis, C. A., & Kazee, A. R. (2011). Using antecedent exercise to decrease challenging behavior in boys with developmental disabilities and an emotional disorder. *Journal of Positive Behavioral Interventions, 13*, 230–239.

Carroll, D. D., Courtney-Long, E. A., Stevens, A. C., Sloan, M. L., Lullo, C., Visser, S. N., et al. (2015). Vital signs: Disability and physical activity-United States, 2009–2012. *Centers for Disease Control and Prevention Morbidity and Mortality Weekly Report, 63*, 1–7.

Celiberti, D. A., Bobo, H. E., Kelly, K. S., Harris, S. L., & Handleman, J. S. (1997). The differential and temporal effects of antecedent exercise on the self-stimulatory behavior of a child with autism. *Research in Developmental Disabilities, 18*, 139–150.

Centers for Disease Control and Prevention. (2008). *Physical activity for everyone.* Retrieved from www.cdc.gov/physicalactivity/everyone/guidelines/adults.html.

Darden-Brunson, F., Green, A., & Goldstein, H. (2008). Video-based instruction for children with autism. In J. K. Luiselli, D. C. Russo, W. P. Christin & S. Wilczynski (Eds.), *Effective practices for children with autism: Educational and behavior support interventions that work* (pp. 241–268). New York: Oxford University Press.

Dickinson, K., & Place, M. (2014). A randomized control trial of the impact of a computer-based activity programme upon the fitness of children with autism. *Autism Research and Treatment, 2*, 1–9.

DiGennaro Reed, F. L., & Codding, R. S. (2011). Intervention integrity assessment. In J. K. Luiselli (Ed.), *Teaching and behavior support for children and adults with autism spectrum disorder: A practitioner's guide* (pp. 38–47). New York: Oxford University Press.

Dowda, M., Pate, R. R., Trost, S. G., Almeida, M. J., & Sirad, J. R. (2004). Influences of preschool policies and practices on children's physical activity. *Journal of Community Health, 29*, 183–196.

Dowrick, P. W., & Dove, C. (1980). The use of self-modeling to improve the swimming performance of spina bifida children. *Journal of Applied Behavior Analysis, 13*, 51–56.

Ekelund, U., Luan, J., Sherar, L. B., Esliger, D. W., Griew, P., & Cooper, A. (2012). Moderate to vigorous physical activity and sedentary time and cardiometabolic risk factors in children and adolescents. *Journal of the American Medical Association, 307*, 704–712.

Elliot, R. O., Dobbin, A. R., Rose, G. D., & Soper, H. V. (1994). Vigorous, aerobic exercise versus general motor training activities: Effects on maladaptive and stereotypic behaviors of adults with both autism and mental retardation. *Journal of Autism and Developmental Disorders, 24*, 565–576.

Emerson, E. (2007). Poverty and people with intellectual disabilities. *Mental Retardation and Developmental Disabilities Research Reviews, 13*, 107–113.

Finkelstein, E. A., Brown, D. S., Brown, D. R., & Buchner, D. M. (2008). A randomized study of financial incentives to increase physical activity among sedentary adults. *Preventive Medicine, 47*, 182–187.

Fleming, R. K. (2011). Obesity and weight regulation. In J. K. Luiselli (Ed.), *The handbook of high-risk challenging behaviors in people with developmental disabilities* (pp. 195–207). Baltimore, MD: Brookes.

Fogel, V. A., Miltenberger, R. G., Graves, R., & Koehler, S. (2010). The effects of exergaming on physical activity among inactive children in a physical education classroom. *Journal of Applied Behavior Analysis, 43*, 591–600.

Gabler-Halle, D., Halle, J. W., & Chung, Y. B. (1993a). The effects of aerobic exercise on psychological and behavioral variables of individuals with developmental disabilities: A critical review. *Research in Developmental Disabilities, 14*, 359–386.

Gabler-Halle, D., Halle, J. W., & Chung, Y. B. (1993b). The effects of aerobic exercise on psychological and behavioral variables of individuals with developmental disabilities: A critical review. *Research in Developmental Disabilities, 14*, 359–386.

Glidden, L. M., Bamberger, K. T., Draheim, A. R., & Kersh, J. (2011). Parent and athlete perceptions of Special Olympics participation: Utility and danger of proxy responding. *Intellectual and Developmental Disabilities, 49*, 37–45.

Gordon, R., Handleman, J. S., & Harris, S. L. (1986). The effects of continent versus non-contingent running on the out-of-seat behavior of an autistic boy. *Child & Family Behavior Therapy, 8*, 37–44.

Graf, D., Pratt, L., Hester, C., & Short, K. (2009). Playing active video games increases energy expenditure in children. *Pediatrics, 124*, 534–540.

Hagermoser Sanetti, L., & Kratochwill, T. (2014). *Treatment integrity: A foundation for evidence-based practice in applied psychology*. Washington, DC: American Psychological Press.

Haskell, W. L., lee, I., Pate, R. R., Powell, K. E., Blair, S. N., Franklin, B. A., et al. (2007). Physical activity and public health: Updated recommendation for adults from the American College of Sports Medicine and the American Heart Association. *Circulation, 116*, 1081–1093.

Heath, G., & Fentem, P. (1997). Physical activity among persons with disabilities: A public health perspective. *Exercise and Sport Science Review, 25*, 195–234.

Hustyi, K. M., Normand, M. P., & Larson, T. A. (2011). Behavioral assessment of physical activity in obese preschool children. *Journal of Applied Behavior Analysis, 44*, 635–639.

Hustyi, K. M., Normand, M. P., Larson, T. A., & Morely, A. J. (2012). The effect of outdoor activity context on physical activity in preschool children. *Journal of Applied Behavior Analysis, 41*, 401–405.

Kazdin, A. E. (1977). Assessing the clinical or applied importance of behavior change through social validation. *Behavior Modification, 1*, 427–452.

Kennedy, C. H. (2002). The maintenance of behavior change as an indicator of social validity. *Behavior Modification, 26*, 594–604.

Knights, S., Graham, N., Switzer, L., Hernandex, H., Ye, Z., Findlay, B., Xie, W., Wright, V., & Fehlings, D. (2014). An innovative cycling exergame to promote cardiovascular fitness in youth with cerebral palsy: A brief report. *Developmental Neurorehabilitation*.

Krahn, G. L., Hammond, L., & Turner, A. (2006). A cascade of disparities: Health and health care access for people with intellectual disabilities. *Mental retardation and Developmental Disabilities Research Reviews, 12*, 70–82.

Kurti, A. N., & Dallery, J. (2013). Internet-based contingency management increases walking in sedentary adults. *Journal of Applied Behavior Analysis, 46*, 568–581.

LaLonde, K. B., MacNeill, B. R., Eversole, L. W., Ragotzy, S. P., & Poling, A. (2014). Increasing physical activity in young adults with autism spectrum disorders. *Research in Autism Spectrum Disorders, 8*, 1679–1684.

Lancioni, G. E., Sigafoos, J., O'Reilly, M. F., & Singh, N. N. (2012a). *Assistive technology: Interventions for individuals with severe-profound and multiple disabilities*. New York: Springer.

Lancioni, G. E., Singh, N. N., O'Reilly, M. F., Sigafoos, J., Alberti, G., Boccasini, A., et al. (2013). Technology-based programs to improve walking behavior of persons with multiple disabilities: Two single-case studies. *Disability and Rehabilitation: Assistive Technology, 8*, 92–98.

Lancioni, G. E., Singh, N. N., O'Reilly, M. F., Sigafoos, J., Alberti, G., Perilli, V., et al. (2014). Microswitch-aided programs to support physical exercise or adequate ambulation in persons with multiple disabilities. *Research in Developmental Disabilities, 35*, 2190–2198.

Lancioni, G. E., Singh, N. N., O'Reilly, M. F., Sigafoos, J., Didden, R., Manfredi, F., et al. (2009). Fostering locomotor behavior of children with developmental disabilities: An overview of studies using treadmills and walkers with microswitches. *Research in Developmental Disabilities, 30*, 308–322.

Lancioni, G. E., Singh, N. N., O'Reilly, M. F., Sigafoos, J., La Martire, M. L., Oliva, D., et al. (2012b). Technology-based programs to promote walking fluency or improve foot-ground contact during walking: Two case studies of adults with multiple disabilities. *Research in Developmental Disabilities, 33*, 111–118.

Lancioni, G. E., Singh, N. N., O'Reilly, M. F., Sigafoos, J., Oliva, D., Smaldone, A., et al. (2010). Promoting ambulation responses among children with multiple disabilities through walkers and micoswitches with contingent stimuli. *Research in Developmental Disabilities, 31*, 811–816.

Lang, R., Koegel, L. K., Ashbaugh, K., Regester, A., Ence, W., & Smith, W. (2010). Physical exercise in individuals with autism spectrum disorder: A systematic review. *Research in Autism Spectrum Disorders, 4*, 565–576.

Larson, T. A., Normand, M. P., & Hustyi, K. M. (2011). Preliminary evaluation of an observation system for recording physical activity in children. *Behavioral Interventions, 26*, 193–203.

Larson, T. A., Normand, M. P., Morley, A. J., & Hustyi, K. M. (2014a). The role of the physical environment in promoting physical activity in children across different group compositions. *Behavior Modification, 38*, 837–851.

Larson, T. A., Normand, M. P., Morley, A. J., & Miller, B. G. (2013). A functional analysis of moderate-to-vigorous physical activity in young children. *Journal of Applied Behavior Analysis, 46*, 199–207.

Larson, T. A., Normand, M. P., Morley, A. J., & Miller, B. G. (2014b). Further evaluation of a functional analysis of moderate-to-vigorous physical activity in young children. *Journal of Applied Behavior Analysis, 47*, 219–230.

Leininger, L., Coles, M., & Gilbert, J. (2010). Comparing enjoyment and perceived exertion between equivalent bouts of physically interactive video gaming and treadmill walking. *Health Fitness Journal of Canada, 3*, 12–18.

Lo, Y., Burk, B., & Anderson, A. L. (2014). Using progressive video prompting to teach students with moderate intellectual disability to shoot a basketball. *Education and Training in Autism and Developmental Disabilities, 49*, 354–367.

Lotan, M., Yalon-Chamovitz, S., & Weiss, P. L. T. (2009). Improving physical fitness of individuals with intellectual and developmental disability through a virtual realty intervention program. *Research in Developmental Disabilities, 30*, 229–239.

Luiselli, J. K. (2011). Training parents and other care providers. In J. K. Luiselli (Ed.), *Teaching and behavior support for children and adults with autism spectrum disorder: A practitioner's guide* (pp. 212–216). New York: Oxford University Press.

Luiselli, J. K. (2014). Exercise, physical activity, and sports. In J. K. Luiselli (Ed.), *Children and youth with autism spectrum disorder (ASD): Recent Advances and Innovations in Assessment, Education, and Intervention* (pp. 194–204). New York: Oxford University Press.

Luiselli, J. K. (2015a). Health and wellness. In N. N. Singh (Ed.). *Clinical handbook of evidence-based practices for individuals with intellectual disabilities.* New York: Springer (in press).

Luiselli, J. K. (2015b). Performance management and staff preparation. In F. D. Reed & D. D. Reed (Eds.), *Bridging the gap between science and practice in autism service delivery.* New York: Springer.

Luiselli, J. K., Duncan, N. G., Keary, P., Godbold-Nelson, E., Parenteau, R. E., & Woods, K. E. (2013a). Behavioral coaching of track athletes with developmental disabilities: Evaluation of sprint performance during training and Special Olympics competition. *Journal of Clinical Sport Psychology, 7*, 264–274.

Luiselli, J. K., & Fischer, A. J. (Eds.). (2015). *Computer-assisted and web-based innovations in psychology, special education, and health.* New York: Elsevier.

Luiselli, J. K., & Reed, D. D. (Eds.). (2011). *Behavioral sport psychology: Evidence-based approaches to performance enhancement.* New York: Springer.

Luiselli, J. K., Woods, K. E., Keary, P., & Parenteau, R. E. (2013b). Practitioner beliefs about athletic and health promoting activities for children and youth with intellectual and developmental disabilities: A social validation survey. *Journal of Developmental and Physical Disabilities.*

Luiselli, J. K., Woods, K. E., & Reed, D. D. (2011). Review of sports performance research with youth, collegiate, and elite athletes. *Journal of Applied Behavior Analysis, 44*, 999–1002.

Luyben, P. D., Funk, D. M., Morgan, J. K., Clark, K. A., & Delulio, D. W. (1986). Team sports for the severely retarded: Training a side-of-the-foot soccer pass using a maximum-to-minimum prompt reduction strategy. *Journal of Applied Behavior Analysis, 19*, 431–436.

Mann, J., Zhou, H., McDermott, S., & Poston, M. B. (2006). Healthy behavior change of adults with mental retardation: Attendance in a health promotion program. *American Journal of Mental Retardation, 111*, 62–73.

McIver, K. L., Brown, W. H., Pfeiffer, K. A., Dowda, M., & Pate, R. R. (2009). Assessing children's physical activity in their homes: The Observational System for Recording Physical Activity in Children-Home. *Journal of Applied Behavior Analysis, 42*, 1–16.

McKenzie, T. L., Marshall, M. A., Sallis, J. F., & Conway, T. L. (2000). Leisure-time physical activity in school environments: An observational study using SO-PLAY. *Preventive Medicine, 30*, 70–77.

McKenzie, T. L., Sallis, J. F., Patterson, T. L., Elder, J. P., Berry, C. C., & Rupp, J. W. (1991). BEACHES: An observational system for assessing children's eating and physical activity behaviors and associated events. *Journal of Applied Behavior Analysis, 24*, 141–151.

Mhurchu, C. N., Maddison, R., Jiang, Y., Jull, A., Prapavessis, H., & Rodgers, A. (2008). Coach potatoes and jumping beans: A pilot study of the effects of active video games on physical activity in children. *International Journal of Behavior, Nutrition, and Physical Activity, 5*, 8.

Morrison, H., Roscoe, E. M., & Atwell, A. (2011). An evaluation of antecedent exercise on behavior maintained by automatic reinforcement using a three-component schedule. *Journal of Applied Behavior Analysis, 44*, 523–541.

Nikopoulos, C., Luiselli, J. K., & Fischer, A. J. (2015). Video modeling. In J. K. Luiselli & A. J. Fischer (Eds.), *Computer-assisted and web-based innovations in psychology, special education, and health.* Elsevier, Amsterdam (in press).

Oriel, K., George, C., Peckus, R., & Semon, A. (2011). The effects of aerobic exercise on academic engagement in young children with autism spectrum disorder. *Pediatric Physical Therapy, 23*, 187–193.

Otto, M. W., & Smits, J. A. J. (2011). *Exercise for mood and anxiety: Proven strategies for overcoming depression and enhancing wellbeing*. New York: Oxford University Press.

Parsons, M. B., Rollyson, J. H., & Reid, D. H. (2013). Evidence-based staff training: A guide for practitioners. *Behavior Analysis in Practice, 5*, 2–11.

Peterson, J. J., Janz, K. F., & Lowe, J. B. (2008). Physical activity among adults with intellectual disabilities living in community settings. *Preventive Medicine, 47*, 101–106.

Petry, N. M., Andrade, L. F., Barry, D., & Byrne, S. (2013). A randomized study of reinforcing walking in older adults. *Psychology and Aging, 28*, 1164–1173.

Reilly, J. J., & Kelly, J. (2011). Long-term impact of overweight and obesity in childhood and adolescence on morbidity and premature morbidity in adulthood: Systematic review. *International Journal of Obesity, 35*, 891–898.

Reimers, T., Wacker, D. P., Coopers, L. J., & Raad, A. O. (1992). Acceptability of behavioral treatments for children: Analog and naturalistic evaluations by parents. *School Psychology Review, 21*, 639–640.

Rimmer, J. H. (1999). Health promotion for people with disabilities: The emerging paradigm shift from disability prevention to prevention of secondary conditions. *Physical Therapy, 79*, 495–502.

Rimmer, J. H., Riley, B., Wang, E., Rauworth, A., & Jurkowski, J. (2004). Physical activity participation among persons with disabilities: Barriers and facilitators. *American Journal of Preventive Medicine, 26*, 419–425.

Rogers, L., Hemmeter, M. L., & Wolery, M. (2010). Using a constant time delay procedure to teach foundational swimming skills to children with autism. *Topics in Early Childhood Special Education*, 30, 102–111.

Rosenthal-Malek, A., & Mitchell, S. (1997). Brief report: The effects of exercise on the self-stimulatory behaviors and positive responding of adolescents with autism. *Journal of Autism and Developmental Disorders, 27*, 193–202.

Ross, R., Dagone, D., Jones, P. J., Smith, H., Paddags, A., Hudson, R., et al. (2000). Reduction in obesity and related comorbid conditions after diet-induced weight loss in men: A randomized, controlled trial. *Annals of Internal Medicine, 133*, 92–103.

Scepters, M., Kerr, M., O'Hara, D., Bainbridge, D., Cooper, S. A., Davis, R., et al. (2005). Reducing disparity in people with intellectual disabilities. *Journal of policy and Practice in Intellectual Disability, 2*, 249–255.

Seekins, T., Traci, M. A., Bainbridge, D., & Humphries, K. (2005). Secondary conditions risk appraisal for adults. In W. M. Nehring (Ed.), *Health promotion for persons with intellectual and developmental disabilities* (pp. 325–342). Washington, DC: AAMR.

Shayne, R. K., Fogel, V. A., Miltenberger, R. G., & Koehler, S. (2012). The effects of exergaming on physical activity in a third-grade physical education class. *Journal of Applied Behavior Analysis, 45*, 211–215.

Sorensen, C., & Zarrett, N. (2014). Benefits of physical activity for adolescents with autism spectrum disorders: A comprehensive review. *Review Journal of Autism and Developmental Disorders, 1*, 344–353.

Sowa, M., & Meulenbroek, R. (2012). Effects of physical exercise on autism spectrum disorders: A meta-analysis. *Research in Autism Spectrum Disorders, 27*, 193–202.

Tiger, J. H., & Kliebert, M. L. (2011). Stimulus preference assessment. In J. K. Luiselli (Ed.), *Teaching and behavior support for children and adults with autism spectrum disorder: A practitioner's guide* (pp. 30–37). New York: Oxford University Press.

Troiano, R. P., Berrigani, D., Dodd, K. W., Masse, L. C., Tilert, T., & McDowell, M. (2008). Physical activity in the United States measured by accelerometer. *Medicine and Science in Sports and Exercise, 40*, 181–189.

Tryon, W. W. (2011). Actigraphy: The ambulatory measurement of physical activity. In J. K. Luiselli & D. D. Reed (Eds.), *Behavioral sport psychology: Evidence-based approaches to performance enhancement* (pp. 25–41). New York: Springer.

Tyler, K., MacDonald, M., & Menear, K. (2014). Physical activity and physical fitness of school-age children and youth with autism spectrum disorders. *Autism Research and Treatment, 2*, 1–6.

U.S. Department of Health and Human Services. (2005). The Surgeon General's call to action to improve the health and wellness of persons with disabilities. Rockville, MD. Available at http://www.surgeongeneral.gov/library/calls/index.html.

U.S. Public Health Service (USPHS). (2002). *Closing the gap: A national blueprint for improving the health of individuals with mental retardation. Report of the surgeon general's conference on health disparities and mental retardation.* Washington, DC: U.S. Department of Health and Human Services, Office of the Surgeon General.

Van Camp, C. M., & Hayes, L. B. (2012). Assessing and increasing physical activity. *Journal of Applied Behavior Analysis, 45*, 871–875.

VanWormer, J. J. (2004). Pedometers and brief E-counseling: Increasing physical activity for overweight adults. *Journal of Applied Behavior Analysis, 37*, 421–425.

Wack, S. R., Crosland, K. A., & Miltenberger, R. G. (2014). Using goal setting and feedback to increase weekly running distance. *Journal of Applied Behavior Analysis, 47*, 181–185.

Washington, W. D., Banna, K. M., & Gibson, A. L. (2014). Preliminary efficacy of prize-based contingency management to increase activity levels in healthy adults. *Journal of Applied Behavior Analysis, 47*, 231–245.

Wolf, M. M. (1978). Social validity: The case for subjective measurement or how applied behavior analysis is finding its heart. *Journal of Applied Behavior Analysis, 11*, 202–214.

Wysocki, T., Hall, G., Iwata, B., & Riordan, M. (1979). Behavioral management of exercise: Contracting for aerobic points. *Journal of Applied Behavior Analysis, 12*, 55–64.

Yamaki, K., Rimmer, J. H., Lowry, L. C., & Vogel, T. (2011). Prevalence of obesity-related chronic health conditions in overweight adolescents with disabilities. *Research in Developmental Disabilities, 32*, 280–288.

Chapter 5
Assistive Technology in Severe and Multiple Disabilities

Giulio E. Lancioni, Nirbhay N. Singh, Mark F. O'Reilly, Jeff Sigafoos and Doretta Oliva

Summary

This chapter is aimed at providing a general picture of basic technology resources and intervention programs developed and assessed for improving the situation of persons with intellectual and multiple disabilities. In particular, the chapter focuses on technology and programs used to help those persons (a) develop control of environmental stimulation and strengthen adaptive behavior, (b) improve their ambulation (i.e., enhance their continuity and increase their adequate foot positioning), (c) manage stimulus choice opportunities, (d) increase adaptive responding (and stimulation control) and curb inappropriate behavior or posture, (e) access environmental stimulation and caregiver attention, (f) formulate requests, and (g) manage indoor orientation and travel. In order to offer an illustrative view of the technology resources and intervention programs used within each of the aforementioned areas, a few studies published in those areas are summarized in

G.E. Lancioni (✉)
Department of Neuroscience and Sense Organs, University of Bari,
Corso Italia 23, 70121 Bari, Italy
e-mail: giulio.lancioni@uniba.it

N.N. Singh
Medical College of Georgia, Augusta University, Augusta, GA, USA

M.F. O'Reilly
University of Texas at Austin, Austin, TX, USA

J. Sigafoos
Victoria University of Wellington, Wellington, New Zealand

D. Oliva
Lega F. D'Oro Research Center, Osimo, Italy

J.K. Luiselli (ed.), *Behavioral Health Promotion and Intervention in Intellectual and Developmental Disabilities*, Evidence-Based Practices in Behavioral Health,
DOI 10.1007/978-3-319-27297-9_5

detail. Eventually, considerations are made with regard to the results of the studies and their practical implications for daily contexts. New issues for future research are also suggested.

Introduction

Education, rehabilitation and care contexts for persons with severe or profound intellectual and multiple disabilities are becoming increasingly familiar with the notion and use of "assistive technology" (i.e., technical devices aimed at helping persons with disabilities improve their general performance and thus decrease the negative effects of their disabling conditions) (Bauer et al. 2011; Belva and Matson 2013; Brown et al. 2009; Lancioni et al. 2014b; Reichle 2011; Shih 2011). In practice, the use of assistive technology is viewed as a way to enhance the rehabilitation perspectives or care quality for those persons who, without the help of such technology, would have a more difficult daily existence and a gloomier future (Brown et al. 2009; Holburn et al. 2004; Lui et al. 2012; Moisey 2007; Moisey and van de Keere 2007; Ripat and Woodgate 2011; Scherer et al. 2011; Tam et al. 2011).

The devices referred to with the assistive technology label can vary widely, in line with the characteristics of the persons served and the objectives targeted within their programs (Bauer et al. 2011; Borg et al. 2011; Burne et al. 2011; Lancioni et al. 2013b). For example, microswitches (i.e., sensors for detecting responses even if minimal) linked to computer technology have been used for helping persons with and without extensive motor impairment and severe/profound intellectual and multiple disabilities interact with (control) stimulation events in their immediate surroundings (Holburn et al. 2004; Gutowski 1996; Mechling 2006; Saunders et al. 2003). Speech Generating Devices (SGDs) have been used to enable persons with intellectual and communication disabilities make requests and gain access to preferred stimulation events (Van der Meer et al. 2012a, b). Combinations of microswitches and SGDs have been used to allow persons with multiple disabilities to control environmental stimulation and also call for caregiver attention (Lancioni et al. 2009a, b). Computer-aided packages have been used to provide pictorial instructions for activity steps and to help the participants reach different workstations and carry out object assembling (Furniss et al. 2001; Lancioni et al. 2013c, 2014a).

Obviously, the technology has to be adapted to the characteristics of the participants and needs to be introduced through carefully planned intervention programs (Bauer et al. 2011; Borg et al. 2011; Burne et al. 2011; Lancioni et al. 2013b). The implications of the first point are that the development/choice of the technology should be a joint initiative of technical experts and education/rehabilitation personnel (Borg et al. 2011; Burne et al. 2011; Lancioni et al. 2013b, 2014b; Rispoli et al. 2010). The implications of the second point are that carefully designed intervention programs are needed to ensure that the participants learn how to use the technology solution selected for them effectively (Banda et al. 2011; Lancioni et al. 2011d, 2013b; Mechling and Gustafson 2009).

This chapter is aimed at providing a general picture of basic technology resources and intervention programs developed and assessed for improving the situation of persons with intellectual and multiple disabilities (Bauer et al. 2011; Lancioni et al. 2013b). In particular, the chapter focuses on technology and programs used to help those persons (a) develop control of environmental stimulation and strengthen adaptive behavior, (b) improve their ambulation (i.e., enhance their continuity and increase their adequate foot positioning), (c) manage stimulus choice opportunities, (d) increase adaptive responding (and stimulation control) and curb inappropriate behavior or posture, (e) access environmental stimulation and caregiver attention, (f) formulate requests, and (g) manage indoor orientation and travel. In order to provide an illustrative view of the technology resources and intervention programs used within each of the aforementioned areas, a few studies published in those areas are summarized in detail. Eventually, considerations are made with regard to the results of the studies and their practical implications for daily contexts. New issues for future research are also suggested (cf. Lancioni et al. 2007a, 2014d, e; Rispoli et al. 2010; Sigafoos et al. 2014a; Thunberg et al. 2007). Table 5.1 is a brief map of the chapter and lists (a) the research areas covered in the chapter as well as (b) the studies summarized in the text as illustrations of the technology and intervention conditions available within those areas.

Table 5.1 Chapter summary map

Areas			
Studies	Participants (number)	Age (years)	Technology to detect responses or provide instructions
Developing stimulation control and adaptive responding			
Mechling (2006)	3	6–19	Pressure microswitches to detect hand/arm responses
Lancioni et al. (2013d)	2	21, 26	Optic microswitch to detect forehead skin movement
Lancioni et al. (2014c)	2	21, 16	Optic microswitch to detect head responses and tilt microswitch to detect hand responses
Lancioni et al. (2014a)	2	13, 30	Optic microswitches to detect object-manipulation responses
Improving ambulation			
Lancioni et al. (2010c)	5	5.5–11	Optic microswitches to detect step responses
Lancioni et al. (2014b)	1	23	Optic microswitches to detect step responses
	1	10	Optic microswitches to detect foot positions
Promoting stimulus choice			
Lancioni et al. (2011c)	2	34, 31	Pressure microswitch for hand closure and stimulus presentation system
Lancioni et al. (2013g)	1	9	Optic microswitch for smile response and stimulus presentation system

(continued)

Table 5.1 (continued)

Areas			
Studies	Participants (number)	Age (years)	Technology to detect responses or provide instructions
	1	56	Optic microswitch for tongue response and stimulus presentation system
Promoting adaptive responding and reducing problem behavior or posture			
Lancioni et al. (2008a)	1	29	Optic microswitch for the adaptive response and tilt microswitch for hand stereotypies
Lancioni et al. (2013e)	1	10	Optic microswitches for the adaptive response and problem head posture
Promoting control of environmental stimulation and caregiver attention			
Lancioni et al. (2009a)	11	5–18	Microswitch and SGD-related sensor for two different responses
Lancioni et al. (2009b)	8	5–18	Microswitch and SGD-related sensor for two different responses
Promoting active communication (requests) via SGDs			
Lancioni et al. (2011e)	1	33	SGD with five requests activated with touch response
Sigafoos et al. (2013)	2	4, 5	SGD with one request activated with touch response
Promoting orientation and activity engagement			
Lancioni et al. (2010b)	2	38, 32	Orientation technology providing verbal instructions

Developing Stimulation Control and Adaptive Responding

Two groups of participants may be involved in programs aimed at developing stimulation control and adaptive responding and relying on the use of microswitches, that is, (a) persons with very extensive motor impairment and severe/profound intellectual or multiple disabilities, and (b) persons with severe/profound intellectual or multiple disabilities and moderate or no specific motor impairment (Holburn et al. 2004; Lancioni et al. 2014a, d, e). For example, Mechling (2006) worked with three participants of 6–19 years of age who were diagnosed with profound intellectual disabilities and serious motor impairment. The participants were taught to activate pressure microswitches to access environmental stimulation through small hand/arm or head movements. Sessions lasted 9 min and were divided into three sections of 3 min, each of which involved a specific type of stimulation for the participants' responses. The use of the different types of stimulation served to determine which of the three had the greatest impact. Once this information was acquired, the rest of the sessions only involved the stimulation considered most preferred/effective. The results showed that all three participants had clear preference for a stimulation that involved visual images/inputs prepared by their instructors. When this stimulation was available, their response frequencies varied between five and nine per 3-min periods. The participants continued to have relatively high response frequencies during the final intervention sessions, in which only the most preferred stimulation was available for their responses.

Lancioni et al. (2013d) worked with two young men of 21 and 26 years of age who were affected by multiple (i.e., intellectual, motor, and sensory) disabilities. The two men did not possess any interaction with objects, and the purpose of the study was to enable them to seek preferred environmental stimulation through a small upward movement of the forehead skin. Such movement activated an optic sensor/microswitch, which was positioned above the participant's left or right eyebrow, about 2 mm above a black mini sticker. An upward movement of the forehead skin caused the optic sensor to see (overlap with the sticker), and thus to be activated. Any activation allowed the men to access preferred stimuli for 8–10 s, except during the baseline phases of the study. Data showed that both men learned to use the forehead response (movement) efficiently and performed it quite frequently during (a) the intervention phases of the study (i.e., when it was followed by the preferred stimulation) as well as (b) the post-intervention check when the preferred stimulation was still in use.

Lancioni et al. (2014c) carried out a study with a woman with Rett syndrome and an adolescent with extensive neuro-motor and intellectual disabilities who were 21 and 16 years old. The woman could activate optic sensors placed on her shoulder by rotating/bending her head to the right or the left. Sensor/microswitch activation enabled her to access animation films with music for 10–15 s. The adolescent could activate mini shock absorbers and tilt devices (i.e., the microswitch) by forward, sideward and downward movements of his right hand. Any microswitch activation gained him access to 10–15 s of home videos with songs. The stimulation selected for the two participants was considered highly preferred/enjoyable for them. The study involved an ABAB sequence. The initial baseline (A) assessment showed that both participants had low levels of head or hand responses. The intervention (B) phases showed a clear increase in the response frequencies with considerably high access to their preferred stimulation and the occurrence of frequent indices of happiness (i.e., expressions such as smiling associated with an apparent enjoyment of the situation; see Dillon and Carr 2007).

Lancioni et al. (2014a) carried out a program to help two participants of 13 and 30 years of age, with multiple (i.e., intellectual, sensory, motor, and communication) disabilities and minimal object interaction, to develop an object-manipulation (adaptive) response. Such response consisted of taking objects from a table and placing them into a container. The response activated an optic sensor (microswitch), which was placed at the opening of the container. Microswitch activation led the participants to obtain 5 or 6 s of preferred stimulation. Data were very encouraging. Both participants learned to perform the adaptive response and continued to execute it also when the objects were moved slightly more distant from the container and thus the participants were to make a greater effort to maintain their performance.

Improving Ambulation

Ambulation (walking) is a critical skill with a multitude of practical and social implications. In fact, ambulation can be instrumental to allow a person to reach different places in order to get involved in different activities and/or meet different people (Hayakawa and Kobayashi 2011; Lancioni et al. 2009d). A number of persons with severe/profound intellectual and multiple disabilities present ambulation problems even in absence of specific or very serious motor impairments. The most recurrent problem is discontinuity (breaks) in the ambulation process that these persons tend to display when using a walker device as well as when following a rail or other spatial/physical reference (Lancioni et al. 2010c, 2013f). Another problem that might be encountered is toe walking (Lancioni et al. 2014b). Lancioni et al. (2010c) conducted a study with five children who used walker devices but tended to be largely discontinuous in their ambulation. The technology used for the study consisted of (a) microswitches monitoring the participants' step responses and (b) a computer device serving to activate stimulation sources attached to the walkers or the children's body (e.g., vibration devices). The children were reported to be in the severe or profound intellectual disability range and were affected by spastic tetraparesis. Four of them also presented with visual impairment. Although the walker represented a sufficiently secure support, they performed only a few steps and did not seem to be motivated to do more. In light of this situation, the use of microswitches to monitor step responses and trigger the occurrence of preferred stimulation contingent on (immediately after) the performance of those steps was considered to be critically important. The study involved an ABAB sequence for four children and an AB sequence for one child. The A and B represented baseline and intervention phases. Sessions lasted 5 min for all participants and were generally implemented several times a day. Preferred stimulation for the step responses was available only during the B phases. The stimulation was activated for 3–5 s if the child received it at each (right- and left-foot) step, and for about 8 s if the child received it only in relation to his right-foot steps. During the initial baseline, the participants showed mean frequencies of 7–26 steps per session. During the first intervention phase, their mean frequencies of steps increased to between 23 and 110 per session. These frequencies increased further during the second intervention phase for each of the four children who had such a phase.

Lancioni et al. (2014b) reported a study in which a 23-year-old man with multiple disabilities (i.e., intellectual disability, blindness, and moderate hearing loss) who was to walk along a rail in a corridor (transporting objects) displayed breaks in his ambulation. The ambulation sessions programmed for him involved five travels that were to be carried out using the aforementioned rail. The length of each travel was nearly 7 m. The man was fitted with optic sensors (microswitches) at the heels of his shoes and vibratory devices at his waist, shoulders, and wrists. Each step turned on two vibratory devices for about 1 s during the intervention phases of the study, which included an ABAB sequence. At the end of each travel (i.e., after the man put away the object he had transported), a brief hand massage was also available. During the initial baseline (A) phase, about 25 % of the travels were carried out independently. During the first intervention (B) phase, the percentage increased to about 80. The percentage declined during the second baseline and increased to nearly 90 by the second intervention phase. Moreover, the time required for the travels decreased during the intervention phases.

Lancioni et al. (2014b) also worked with a girl of 10 years of age, who was affected by multiple (intellectual and sensory) disabilities and emotional instability, and displayed toe walking. The ambulation sessions programmed for her included five travels each of which was about 25-m long. The girl was provided with optic sensors at the heels of her shoes, an MP3 fitted with preferred songs and brief verbal reminders, and a bracelet that could light up with flickering lights. An optic microswitch was activated when the girl's heel was close to (less than 2 mm from) the ground. Microswitch activation turned on the MP3 with preferred songs and the flickering light for about 1 s (during the intervention phases of the study). The stimulation could be almost continuous if the girl ambulated with adequate foot position. During the first baseline phase, the percentage of steps with adequate foot position was about 10. During the first intervention phase, it increased to about 70. It declined during the second baseline and increased again (to about 90) during the second intervention phase. This last percentage was maintained also when the walking conditions were slightly changed, asking the girl more independence.

Promoting Stimulus Choice

The use of microswitches and computer systems can also help participants to have an active role in deciding about the type of environmental stimulation they want to have (Lancioni et al. 2006a, b, 2013b; Sullivan et al. 1995). One way to exercise choice for persons with extensive motor impairment and intellectual disabilities could involve the (a) activation of a microswitch (i.e., the performance of an affirmative/selection response) in relation to a computer's presentation of samples (previews) of stimuli that the participant wants to access, and (b) abstention from microswitch activation (i.e., abstention from the affirmative/selection response) in relation to the computer's presentation of samples of stimuli that the participant does not want to access.

Lancioni et al. (2011c) evaluated a stimulus choice program with two adults of 34 and 31 years of age who were diagnosed with multiple disabilities and were sedentary and typically passive. At each session, a computer system presented 16 stimulus samples. Twelve of them represented stimuli/events considered to be preferred (e.g., songs and music, familiar voices, and noises) and four represented stimuli considered to be non-preferred (e.g., white noise or distorted sounds). A sample was presented for about 5 s. If the participants performed an affirmative/selection response within 6 s from the end of the sample, the computer system presented the corresponding stimulus for 20 s. Performance of the response within 6 s from the end of a 20-s stimulation period caused the system to continue the presentation of the same stimulus for another 20-s period. The response (i.e., a slight hand closure) activated a pressure microswitch, which was placed inside the participants' hand. Abstention from the aforementioned response after a stimulus sample or the end of a 20-s stimulation period amounted to participant's lack of positive interest in (rejection of) that particular stimulus situation and caused the system to pause briefly and then present the next stimulus sample of the sequence available. Data showed that both participants (a) selected an average of about seven or eight of the preferred stimuli available in the sessions, (b) requested several repetitions of many of the stimuli chosen (i.e., thus increasing considerably the number of stimulation events experienced), and (c) abstained from responding almost consistently in relation to the non-preferred stimuli. Interestingly, the participants' mood during the sessions showed a clear improvement, with multiple indices of happiness.

Lancioni et al. (2013g) carried out two studies aimed at enabling a child and a man to make stimulus choices through programs matching the one just described (Lancioni et al. 2011c). The child participating in the first study was 9 years old, presented with pervasive motor impairment, lack of speech and minimal residual vision, and was considered to function within the moderate/severe intellectual disability range. Procedural conditions, stimulus samples and stimulation periods were comparable to those described for the aforementioned study on choice (Lancioni et al. 2011c). The response for making choices was however different. It consisted of a smile expression, which entailed widening the mouth and expanding/lifting the cheekbone areas. This response activated an optic microswitch, which was held across the area before his left cheekbone. The man participating in the second study was 56 years old, presented with pervasive motor impairment and lack of speech due to acquired brain injury. Procedural conditions matched those described above. The response for making choices consisted of a tongue movement toward the right corner of his mouth. Such response activated a light-dependent resistor (i.e., a specific form of optic microswitch). Data showed that both participants were successful in choosing stimuli considered to be preferred (and asking for repeated presentations of many of those stimuli) and avoiding stimuli considered non-preferred.

Promoting Adaptive Responding and Reducing Problem Behavior or Posture

The primary worry about persons with extensive intellectual and multiple disabilities concerns their narrow repertoire of adaptive responses and their apparent inability to interact with their environment and consequently to enrich their input and enhance their development (Lancioni et al. 2013a; Zucker et al. 2013). The studies reviewed in the previous sections of this chapter were attempts to deal with such worry. Another worry concerns the possible presence of problem behavior (e.g., hand mouthing and eye poking) or problem postures (e.g., head forward bending). Conventional intervention approaches have generally dealt with the two types of worries separately, that is, different programs were developed for promoting adaptive responding (with independent access to environmental stimulation) and for reducing problem behavior or postures (Lancioni et al. 2009c). During the last 10 years, several studies have been reported showing the possibility of targeting both types of worries within single intervention programs. Those programs combine microswitches for monitoring the positive/adaptive responding and the problem posture/behavior (Lancioni et al. 2007c, 2008a, d, 2013a, e).

For example, Lancioni et al. (2008a) carried out a study with a man of 29 years of age who presented with intellectual disability, lack of speech and other specific forms of communication, minimal interest in objects, paresis of the lower limbs, and hand stereotypies. The stereotypies were apparently maintained by automatic reinforcement. The adaptive responses targeted within the program were object-contact responses, which entailed putting one or both hands inside a box with vibrating objects and touching one or more of those objects. Such response would activate optic sensors inside the box. The stereotypies consisted of rotating the left hand and wrist back and forth in connection with the right hand or away from it. The presence of stereotypies activated tilt microswitches, which were fixed on a wristband that the man wore on his left wrist. The study involved an ABAB sequence. During the A (baseline) phases, the microswitches were used and connected to a computer system, but no consequences were available for adaptive responses and stereotypies. During the intervention phases, object-contact responses performed in absence of stereotypies produced preferred stimulation, which involved vibration, music, voices, noises or lights. The stimulation lasted 8 s if stereotypies did not occur during that time. Otherwise, it was interrupted. During the baseline phases, the man showed low or declining frequencies of adaptive responses and relatively high levels of stereotypies. During the intervention phases, the frequencies of adaptive responses increased largely and the levels of stereotypies dropped very visibly.

Lancioni et al. (2013e) directed one of their programs to a child of 10 years of age who was affected by intellectual, sensory and motor disabilities. The goals of the program set up for this child were those of (a) promoting and strengthening adaptive hand engagement (i.e., interaction with objects) and (b) reducing a problem head posture (i.e., head forward bending). The hand engagement targeted as first objective of the study was considered critical for fostering the child's acquisition of new information and basic development. The problem posture was targeted for reduction because it was considered harmful for his physical condition and social status. Performance of the adaptive response activated tilt and optic microswitches, which were linked to the objects in front of the child. Problem head posture activated an optic microswitch, which was placed on the headrest of the child's wheelchair. The study included a sequence of five phases. The first phase was a baseline, in which the adaptive response and problem posture were monitored but no consequences were scheduled for them. The second phase was aimed at promoting the adaptive response. Each occurrence of the response was followed by a brief period of preferred stimulation irrespective of the head posture. The third phase entailed the occurrence of preferred stimulation for each adaptive response performed in the absence of the problem posture. The stimulation, moreover, lasted the scheduled time only if the problem posture did not appear during that time. The fourth and fifth phases of the study corresponded to the first and third phases just described. Data showed that the program was largely successful. Indeed, the child displayed large increases in the frequency of adaptive responses and critical decreases in the presence of the problem posture during the third and fifth phases of the study (i.e., when stimulation for adaptive responses was available only if the child controlled his head posture).

Promoting Control of Environmental Stimulation and Caregiver Attention

The use of microswitches, as described above, provides encouraging evidence as to the potential of these devices in helping persons with severe/profound and multiple disabilities manage stimulation control and choice situations (including also those in which they can choose to refrain from problem behavior/postures in order to obtain preferred stimulation). While the use of microswitch-aided programs can be considered a critical supplement to direct staff intervention, even for extended periods of time within the daily contexts, circumstances may be envisaged in which an extension of these programs would be desirable/warranted. One of those circumstances could be represented by the possible need of persons involved in microswitch-aided programs for contact with (attention from) their caregivers. These programs in their standard format are geared to allow the persons to access environmental stimulation but do not entail calls for staff/caregiver attention. An extension of those programs to entail such a possibility has been assessed in a number of studies (Lancioni et al. 2008b, c, 2009a, b).

For example, Lancioni et al. (2009a, b) carried out two studies, which involved 11 and 8 participants with multiple disabilities, respectively. The participants' ages ranged from about 5 to 18 years. In both studies, the participants were taught to use a microswitch to access preferred stimulation and a Speech Generating Device (SGD) to call for caregiver attention. The microswitches included, among others, pressure sensors, tilt devices, and optic sensors. The responses used for activating them and thus accessing environmental stimulation independently included, among others, hand, head, and eyelid movements. The SGDs (also known as VOCAs, that is, Voice Output Communication Aids) were devices that emitted verbal calls for caregiver attention when the participants activated a sensor (similar to the aforementioned microswitches). In relation to those calls, the caregiver could respond with different levels of attention/involvement, that is, (a) verbal attention accompanied by hand clapping and other pleasant sounds/noises or (b) all the above plus various forms of physical contact. The studies were carried out according to a multiple probe design across responses (technology devices). Initially, baseline sessions concerned the microswitch and the SGD devices. Then intervention focused on teaching the participants to activate the microswitch and access preferred stimulation (e.g., music, audio-recording of familiar voices, and vibration) independently. Once the participants had managed the use of the microswitch, the intervention concentrated on the use of SGD device/response. Activation of this device caused the request of caregiver attention and was followed by one of the levels of attention mentioned above. By the last phase of the program, the microswitch and the SGD were simultaneously available to the participants and they could use either of the two devices at will. Data showed that all participants learned to use the microswitch and the SGD during the intervention phases focused on each of them individually. Moreover, they continued to use both devices during the last phase of the program (i.e., when both devices were simultaneously available). It may be relevant to note, however, that the use of the SGD was relatively moderate compared to the use of the microswitch for most of the participants.

Promoting Active Communication (Requests) Via SGDs

The previous section has indicated how SGDs can be combined with microswitches for helping participants access stimulation and call for caregiver attention independently. SGDs can also be used alone, that is, as a tool to allow the participants an effective form of active communication, the opportunity to make requests. Participants can benefit immediately and extensively from this technology if they (a) have failed to develop any (sufficient) speech abilities, (b) do not possess adequate non-verbal communication means (Lancioni et al. 2011e, 2013b; Sigafoos et al. 2013, 2014a; Van der Meer et al. 2012a), and (c) are interested in their environment and the stimuli that it contains (i.e., want to gain access to some of the stimuli and need help to do so; Gevarter et al. 2013a; Kagohara et al. 2013). Obviously, the participants should also possess the motor skills required for the activation of the device chosen. With regard to the last point, one may envisage a device that requires responses such as touching or pressing specific panels/cells with different stimulus images for participants who have sufficient fine motor skills for those responses. A different type of device may be required for participants who cannot afford the aforementioned responses (Lancioni et al. 2013b).

For example, Lancioni et al. (2011e) assessed the use of a SGD with a woman who presented with intellectual disabilities, lack of speech, and respiratory problems. The woman used the SGD to request about five different stimuli (i.e., activities considered fairly interesting for her; e.g., listening to music/songs, watching videos, and using make-up material). Pictorial representations of those activities were visible on five different cells of the SGD. The participant could request any activity by touching the cell showing the representation of such activity. The touch/pressure response triggered the verbalization of a request message concerning that specific activity. The first intervention phase focused on introducing the pictorial representations used to indicate the activities, one at a time. During the following intervention phase, all five representations were visible on the SGD and the participant could select/request any of them. Data showed that the participant used the device successfully and made a mean of about eight requests per session (i.e., periods of 20-25 min).

Sigafoos et al. (2013) used an Apple iPad device with Proloquo2Go software with two children of 4 and 5 years of age, who were diagnosed with autism spectrum disorder and marked developmental delays. The children were taught to use the device to request continuation of their toy play. The children were provided with 3–10 request trials per session. A trial started with the child selecting a toy and playing with it. Shortly after, the experimenter gently took the toy away. The child could have the toy back by touching its representation on the iPad (i.e., by requesting it). Both children learned to request the toy very rapidly and this new communication skill reduced/eliminated inappropriate behaviors that they previously used to get the toy back. The new skill was maintained over time and generalized to other stimuli.

Promoting Orientation and Activity Engagement

Persons with blindness (or minimal residual vision) and intellectual disabilities may have serious problems orienting and traveling even within their daily contexts. Providing those persons with maps of the areas may be of little or no help, given the difficulties of the persons to generalize their basic information to the real context. Similarly, using some landmarks as orientation cues may only occasionally be helpful, given the difficulties in discriminating the landmarks and associating them with different activities and travel directions (Lancioni et al. 2013b; Martinsen et al. 2007; Ross and Kelly 2009). One way to reduce these difficulties involves the use of orientation technology. A basic version of such technology relies on the use of auditory or auditory and tactile direction cues, that is, cues that direct/call the person to the destinations targeted for his or her travels (Lancioni et al. 2010b, 2013b).

For example, Lancioni et al. (2010b) carried out two studies, one of which was directed at a man and a woman of 38 and 32 years of age, respectively. The man had minimal residual vision while the woman was totally blind. Both were rated in the moderate to severe intellectual disability range, had ambulation skills and could also understand and produce basic sentences for communication within their context. Yet, they had difficulties orienting and moving within the day center that they attended, that is, they often failed to reach the rooms where they were expected to carry out small activities and meet staff or other people. The orientation technology employed with these participants provided them with (a) an instruction to turn to their right or to their left immediately after they walked out of a room (i.e., an instruction that was to orient their travel within the hallway) and (b) a similar instruction to turn right or left and enter a room when they reached the entrance of the room where the activity or meeting was to occur. The instruction consisted of a verbal utterance or a combination of a vibratory cue and a verbal utterance. Both participants benefited from the technology and travelled virtually without errors. Moreover, they became much faster in reaching the target destinations.

Considerations on the Technological Resources and Intervention Outcomes Reviewed

Microswitch-aided programs. Programs based on the use of microswitches can be highly effective in helping persons with severe/profound and multiple disabilities (a) control environmental stimulation and strengthen adaptive responding, (b) improve ambulation, (c) achieve choice-making abilities, and (d) combine an increase in adaptive responding with a reduction of problem posture/behavior. Microswitch-aided programs can also be extended with the use of a SGD allowing the participants to call for caregiver attention. The effectiveness of the aforementioned programs represents an important piece of evidence, a strong and encouraging reference for daily contexts dealing with persons with severe/profound and multiple disabilities. A successful use of those programs within those contexts would depend on the respect of at least two basic criteria.

The first criterion is the use of a suitable response-microswitch combination. The response should be in the person's repertoire, simple to perform (i.e., not excessively demanding in terms of effort required) and reliable. At the same time, it should have a low frequency under normal conditions. Only a spontaneous low frequency would allow the person to develop a performance increase in relation to his or her association of the response with positive environmental consequences. In other words, only a low frequency would allow the person to show evidence of response learning and consolidation. The response can vary from a relatively large/obvious piece of behavior (e.g., hand or head movements) to a minimal expression (e.g., forehead skin or eyelid movements). Minimal expressions may represent one of the few usable solutions for persons with pervasive motor impairment who would not be able to display more obvious, marked responses.

The microswitch can only be chosen in relation to the response and needs to be appropriate for it, that is, able to detect it with high accuracy and without creating any sense of discomfort to the person or causing the person an awkward (negatively discriminating) appearance. Pressure and tilt devices represent the most conventional microswitches that can be arranged in different ways and used successfully with more obvious types of responses (i.e., responses that involve a relatively ample, easily observable movement). A variety of other devices have been developed for minimal types of responses. These devices include, among others, optic sensors and camera-based instruments that can be adapted to different forms of subtle responses that require careful monitoring (e.g., eyelid, mouth, and forehead skin movements; see Lancioni et al. 2007a, 2010a, 2011a, b, 2013b, 2014b, c; Lui et al. 2012).

The second criterion is the availability of highly preferred environmental stimulation that the participants can access through their responses (microswitch activations) (Kazdin 2001; Lancioni et al. 2013b). In practice, the possibility of accessing motivating/reinforcing stimulation is a necessary condition for justifying the participants' efforts to produce responses and maintain their active engagement over time (Catania 2012; Kazdin 2001). Absence of relevant stimulation events is most likely to preclude any increase in the participant's responding and thus any positive change in their level of engagement.

It might be important to note that satisfaction of the aforementioned criteria can also be critical to help the participants achieve relevant forms of self-control and improve their mood. Evidence of self-control can be observed in the programs in which microswitches are used for an adaptive response as well as for problem behavior or problem posture. When the participant has strengthened the adaptive response in relation to the positive stimulation that is available for it, the programs confront him or her with a new situation. The stimulation can only be maintained if he or she refrains from the problem behavior/posture. The decision to maintain the stimulation involves the participant's willingness to control his or her problem behavior/posture independent of external forms of restraint (Lancioni et al. 2009c). Evidence of improved mood (i.e., indices of happiness) has been provided by a number of studies in which microswitch activation allows the person access to preferred stimulation (Dillon and Carr 2007; Lancioni et al. 2005, 2007b, 2013b). This evidence underlines the participants' enjoyment of the programs. This enjoyment can be considered as important as, or even more important than, the development of adaptive responding per se (Lancioni et al. 2005, 2007b; Petry et al. 2005, 2009; Szymanski 2000).

SGDs and communication. SGDs can be used in combination with microswitches or as single intervention solutions. Programs combining a SGD and one or more microswitches can be considered practically interesting solutions particularly in those situations in which the participants are expected to engage independently in periods of positive occupation. In those situations, they are likely to display adaptive responding to activate the microswitch(es) available and access preferred environmental stimulation with high levels of satisfaction/enjoyment. Yet, it is also possible that they could feel the desire for caregiver attention. The presence of the SGD is a guarantee for the participants and the caregivers that a personal interaction can be established any time the need/desire for it arises (Lancioni et al. 2008b, 2009a, b, 2013b).

The use of SGDs as communication (request) instruments can be considered critically important for all those participants who have interests in environmental stimulation events, but lack the ability to make those interests known (i.e., do not possess recognizable communication means), given their disabilities (Sigafoos et al. 2013, 2014a). SGDs can be employed in all those situations in which the participants are known to have communication (request) interests to satisfy. For example, one could schedule this kind of approach during snack periods as well as during play or occupational situations (Sigafoos et al. 2013, 2014a, b; Van der Meer et al. 2012a, b). The characteristics of the devices used and the number of requests involved in the communication exchanges should be arranged on the basis of the situations targeted and the participants' levels of functioning (e.g., Lancioni et al. 2011d; Van der Meer et al. 2012a).

One might foresee the use of a basic device with one specific request when the participants are starting a communication program and the situation is simple such as that of a snack (Kagohara et al. 2013; Sigafoos et al. 2013, 2014a). The same snack situation could easily become suitable for a more complex communication exchange when the participants' abilities grow. For these types of participants, one could imagine a device with two or more request options related to two or more snack alternatives (Kagohara et al. 2013; Sigafoos et al. 2014a, b). The way one can progress from a basic device to a more complex one with two or more requests options may change across different participants and situations. New research could be very helpful in clarifying this issue (Gevarter et al. 2013a, b). New research could also help clarify how one can progress from the use of the devices within specific communication situations (e.g., snack and activity) to the use of the devices throughout the day. Obviously, this latter point is closely connected with the expansion of the participants' communication repertoire and topics. In practice, one could imagine of fitting any daily context with a device providing the opportunity to make requests in line with the participant's development (Lancioni et al. 2013b; Sigafoos et al. 2014a, b).

Orientation and travel. Technology for promoting indoor orientation and travel can be considered practically relevant in programs for persons with visual and severe to profound intellectual disabilities as well as for persons with only profound intellectual disabilities. Indeed, orientation and travel require the ability to develop a map of the area within which one has to move and identify landmarks to use efficiently. Such an achievement may be quite difficult to manage for persons with the aforementioned levels of disabilities. For those persons, the availability of environmental cues that directs them to the destinations may be viewed as the best and most effective approach. Indeed such an approach would be easily implemented and the persons could become rapidly capable of reaching destinations and avoiding the frustration of failure. The technology necessary for such an approach can vary depending upon the intellectual and sensory situation of the persons involved. The example described above (Lancioni et al. 2010b) may be considered practical and respectful for persons with visual impairment and moderate/severe intellectual disabilities. A more basic approach could involve sound or vocal cues that are repeatedly, but briefly presented at the destinations until the participants reach them. The use of visual cues marking the route to the destinations can also be considered a viable solution for persons with residual vision (Lancioni et al. 2013b).

Conclusions

The studies reviewed and the considerations previously formulated underline the usability and effectiveness of various forms of technology-aided programs to help persons with intellectual and multiple disabilities pursue functional objectives.

This encouraging picture can be taken as an important piece of evidence and provide essential guidelines for daily contexts dealing with the education and care of these persons. It can also be viewed as a basis for new research in the area. Such research could tackle a number of questions left unanswered by the studies so far carried out. For example, while a number of microswitch devices have been assessed to detect minimal responses, additional efforts are required to find new solutions to help those persons who are considered unable to benefit from currently available microswitch technology (Lancioni et al. 2013b, d, 2014c, e; Leung and Chau 2010; Lui et al. 2012).

The use of SGDs to promote active communication has been shown to be highly useful and has also attracted a sizeable body of research. New research could be directed at two specific issues. The first issue concerns the evaluation of additional forms of technology and/or of representations of the request items. For example, one could imagine that the use of video clips are likely to be more illustrative than static pictures for some participants and thus more helpful for them to start making requests (Mechling and Gustafson 2009). Similarly, SGDs in which the requests are represented by small object replicas could be evaluated to help persons who are affected by blindness in addition to intellectual disabilities. The second issue concerns ways of making the technology consistently available and the communication of the person involved in the program plausible throughout the day (Sigafoos et al. 2014a, b).

While independent orientation and travel can be seen as a valuable educational objective by itself, the possibility of combining this objective with functional occupation might be seen as an important goal. Accordingly, research aimed at assessing technology-aided programs that combine ways to help the persons make their travel functional for the performance of daily activities or other forms of occupational engagements could be encouraged (Lancioni et al. 2013b).

The value of technology and technology-aided programs cannot be measured only in terms of whether they are effective to produce changes in the participants' behavior. Two other relevant measures would be (a) the participants' level of satisfaction with (or preference for) those resources and (b) the level of support/approval provided to those resources by parents, staff, and service providers (Callahan et al. 2008; Lancioni et al. 2013b; Luiselli et al. 2010; Tullis et al. 2011). Research on these two measures would be considered highly desirable and even warranted.

References

Banda, D. R., Dogoe, M. S., & Matuszny, R. M. (2011). Review of video prompting studies with persons with developmental disabilities. *Education and Training in Autism and Developmental Disabilities, 46*, 514–527.

Bauer, S. M., Elsaesser, L.-J., & Arthanat, S. (2011). Assistive technology device classification based upon the World Health Organization's, International Classification of Functioning, Disability and Health (ICF). *Disability and Rehabilitation: Assistive Technology, 6*, 243–259.

Belva, B. C., & Matson, J. L. (2013). An examination of specific daily living skills deficits in adults with profound intellectual disabilities. *Research in Developmental Disabilities, 34*, 596–604.

Borg, J., Larson, S., & Östegren, P. O. (2011). The right to assistive technology: For whom, for what, and by whom? *Disability and Society, 26*, 151–167.

Brown, R. I., Schalock, R. L., & Brown, I. (2009). Quality of life: Its application to persons with intellectual disabilities and their families—Introduction and overview. *Journal of Policy and Practice in Intellectual Disabilities, 6*, 2–6.

Burne, B., Knafelc, V., Melonis, M., & Heyn, P. C. (2011). The use and application of assistive technology to promote literacy in early childhood: A systematic review. *Disability and Rehabilitation: Assistive Technology, 6*, 207–213.

Callahan, K., Henson, R., & Cowan, A. K. (2008). Social validation of evidence-based practices in autism by parents, teachers, and administrators. *Journal of Autism and Developmental Disorders, 38*, 678–692.

Catania, A. C. (2012). *Learning* (5th ed.). New York: Sloan.

Dillon, C. M., & Carr, J. E. (2007). Assessing indices of happiness and unhappiness in individuals with developmental disabilities: A review. *Behavioral Interventions, 22*, 229–244.

Furniss, F., Lancioni, G., Rocha, N., Cunha, B., Seedhouse, P., Morato, P., et al. (2001). VICAID: Development and evaluation of a palmtop-based job aid for workers with severe developmental disabilities. *British Journal of Educational Technology, 32*, 277–287.

Gevarter, C., O'Reilly, M. F., Rojeski, L., Sammarco, N., Lang, R., Lancioni, G. E., et al. (2013a). Comparing communication systems for individuals with developmental disabilities: A review of single-case research studies. *Research in Developmental Disabilities, 34*, 4415–4432.

Gevarter, C., O'Reilly, M. F., Rojeski, L., Sammarco, N., Lang, R., Lancioni, G. E., et al. (2013b). Comparisons of intervention components with augmentative and alternative communication systems for individuals with developmental disabilities: A review of the literature. *Research in Developmental Disabilities, 34*, 4404–4414.

Gutowski, S. J. (1996). Response acquisition for music or beverages in adults with profound multiple handicaps. *Journal of Developmental and Physical Disabilities, 8*, 221–231.

Hayakawa, K., & Kobayashi, K. (2011). Physical and motor skill training for children with intellectual disabilities. *Perceptual and Motor Skills, 112*, 573–580.

Holburn, S., Nguyen, D., & Vietze, P. M. (2004). Computer-assisted learning for adults with profound multiple disabilities. *Behavioral Interventions, 19*, 25–37.

Kagohara, D. M., Van der Meer, L., Ramdoss, S., O'Reilly, M. F., Lancioni, G. E., Davis, T. N., et al. (2013). Using iPods® and iPads® in teaching programs for individuals with developmental disabilities: A systematic review. *Research in Developmental Disabilities, 34*, 147–156.

Kazdin, A. E. (2001). *Behavior modification in applied settings* (6th ed.). New York: Wadsworth.

Lancioni, G. E., Bellini, D., Oliva, D., Singh, N. N., O'Reilly, M. F., Lang, R., et al. (2011a). Camera-based microswitch technology to monitor mouth, eyebrow, and eyelid responses of children with profound multiple disabilities. *Journal of Behavioral Education, 20*, 4–14.

Lancioni, G. E., Bellini, D., Oliva, D., Singh, N. N., O'Reilly, M. F., Lang, R., et al. (2011b). Persons with multiple disabilities select environmental stimuli through a smile response monitored via camera-based technology. *Developmental Neurorehabilitation, 14*, 267–273.

Lancioni, G. E., Bellini, D., Oliva, D., Singh, N. N., O'Reilly, M. F., & Sigafoos, J. (2010a). Camera-based microswitch technology for eyelid and mouth responses of persons with profound multiple disabilities: Two case studies. *Research in Developmental Disabilities, 31*, 1509–1514.

Lancioni, G. E., O'Reilly, M. F., Singh, N. N., Oliva, D., Baccani, S., Severini, L., et al. (2006a). Micro-switch programmes for students with multiple disabilities and minimal motor behaviour: Assessing response acquisition and choice. *Pediatric Rehabilitation, 9*, 137–143.

Lancioni, G. E., O'Reilly, M. F., Singh, N. N., Sigafoos, J., Didden, R., Oliva, D., et al. (2009a). Persons with multiple disabilities accessing stimulation and requesting social contact via microswitch and VOCA devices: New research evaluation and social validation. *Research in Developmental Disabilities, 30*, 1084–1094.

Lancioni, G. E., O'Reilly, M. F., Singh, N. N., Sigafoos, J., Didden, R., Oliva, D., et al. (2007a). Persons with multiple disabilities and minimal motor behavior using small forehead movements and new microswitch technology to control environmental stimuli. *Perceptual and Motor Skills, 104*, 870–878.

Lancioni, G. E., O'Reilly, M. F., Singh, N. N., Sigafoos, J., Didden, R., Smaldone, A., et al. (2008a). Helping a man with multiple disabilities increase object-contact responses and reduce hand stereotypy via a microswitch cluster program. *Journal of Intellectual and Developmental Disability, 33*, 349–353.

Lancioni, G. E., O'Reilly, M. F., Singh, N. N., Sigafoos, J., Oliva, D., Alberti, G., et al. (2013a). Technology-based programs to support adaptive responding and reduce hand mouthing in two persons with multiple disabilities. *Journal of Developmental and Physical Disabilities, 25*, 65–77.

Lancioni, G. E., O'Reilly, M. F., Singh, N. N., Sigafoos, J., Oliva, D., & Severini, L. (2006b). Enabling persons with multiple disabilities to choose among environmental stimuli and request stimulus repetitions through microswitch and computer technology. *Perceptual and Motor Skills, 103*, 354–362.

Lancioni, G. E., O'Reilly, M. F., Singh, N. N., Sigafoos, J., Oliva, D., & Severini, L. (2008b). Enabling two persons with multiple disabilities to access environmental stimuli and ask for social contact through microswitches and a VOCA. *Research in Developmental Disabilities, 29*, 21–28.

Lancioni, G. E., O'Reilly, M. F., Singh, N. N., Sigafoos, J., Oliva, D., & Severini, L. (2008c). Three persons with multiple disabilities accessing environmental stimuli and asking for social contact through microswitch and VOCA technology. *Journal of Intellectual Disability Research, 52*, 327–336.

Lancioni, G. E., O'Reilly, M. F., Singh, N. N., Sigafoos, J., Oliva, D., Smaldone, A., et al. (2009b). Persons with multiple disabilities access stimulation and contact the caregiver via microswitch and VOCA technology. *Life Span and Disability, 12*, 119–128.

Lancioni, G. E., Sigafoos, J., O'Reilly, M. F., & Singh, N. N. (2013b). *Assistive technology: Interventions for individuals with severe/profound and multiple disabilities*. New York: Springer.

Lancioni, G. E., Singh, N. N., O'Reilly, M. F., Green, V. A., Oliva, D., & Campodonico, F. (2013c). Two men with multiple disabilities carry out an assembly work activity with the support of a technology system. *Developmental Neurorehabilitation, 16*, 332–339.

Lancioni, G. E., Singh, N. N., O'Reilly, M. F., Oliva, D., & Basili, G. (2005). An overview of research on increasing indices of happiness of people with severe/profound intellectual and multiple disabilities. *Disability and Rehabilitation, 27*, 83–93.

Lancioni, G. E., Singh, N. N., O'Reilly, M. F., & Sigafoos, J. (2009c). An overview of behavioral strategies for reducing hand-related stereotypies of persons with severe to profound intellectual and multiple disabilities. *Research in Developmental Disabilities, 30*, 20–43.

Lancioni, G. E., Singh, N. N., O'Reilly, M. F., Sigafoos, J., Alberti, G., Bellini, D., et al. (2013d). Persons with multiple disabilities use forehead and smile responses to access or choose among technology-aided stimulation events. *Research in Developmental Disabilities, 34*, 1749–1757.

Lancioni, G. E., Singh, N. N., O'Reilly, M. F., Sigafoos, J., Alberti, G., Oliva, D., et al. (2011c). A technology-aided stimulus choice program for two adults with multiple disabilities: Choice responses and mood. *Research in Developmental Disabilities, 32*, 2602–2607.

Lancioni, G. E., Singh, N. N., O'Reilly, M. F., Sigafoos, J., Alberti, G., Perilli, V., et al. (2014a). People with multiple disabilities learn to engage in occupation and work activities with the support of technology-aided programs. *Research in Developmental Disabilities, 35*, 1264–1271.

Lancioni, G. E., Singh, N. N., O'Reilly, M. F., Sigafoos, J., Alberti, G., Perilli, V., et al. (2014b). Microswitch-aided programs to support physical exercise or adequate ambulation in persons with multiple disabilities. *Research in Developmental Disabilities, 35*, 2190–2198.

Lancioni, G. E., Singh, N. N., O'Reilly, M. F., Sigafoos, J., Alberti, G., Scigliuzzo, F., et al. (2010b). Persons with multiple disabilities use orientation technology to find room entrances during indoor traveling. *Research in Developmental Disabilities, 31*, 1577–1584.

Lancioni, G. E., Singh, N. N., O'Reilly, M. F., Sigafoos, J., Boccasini, A., La Martire, M. L., et al. (2014c). Microswitch-aided programs for a woman with Rett syndrome and a boy with extensive neuro-motor and intellectual disabilities. *Journal of Developmental and Physical Disabilities, 26*, 135–143.

Lancioni, G. E., Singh, N. N., O'Reilly, M. F., Sigafoos, J., Didden, R., Manfredi, F., et al. (2009d). Fostering locomotor behavior of children with developmental disabilities: An overview of studies using treadmills and walkers with microswitches. *Research in Developmental Disabilities, 30*, 308–322.

Lancioni, G. E., Singh, N. N., O'Reilly, M. F., Sigafoos, J., Didden, R., Oliva, D., et al. (2007b). Effects of microswitch-based programs on indices of happiness of students with multiple disabilities: A new research evaluation. *American Journal on Mental Retardation, 112*, 167–176.

Lancioni, G. E., Singh, N. N., O'Reilly, M. F., Sigafoos, J., & Oliva, D. (2014d). Assistive technology for people with severe/profound intellectual and multiple disabilities. In G. E. Lancioni & N. N. Singh (Eds.), *Assistive technology for people with diverse abilities* (pp. 277–313). New York: Springer.

Lancioni, G. E., Singh, N. N., O'Reilly, M. F., Sigafoos, J., & Oliva, D. (2014e). Intervention programs based on microswitch technology for persons with multiple disabilities: An overview. *Current Developmental Disorders Reports, 1*, 67–73.

Lancioni, G. E., Singh, N. N., O'Reilly, M. F., Sigafoos, J., Oliva, D., Boccasini, A., et al. (2013e). Persons with multiple disabilities increase adaptive responding and control inadequate posture or behavior through programs based on microswitch-cluster technology. *Research in Developmental Disabilities, 34*, 3411–3420.

Lancioni, G. E., Singh, N. N., O'Reilly, M. F., Sigafoos, J., Oliva, D., Campodonico, F., et al. (2013f). Walker devices and microswitch technology to enhance assisted indoor ambulation by persons with multiple disabilities: Three single-case studies. *Research in Developmental Disabilities, 34*, 2191–2199.

Lancioni, G. E., Singh, N. N., O'Reilly, M. F., Sigafoos, J., Oliva, D., & D'Amico, (2013g). Technology-aided programs to enable persons with multiple disabilities to choose among environmental stimuli using a smile or a tongue response. *Research in Developmental Disabilities, 34*, 4232–4238.

Lancioni, G. E., Singh, N. N., O'Reilly, M. F., Sigafoos, J., Oliva, D., Gatti, M., et al. (2008d). A microswitch-cluster program to foster adaptive responses and head control in students with multiple disabilities: Replication and validation assessment. *Research in Developmental Disabilities, 29*, 373–384.

Lancioni, G. E., Singh, N. N., O'Reilly, M. F., Sigafoos, J., Oliva, D., Severini, L., et al. (2007c). Microswitch technology to promote adaptive responses and reduce mouthing in two children with multiple disabilities. *Journal of Visual Impairment and Blindness, 101*, 628–636.

Lancioni, G. E., Singh, N. N., O'Reilly, M. F., Sigafoos, J., Oliva, D., Smaldone, A., et al. (2011d). A verbal-instruction system to help persons with multiple disabilities perform complex food- and drink-preparation tasks independently. *Research in Developmental Disabilities, 32*, 2739–2747.

Lancioni, G. E., Singh, N. N., O'Reilly, M. F., Sigafoos, J., Oliva, D., Smaldone, A., et al. (2010c). Promoting ambulation responses among children with multiple disabilities through walkers and microswitches with contingent stimuli. *Research in Developmental Disabilities, 31*, 811–816.

Lancioni, G. E., Singh, N. N., O'Reilly, M. F., Sigafoos, J., Ricci, I., Addante, L. M., et al. (2011e). A woman with multiple disabilities uses a VOCA system to request for and access caregiver-mediated stimulation events. *Life Span and Disability, 14*, 91–99.

Leung, B., & Chau, T. (2010). A multiple camera tongue switch for a child with severe spastic quadriplegic cerebral palsy. *Disability and Rehabilitation: Assistive Technology, 5*, 58–68.

Lui, M., Falk, T. H., & Chau, T. (2012). Development and evaluation of a dual-output vocal cord vibration switch for persons with multiple disabilities. *Disability and Rehabilitation: Assistive Technology, 7*, 82–88.

Luiselli, J. K., Bass, J. D., & Whitcomb, S. A. (2010). Teaching applied behavior analysis knowledge competencies to direct-care service providers: Outcome assessment and social validation of a training program. *Behavior Modification, 34*, 403–414.

Martinsen, H., Tellevik, J. M., Elmerskog, B., & Storliløkken, M. (2007). Mental effort in mobility route learning. *Journal of Visual Impairment and Blindness, 101*, 327–338.

Mechling, L. C. (2006). Comparison of the effects of three approaches on the frequency of stimulus activation, via a single switch, by students with profound intellectual disabilities. *The Journal of Special Education, 40*, 94–102.

Mechling, L. C., & Gustafson, M. (2009). Comparison of the effects of static picture and video prompting on completion of cooking related tasks by students with moderate intellectual disabilities. *Exceptionality, 17*, 103–116.

Moisey, S. D. (2007). The inclusive Libraries initiative: Enhancing the access of persons with developmental disabilities to information and communication technology. *Developmental Disabilities Bulletin, 35*, 56–71.

Moisey, S., & van de Keere, R. (2007). Inclusion and the internet: Teaching adults with developmental disabilities to use information and communication technology. *Developmental Disabilities Bulletin, 35*, 72–102.

Petry, K., Maes, B., & Vlaskamp, C. (2005). Domains of quality of life of people with profound multiple disabilities: The perspective of parents and direct support staff. *Journal of Applied Research in Intellectual Disabilities, 18*, 35–46.

Petry, K., Maes, B., & Vlaskamp, C. (2009). Measuring the quality of life of people with profound multiple disabilities using the QOL-PMD: First results. *Research in Developmental Disabilities, 30*, 1394–1405.

Reichle, J. (2011). Evaluating assistive technology in the education of persons with severe disabilities. *Journal of Behavioral Education, 20*, 77–85.

Ripat, J., & Woodgate, R. (2011). The intersection of culture, disability and assistive technology. *Disability and Rehabilitation: Assistive Technology, 6*, 87–96.

Rispoli, M. J., Franco, J. H., van der Meer, L., Lang, R., & Camargo, S. P. H. (2010). The use of speech generating devices in communication interventions for individuals with developmental disabilities: A review of the literature. *Developmental Neurorehabilitation, 13*, 276–293.

Ross, D. A., & Kelly, G. W. (2009). Filling the gaps for indoor wayfinding. *Journal of Visual Impairment and Blindness, 103*, 229–234.

Saunders, M. D., Smagner, J. P., & Saunders, R. R. (2003). Improving methodological and technological analyses of adaptive switch use of individuals with profound multiple impairments. *Behavioral Interventions, 18*, 227–243.

Scherer, M. J., Craddock, G., & Mackeogh, T. (2011). The relationship of personal factors and subjective well-being to the use of assistive technology devices. *Disability and Rehabilitation, 33*, 811–817.

Shih, C.-H. (2011). Assisting people with developmental disabilities to improve computer pointing efficiency through multiple mice and automatic pointing assistive programs. *Research in Developmental Disabilities, 32*, 1736–1744.

Sigafoos, J., Lancioni, G. E., O'Reilly, M. F., Achmadi, D., Stevens, M., Roche, L., et al. (2013). Teaching two boys with autism spectrum disorders to request the continuation of toy play using an iPad®-based speech-generating device. *Research in Autism Spectrum Disorders, 7*, 923–930.

Sigafoos, J., O'Reilly, M., Lancioni, G. E., & Sutherland, D. (2014a). Augmentative and alternative communication for individuals with autism spectrum disorder and intellectual disability. *Current Developmental Disorders Reports, 1*, 51–57.

Sigafoos, J., Schlosser, R. W., Lancioni, G. E., O'Reilly, M. F., Green, V. A., & Singh, N. N. (2014b). In G. E. Lancioni & N. N. Singh (Eds.), *Assistive technology for people with diverse abilities* (pp. 77–112). New York: Springer.

Sullivan, M. W., Laverick, D. H., & Lewis, M. (1995). Fostering environmental control in a young child with Rett syndrome: A case study. *Journal of Autism and Developmental Disorders, 25*, 215–221.

Szymanski, L. S. (2000). Happiness as a treatment goal. *American Journal on Mental Retardation, 105*, 352–362.

Tam, G. M., Phillips, K. J., & Mudford, O. C. (2011). Teaching individuals with profound multiple disabilities to access preferred stimuli with multiple microswitches. *Research in Developmental Disabilities, 32*, 2352–2361.

Thunberg, G., Ahlsén, E., & Sandberg, A. D. (2007). Children with autistic spectrum disorders and speech-generating devices: Communication in different activities at home. *Clinical Linguistics and Phonetics, 21*, 457–479.

Tullis, C. A., Cannella-Malone, H. I., Basbigill, A. R., Yeager, A., Fleming, C. V., Payne, D., et al. (2011). Review of the choice and preference assessment literature for individuals with severe to profound disabilities. *Education and Training in Autism and Developmental Disabilities, 46*, 576–595.

Van der Meer, L., Kagohara, D., Achmadi, D., O'Reilly, M. F., Lancioni, G. E., Sutherland, D., et al. (2012a). Speech-generating devices versus manual signing for children with developmental disabilities. *Research in Developmental Disabilities, 33*, 1658–1669.

Van der Meer, L., Sutherland, D., O'Reilly, M. F., Lancioni, G. E., & Sigafoos, J. (2012b). A further comparison of manual signing, picture exchange, and speech-generating devices as communication modes for children with autism spectrum disorders. *Research in Autism Spectrum Disorders, 6*, 1247–1257.

Zucker, S. H., Perras, C., Perner, D. E., & Murdick, N. (2013). Best practices for practitioners in autism, intellectual disability, and developmental disabilities. *Education and Training in Autism and Developmental Disabilities, 48*, 439–442.

Chapter 6
Body-Focused Repetitive Behaviors

Raymond G. Miltenberger and Claire A. Spieler

Body-focused repetitive behaviors, including skin picking, skin biting, nail biting, hair pulling, mouth chewing, thumb and finger sucking, and lip biting, are behaviors that involve repetitive movements centered around the body (Teng et al. 2002). These behaviors have the potential to be health and life threatening, producing consequences such as infection, scarring, and other tissue damage (Woods et al. 2001). Skin picking may cause infections that require treatment by antibiotics and tissue damage that requires skin grafts (Odlaug and Grant 2008). Hair pulling may result in serious health complications including hair follicle damage, carpal tunnel syndrome, and even gastrointestinal and dental problems when the hair is pulled and subsequently consumed (Rapp et al. 2000a, b; Woods et al. 2006). Dental problems can also result from body-focused repetitive behaviors such as nail biting, thumb sucking, mouth chewing, and lip biting (Snorrason and Woods 2014; Teng et al. 2002). Not only can body-focused repetitive behaviors produce physical harm, but they also correlate with social distress, stigmatizing perceptions, and lower levels of self-esteem (Joubert 1993; Long et al. 1998; Snorrason and Woods 2014). Body-focused repetitive behaviors occur in people who are typically-developing and people with intellectual and developmental disabilities (IDD) (Lang et al. 2009). Some studies indicate that there is a higher prevalence among people with intellectual disabilities (Didden et al. 2007; Lang et al. 2009; Long et al. 1998).

One of the most effective treatments for decreasing and eliminating body-focused repetitive behaviors in a typical population is habit reversal (Miltenberger et al. 1998a, b; Woods and Miltenberger 1995). Habit reversal was developed as a treatment package for nervous habits and tics (Azrin and Nunn 1973). The original

R.G. Miltenberger (✉) · C.A. Spieler
University of South Florida, Tampa, FL, USA
e-mail: miltenbe@usf.edu

J.K. Luiselli (ed.), *Behavioral Health Promotion and Intervention in Intellectual and Developmental Disabilities*, Evidence-Based Practices in Behavioral Health,
DOI 10.1007/978-3-319-27297-9_6

procedures included awareness training, competing response practice, habit control motivation, and generalization training (Azrin and Nunn 1973). Awareness training for nervous habits involves response description in which the client describes and discusses the unique topography of the habit behavior with the therapist. The next step, response detection, involves practice recognizing when the behavior occurs until the client reliably detects each occurrence. An early warning procedure may also be used which requires the client to practice recognizing the earliest movements of the behavior. The client may also be exposed to situation awareness training in which he or she recalls common situations in which the behavior typically occurs. Competing response practice begins with the identification and selection of a response that is incompatible with (competes with) the habit behavior. The client then practices the competing response and engages in the competing response for a few minutes contingent on the occurrence of the habit behavior. Once the competing response is practiced contingent on the behavior or anticipation of the behavior in treatment sessions, the client is instructed to use the competing response to control the habit behavior outside of the treatment sessions. Habit control motivation typically includes a habit inconvenience review and social support. Habit inconvenience review highlights how the client's habit has inconvenienced the client or impaired his or her functioning and well-being. In social support, family or friends of the client are encouraged to prompt the use of the competing response, praise the client's use of the competing response, and praise the client's improved appearance or lifestyle as a result of using the competing response. Finally, generalization training is incorporated into the habit reversal procedure to ensure that treatment effects will be demonstrated in the client's natural environment.

Although the multi-component habit reversal procedure was shown to be effective in a number of early studies (Azrin et al. 1980a, b, 1982), researchers subsequently evaluated more simplified forms of the procedure (Miltenberger et al. 1998a, b). Simplified habit reversal, consisting of awareness training and competing response training, has successfully decreased and eliminated several habit behaviors in children and adults (Azrin and Peterson 1989; Miltenberger and Fuqua 1985; Miltenberger et al. 1985; Ollendick 1981; Woods and Miltenberger 1995). However, research suggests that habit reversal or simplified habit reversal (hereafter just called habit reversal) may be an ineffective treatment for people with IDD (Miltenberger et al. 1998a, b) because some of the components of habit reversal may require a higher level of functioning or motivation to be successfully completed. In particular, the competing response component is a self-management procedure that must be implemented contingent on the habit behavior across the client's day without direct intervention by staff or parents. In addition, the success of the competing response component is predicated on the success of awareness training and the client's motivation to decrease the habit behavior. Although habit reversal may be ineffective for persons with IDD due to limited skills or motivation, habit reversal may be an effective intervention for people with IDD if it is modified or supplemented with additional procedures (Cavalari et al. 2013; Conlea and Klein-Tasman 2013). Efforts to implement habit reversal procedures with individuals with intellectual disabilities typically require supplemental intervention components such as prompting, differential reinforcement, and response cost (Cavalari et al. 2013; Long et al. 1999; Miltenberger et al. 1998a, b). In addition, given the limited success of habit reversal, other behavioral interventions have been evaluated for habit behaviors exhibited by individuals with intellectual disabilities. This chapter will highlight research findings on interventions for treating body-focused repetitive behaviors and recommend best practices for clinical treatment with people with intellectual disabilities.

Function of Body-Focused Repetitive Behaviors

Identifying the function of problem behavior is important and often necessary for deciding on best treatment practices. Functional treatments, those that address the antecedents and consequences maintaining the problem behavior, are typically the most successful in achieving desired behavioral outcomes. Furthermore, they are comprised of positive practices rather than aversive procedures (e.g., Kurtz et al. 2003; Neef and Iwata 1994; Pelios et al. 1999). Rapp et al. (2000a, b) suggest that identifying the conditions under which habit behaviors are likely to occur contributes to development or selection of an intervention most likely to be effective, particularly with individuals with IDD whom may not respond to interventions (habit reversal) used with a typically developing population. Studies that have conducted functional analyses for various habit behaviors have determined that the function is commonly automatic reinforcement (Cowdery et al. 1990; Deaver et al. 2001; Ellingson et al. 2000; Miltenberger et al. 1998a, b; Rapp et al. 1999, 2000a, b; Roscoe et al. 2013). The majority of studies evaluating treatments for body-focused repetitive behaviors that do not conduct a functional analysis rely on the assumption that the behavior is automatically reinforced from the outcome of other functional assessment strategies (e.g., Lang et al. 2009; Radstaake et al. 2011; Rapp et al. 2000a, b). When a behavior is automatically reinforced, it produces a reinforcing consequence directly (not mediated by other individuals) that strengthens and maintains that behavior (Miltenberger 2016). Behaviors maintained by automatic reinforcement tend to be more difficult to treat because you cannot directly modify the contingencies maintaining the behavior and the reinforcement for engaging in the behavior is constantly available because it results directly from the behavior rather than the actions of others (Piazza et al. 2000). Interventions for automatically reinforced behaviors may involve sensory extinction, achieved by masking the stimulation produced by the behavior, or matching the stimulation produced by the behavior with a more appropriate reinforcer delivered in a noncontingent reinforcement or differential reinforcement procedure (Miltenberger 2016).

Some studies evaluating the effects of particular interventions on body-focused repetitive behaviors suggest that, with the availability of strong reinforcement, addressing the automatic reinforcement function of the behavior may not be necessary. For example, Cowdery et al. (1990) evaluated the effects of a token economy combined with a differential reinforcement of other behavior (DRO) schedule on the self-injurious skin-picking behavior of a 9-year-old boy. Although the subject, Jerry, was not diagnosed with an intellectual disability, he was determined to have low-normal range intelligence and was frequently hospitalized due to the extent of his skin picking and severity of resulting tissue damage. After determining Jerry's skin-picking to be maintained by automatic reinforcement, a DRO and token reinforcement system was implemented due to the impracticality of implementing interventions involving sensory extinction or matched stimulation for the severe behavior. Jerry earned one penny contingent on each interval in which he did not engage in skin picking while alone in a room with no play activities or tangibles available. Additionally, after the reversal phase, if Jerry earned all five available pennies in a session, he also earned a bonus nickel. Coins were exchanged for reinforcing activities or items following the conclusion of each session. The DRO intervals were gradually increased from 2 min to 30 min throughout the study. Results indicated that DRO and token reinforcement decreased Jerry's skin picking to zero or near zero levels across increasing session durations. This study suggests the potential effectiveness of differential reinforcement as an intervention for body-focused repetitive behaviors using reinforcement that is not functionally related to the behavior of concern.

Despite the finding that interventions for body-focused repetitive behaviors may be effective even if they do not address the antecedents and consequences maintaining the behavior, it is nonetheless prudent to conduct a functional assessment before deciding on intervention. A functional assessment will identify or rule out social reinforcement for the behavior. If the behavior is shown to be maintained by social reinforcement, interventions addressing the social contingencies maintaining the behavior would be warranted. If the behavior is not maintained by social reinforcement, functional analysis procedures to identify the nature of the stimulation reinforcing the behavior would be warranted. Functional interventions might then involve masking the stimulation maintaining the behavior (sensory extinction) or providing matched stimulation noncontingently or as a reinforcer for alternative behavior (e.g., Rapp et al. 1999, 2000a, b).

Research Findings

A variety of interventions have been evaluated for body-focused repetitive behaviors exhibited by individuals with disabilities. These interventions include differential reinforcement (with and without response cost), response interruption, redirection, and prevention, punishment, and an awareness enhancement device.

Differential Reinforcement

Differential reinforcement involves providing a reinforcer for a desirable behavior or for the absence of the problem behavior while withholding reinforcement for the problem behaviors (Miltenberger 2016). Interventions utilizing differential reinforcement may be effective in decreasing health-threatening habit behaviors for people with intellectual disabilities when used alone or combined with habit reversal. Long et al. (1999) evaluated the effects of habit reversal and habit reversal combined with other interventions on the oral-digital habit behaviors (i.e., nail-biting, finger sucking) of four individuals with intellectual disabilities. The other interventions included remote prompting, differential reinforcement of nail growth, and differential reinforcement of zero responding (DRO) or differential reinforcement of alternative behaviors (DRA) with response cost. Remote prompting involved the investigator observing the participant through a one-way mirror and verbally prompting the participant through an intercom system to engage in a competing response when the participant was observed to be engaging in his target behavior. Differential reinforcement of nail growth involved distribution of $5 contingent upon healthy fingernail conditions and uniform nail growth or maintenance of length. In the DRA/DRO and response cost procedure, the participants were instructed not to engage in their target behaviors while the investigator left the room. At the end of a 30-s interval, the investigator delivered one dime or piece of candy if the participants did not engage in the target behavior (as observed through an observation window) and three dimes or pieces of candy if the participants were executing a competing response when the experimenter re-entered the room. Whenever a participant engaged in a target behavior, the investigator entered the room, prompted the competing response, removed a dime or piece of candy, and reset the interval timer. The interval was increased by 60 s following the delivery of each reinforcer.

Habit reversal consisted of awareness training, competing response training, and social support. Modifications were made to enhance the effectiveness of habit reversal for the participants. In one modification, awareness training was supplemented with a game in which the participants indicated when the experimenters engaged in approximations of their target behaviors. In another modification, the experimenters pushed against the participants' arms while they approximated their target behaviors to enhance their awareness of the movements. Despite these procedural modifications, results indicated that habit reversal combined with additional contingencies was more effective than habit reversal alone for all participants. Long et al. (1999) offer a couple explanations for the ineffectiveness of habit reversal. First, a lack of reinforcement in the participants' natural environments to maintain their use of the competing responses may have accounted for the failure. Second, the individuals may have been insensitive to social stigma or other negative consequences that may have occurred contingent on their habit behaviors. These potential factors are important to consider when selecting a treatment for body-focused repetitive behaviors exhibited by individuals with intellectual disabilities.

Other studies support the use of differential reinforcement (DRA and DRO) for the reduction of body-focused repetitive behaviors (e.g., Cavalari et al. 2013; Cowdery et al. 1990; Lang et al. 2009; Radstaake et al. 2011; Rapp et al. 2000a, b; Roscoe et al. 2013). In treating body-focused repetitive behaviors, DRA may involve the manipulation of a small toy or other tangible item that is available non-contingently (Cavalari et al. 2013; Radstaake et al. 2011). Cavalari et al. (2013) employed a token economy with an adolescent diagnosed with autism who engaged in self-injurious skin picking on her hands and arms. The token economy consisted of red and blue tokens that could be redeemed for preferred leisure activities. The participant received a red token contingent upon each 15-min interval in which she did not engage in skin picking and independently manipulated fidget toys that were available non-contingently at her desk in her classroom. She earned a blue token following each 15-min interval in which she engaged in skin picking and manipulated the fidget toys immediately following prompting from staff. The authors referred to the use of fidget toys as a competing response because it was an incompatible behavior to skin picking. In a treatment fading phase, the interval for token reinforcement was increased to 30 min, the fidget toys were removed, and the staff provided praise for "calm hands" when the participant was not engaging in skin picking and ignored instances of skin picking. Fewer instances of skin picking were observed during this intervention and the results maintained during treatment fading and months following the intervention as reported by staff.

Radstaake et al. (2011) also utilized differential reinforcement with an adolescent with Prader-Willi syndrome and mild to moderate intellectual disability who engaged in skin picking. She was exposed to two alternative behaviors to skin picking which the authors refer to as differential reinforcement of incompatible behavior (DRI) and DRA. The DRI behaviors were squeezing a small toy with both hands and completing a puzzle. The DRA behavior was requesting lotion to apply to her skin. Caregivers prompted the incompatible and/or alternative behavior contingent upon occurrences of skin picking, situations in which skin picking had previously been observed, and when the participant reported feeling compelled to pick her skin. Meetings with the authors were also arranged throughout the study to rehearse the alternative behaviors and evaluate the condition of her wounds caused by skin picking. Additional praise and small tangible reinforcers were available for attending meetings and more preferred reinforcers were available for noticeable healing of wounds and absence of new wounds. To establish the effectiveness of the procedure, outside observers categorized pictures of the participant's skin from the beginning to the end of the study into a correct timeline (i.e., before treatment, after treatment). Results indicated that the differential reinforcement treatment successfully reduced skin picking and increased healing of wounds.

For body-focused repetitive behaviors that involve one's hands and fingers, such as skin picking, hair pulling, or hand mouthing, manipulating a toy or item with both hands is not only a behavior that is an alternative to the habit, but also a behavior that is incompatible with the habit. In one case, Ladd et al. (2009) reduced self-injurious skin picking in a young girl with autism using only noncontingent access to toys during times in which skin picking was likely to occur. The authors attribute the behavioral reduction to the alternative source of sensory stimulation provided by the toys or to the incompatibility between skin picking and manipulating the toys. Similarly, Realon et al. (1995) reduced self-injurious hand mouthing in an adolescent with a profound intellectual disability simply by providing access to preferred leisure items.

Interventions using differential reinforcement typically require implementation by others who monitor the target behavior and provide the reinforcer contingent on an alternative behavior or on the absence of the problem behavior. However, Tiger et al. (2009) demonstrated maintenance of treatment effects with an individual diagnosed with Asperger syndrome who engaged in self-monitoring of DRO contingencies for his severe skin picking. After a therapist-monitored DRO intervention reduced skin picking to 0 % of intervals, the participant maintained the behavioral reduction by successfully monitoring session intervals, identifying occurrences and nonoccurrences of skin picking, and delivering reinforcement according to his token economy. The results of this study indicate the potential for self-monitoring and differential reinforcement to be used by people with intellectual disabilities who engage in body-focused repetitive behaviors. However, the self-managed intervention was used with one individual with Asperger syndrome, so more research is needed to establish the generality of this type of intervention for individuals with varying types and levels of disabilities.

The success of differential reinforcement suggests that it may be an effective and acceptable treatment for reducing body-focused repetitive behaviors in individuals with intellectual disabilities. Differential reinforcement presents opportunities to use a positive approach to reduce these potentially health-threatening behaviors. If not employed as a stand-alone procedure, differential reinforcement should be a component of any other intervention for body-focused repetitive behaviors in individuals with disabilities.

Response Interruption, Redirection, and Prevention

Response interruption, redirection, and prevention have been used to decrease several types of behaviors including body-focused repetitive behaviors in people with IDD (Lydon et al. 2013). Response interruption and redirection are commonly used to treat stereotypies maintained by automatic reinforcement, but these procedures may also be useful for treating body-focused repetitive behaviors that are maintained by automatic reinforcement. Response interruption involves stopping a response someone is engaging in by physically blocking it with a body part (e.g., the hands) and response redirection involves physically prompting an alternative response (Lydon et al. 2013). Response prevention involves preventing a behavior before it occurs through physical restraint or physical barriers (Van Houton and Rolider 1984). In the case of body-focused repetitive behaviors, response prevention typically involves the application of some device, equipment, or garment as a physical barrier to the body part used to engage in the behavior (e.g., Deaver et al. 2001; Maguire et al. 1995). For example, Deaver et al. (2001) used response prevention when they placed thin cotton mittens on a preschool child's hands to prevent her from engaging in hair pulling during nap times. After first conducting a functional analysis and ruling out social reinforcement for the behavior, Deaver et al. implemented the response prevention intervention at home and at daycare (see Fig. 6.1). The use of mittens eliminated hair twirling (the precursor to hair pulling) each time it was implemented at nap time in the preschool and bedtime in the home. In another example, Rapp et al. (2000a, b) used a hand splint to prevent hair pulling by an adolescent with intellectual disability in the evening when she was in bed. Although response interruption and DRO implemented by the mother were effective during the day, because the mother was not able to implement the procedure while the client was in bed, the response prevention procedure was used. This example illustrates the use of response prevention as an adjunct to other behavioral intervention procedures that is used only when the caregiver cannot implement the other procedure during specified time periods. More intrusive response prevention interventions have also been used for severe behaviors, such as shaving an individual's head to prevent hair pulling (Barrett and Shapiro 1980).

Response prevention might function by eliminating or attenuating the sensory stimulation that comes from certain body-focused repetitive behaviors and, therefore, may be a functional intervention if the behaviors are in fact maintained by automatic reinforcement. For example, Rapp et al. (1999) showed that a latex glove placed on the hand of a young woman who pulled her hair decreased hair pulling and hair manipulation maintained by sensory stimulation. In this case, the latex glove masked the sensory stimulation produced by hair manipulation and thus functioned as sensory extinction. As seen in Fig. 6.2, wearing the latex glove eliminated hair pulling (top panel) and hair manipulation (bottom panel). Although response prevention, interruption, and redirection may address the automatic reinforcement function of some body-focused repetitive behaviors, these procedures might also result in behavior reduction through a punishment process. In one study examining chronic trichotillomania in a woman with a profound intellectual disability, the authors used response interruption (referred to by the authors as response correction), which involved a therapist holding the woman's hands by her side or in her lap for 5 s contingent on occurrences of hair pulling or manipulation (Maguire et al. 1995). This procedure is similar to those used in other studies with body-focused repetitive behaviors such as self-injurious hand-mouthing (Rapp et al. 2000a, b; Turner et al. 1996). Although the response interruption procedure decreased the behavior, Maguire et al. (1995), showed that an intervention using response prevention, placing mitts on the woman's hands contingent on occurrences of the target behaviors, was more successful than the response interruption procedure.

In the literature, response interruption, redirection, or prevention have typically been combined with other procedures such as differential reinforcement (e.g., McEntee et al. 1996; Rapp et al. 2000a, b). Rapp et al. (2000a, b) implemented response interruption (RI) and differential reinforcement (DRO) for a

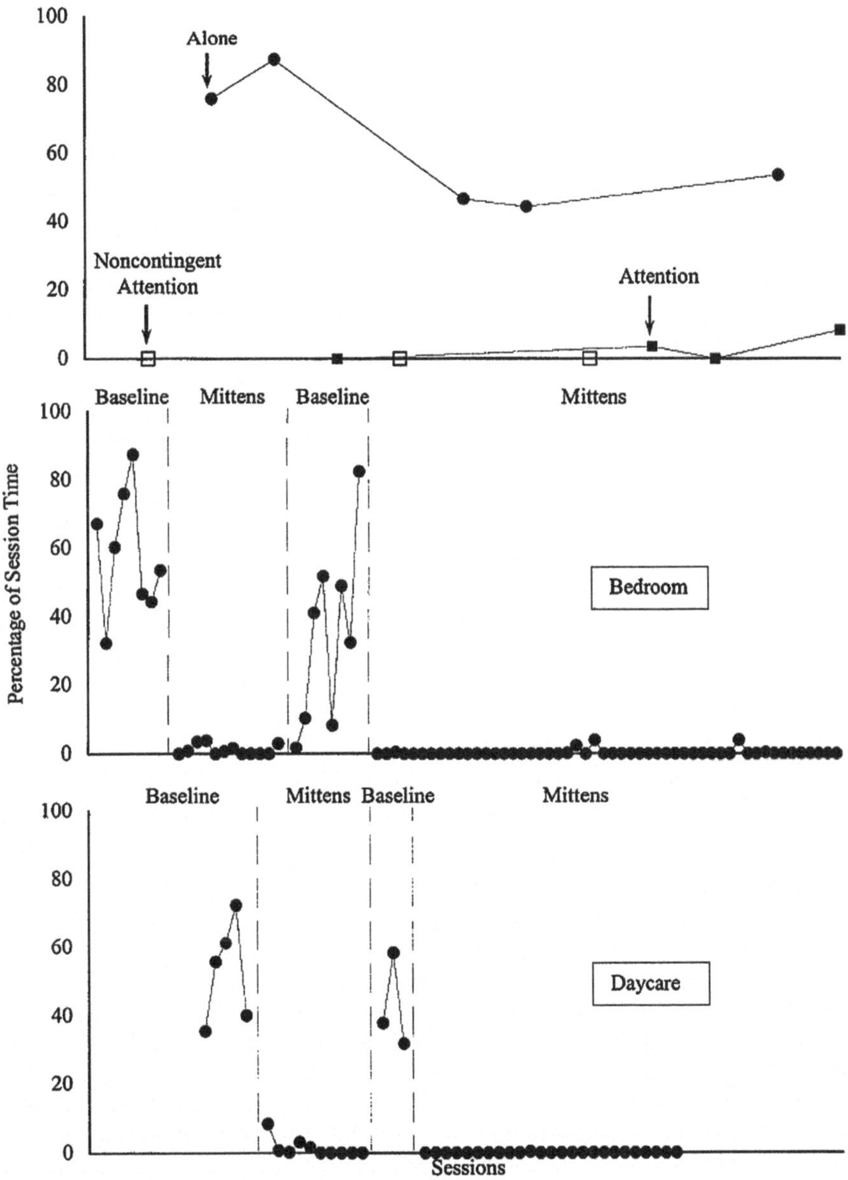

Fig. 6.1 The percentage of session time with hair twirling during the functional analysis (*top panel*). The percentage of session time with hair twirling during baseline and treatment conditions in the home (*middle panel*) and day care settings (*bottom panel*)

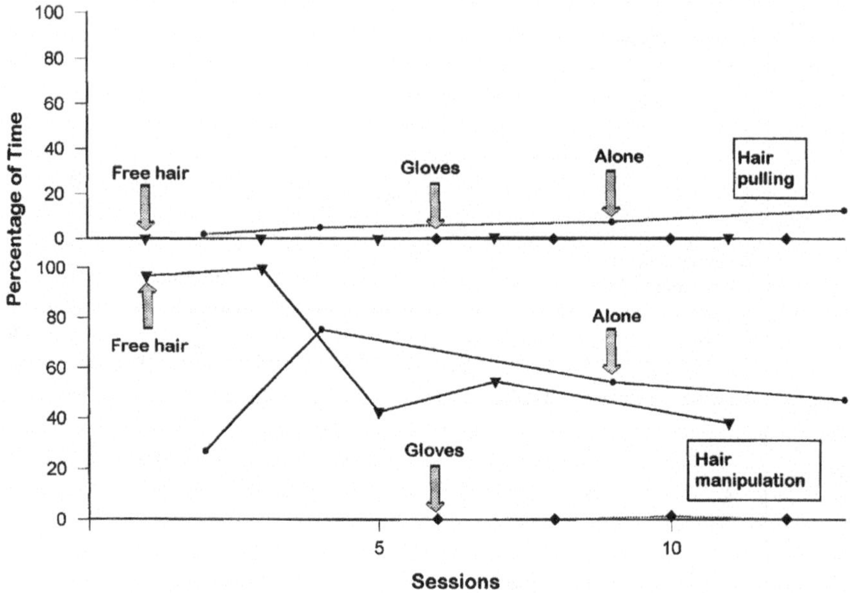

Fig. 6.2 The percentage of session time the participant engaged in hair pulling (*top panel*) and hair manipulation (*bottom panel*) while alone, while wearing the latex glove, and when free hairs were available

woman with intellectual disabilities after wrist weights and non-contingent application of a glove failed to decrease her hair pulling and hair manipulation over several sessions. Response interruption involved the therapist holding the participant's arm at her side for 20 s contingent on hair pulling. Differential reinforcement involved the therapist praising the participant's lack of hair pulling on a resetting interval schedule that was gradually increased from 30 s to 10 min. The RI and DRO intervention immediately decreased hair pulling and hair manipulation to zero or near zero levels. Furthermore, the treatment effects maintained for several sessions and maintained when the participant's mother implemented the intervention in the home.

The findings from the literature suggest that multi-component interventions including some combination of response interruption, response redirection, response prevention, and differential reinforcement is effective for decreasing body-focused repetitive behaviors. However, the lack of component analyses evaluating individual treatment components leads to uncertainty concerning the utility of any one procedure as a treatment for body-focused repetitive behaviors. We believe an initial evaluation of one of the individual treatment components such as response interruption or redirection may be warranted before moving to multi-component interventions that require more effort and time to implement. If the individual treatment component is proven effective, additional procedures can be avoided and if proven ineffective, additional procedures can be added.

Punishment

Punishment is characterized by a reduction in a behavior when a particular consequence follows the behavior (Miltenberger 2016). The two variations of punishment include positive punishment, in which an aversive stimulus is presented following the behavior, or negative punishment, in which a reinforcing stimulus is removed following the behavior (Miltenberger 2016). Various forms of punishment have been used to reduce body-focused repetitive behaviors in individuals with IDD (e.g., Altman et al. 1978; Barmann and Vitali 1982; Barrett and Shapiro 1980; Corte et al. 1971; Gross et al. 1982).

One form of punishment that has been used to decrease body-focused repetitive behaviors is facial screening. Facial screening utilizes the brief application of a bib to cover an individual's face contingent on the problem behavior. Barmann and Vitali (1982) evaluated the effectiveness of facial screening in the treatment of hair pulling exhibited by three young children with intellectual disabilities. The use of the bib in the intervention did not restrict the children's breathing and was considered to be an acceptable and ethical intervention by the caregivers. The results indicated that the facial screening procedure decreased hair pulling to zero for all three children. Furthermore, hair pulling remained at zero across several months for all three children and maintained in an additional school setting for the two children who were in school. Parental reports for two of the children also indicated that tissue damage and bald spots previously resulting from the hair pulling had healed. Because it involves the response-contingent presentation of a stimulus and a subsequent decrease in behavior, facial screening would be considered a form of positive punishment.

Overcorrection is another form of positive punishment that has been used to decrease body-focused repetitive behaviors. In the overcorrection procedure an effortful response is prompted contingent upon the occurrence of a problem behavior (Miltenberger 2016). In the literature on body-focused repetitive behaviors exhibited by individuals with IDD, successful examples of overcorrection include an oral hygiene procedure involving teeth and gum brushing with antiseptic solution for chronic hand mouthing (Foxx and Azrin 1973) and a hair brushing procedure for hair pulling (Barrett and Shapiro 1980). Because overcorrection requires an effortful response that is related to the topography of the undesired behavior or the effect of the behavior on the environment, it might be seen as an acceptable form of punishment. Other positive punishment procedures for body-focused repetitive behaviors, such as contingent aromatic ammonia and electric shock (Altman et al. 1978; Corte et al. 1971), may not be deemed as acceptable. Although Corte et al. (1971) showed that contingent electric shock eliminated self-injurious body-focused repetitive behaviors in individuals with IDD, shock is generally seen as an unacceptable or even unethical procedure and thus unlikely to be used in contemporary practice (Miltenberger et al. 1989). Altman et al. (1978) used contingent aromatic ammonia to reduce hair pulling in a young girl with cerebral palsy, and finger biting in a young boy with a moderate intellectual disability.

The procedure involved waving an open ammonia capsule near the participant's nose contingent on the problem behavior. Altman et al. found the procedure to be effective in reducing the young girl's hair pulling across several settings when applied for 3 s and in reducing the young boy's finger biting when applied for 1 s. These results suggest that varying durations of contingent ammonia exposure may be effective in decreasing body-focused repetitive behaviors. However, similar to the use of shock as an intervention, the use of aromatic ammonia is likely to be judged unacceptable in contemporary practice. If even considered at all, the use of such a procedure would be reserved for dangerous and intractable body-focused repetitive behavior.

Similar to other interventions used to treat body-focused repetitive behaviors, punishment has been used in combinations with other procedures such as differential reinforcement (Altman et al. 1978; Gross et al. 1982). For example, Gross et al. (1982) evaluated the effects of two combination interventions on the hair pulling in a young boy with cerebral palsy and intellectual disability. These interventions were overcorrection and facial screening, each combined with differential reinforcement of other behavior (DRO). In both procedures, praise was delivered contingent upon each 10-s period that passed with no instances of hair pulling. In the DRO and overcorrection procedure, the therapist raised the boy's arms above his head and in front of his body for 2 min contingent upon each occurrence of hair pulling. During the DRO and facial screening procedure, a bib was placed on the boy's face for 15 s contingent upon each occurrence of hair pulling. Gross et al. found that both interventions decreased the participant's hair pulling but that the facial screening procedure was more effective. Furthermore, as the hair pulling decreased to near zero, the child engaged in more appropriate play and participated more in academic activities. In addition, the tissue damage from hair pulling healed by the 6-week follow-up period.

Without a component analysis, only inferences can be made about critical treatment components in studies that utilize a combination of procedures. When treating behavioral excesses that are particularly harmful or health threatening such as body-focused repetitive behaviors that cause serious tissue damage, it is typically in the best interest of the client to treat the behavior as effectively and efficiently as possible, which may supersede the need to evaluate individual treatment components. Therefore, results from these studies demonstrate effective treatments but do not demonstrate a functional relationship between one component and behavioral reduction.

Awareness Enhancement Device

The awareness enhancement device (AED) is an electronic device designed by Rapp et al. (1998) that emits a tone contingent upon proximity of one's hand to one's head. Failure of habit reversal to decrease hair pulling and hair manipulation exhibited by a woman with an intellectual disability led to the development of the AED.

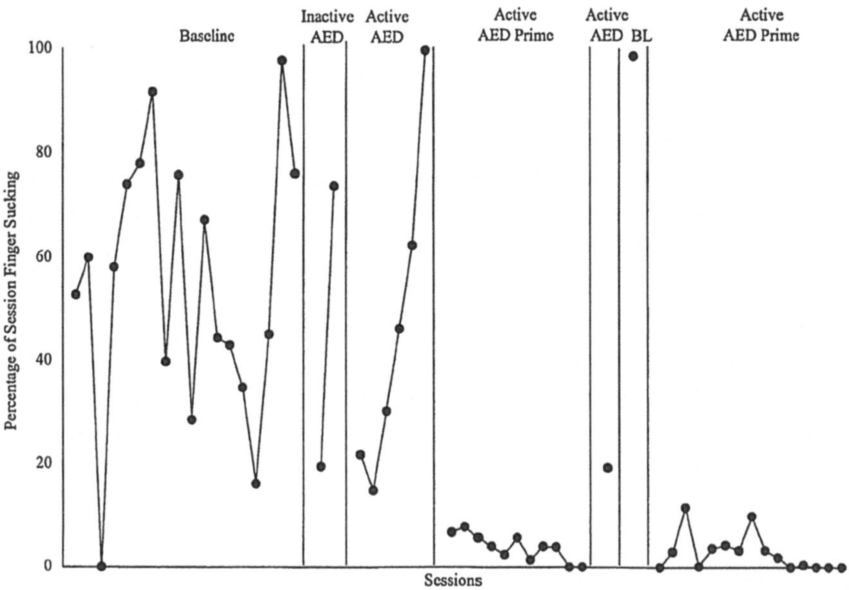

Fig. 6.3 The percentage of session time the participant engaged in finger sucking during baseline (BL), inactive AED, active AED, and active AED prime conditions

The purpose of the AED was to increase awareness of the occurrence of her target behaviors, prompt the use of a competing response (folding her arms across her chest), and provide an aversive auditory stimulus that functioned as positive punishment. The woman was taught to use her competing response for hair pulling when the tone from the AED sounded. The AED emitted the tone contingent upon her hand moving within 6 in of her head. When the AED was activated, the woman's hair pulling and manipulation immediately decreased to near zero and subsequently maintained at zero or near zero levels.

Other studies have demonstrated similar effects using the AED with thumb sucking (Stricker et al. 2001) and finger sucking (Ellingson et al. 2000). One study used the AED to reduce the finger sucking of a young girl diagnosed with attention deficit disorder and found that the AED alone did not eliminate finger sucking (Stricker et al. 2003). However, the addition of a remote-controlled buzzer to the AED and an increase in the decibel level of the buzzer immediately reduced finger sucking to zero and maintained zero or near zero levels of finger sucking in the weeks following treatment. As seen in Fig. 6.3, following baseline and a phase in which the child wore the AED without it being activated (Inactive AED), the use of the AED did not decrease the behavior (active AED). Once the additional buzzer was added (Active AED prime), finger sucking decreased to low levels.

As the name implies, the tone emitted by the AED enhances awareness of the target behaviors as they occur. If the participant has learned a competing response, the tone may then prompt the use of the competing response. The tone emitted by the AED may also function as a positive punisher for the precursor movement of the behavior, making the habit behavior less likely to occur. In addition, moving the hand away from the head may be negatively reinforced by the termination of the tone (Rapp et al. 1998). Regardless of its function, the AED appears to be an effective treatment for reducing health-threatening body-focused repetitive behaviors, and shows promise for individuals with intellectual disabilities. Himle et al. (2008) maintain that being aware of the precursor movements to habit behaviors, the situations in which habit behaviors are likely to occur, and the functions of habit behaviors are necessary for habit reversal to be successful. This emphasis on the importance of awareness may be one explanation for the ineffectiveness of habit reversal with individuals with intellectual disabilities. In addition, it suggests that an automated intervention such as the AED that does not require awareness of the behavior, or a skill set needed to implement a competing response, or the presence of a care giver to implement contingencies, may be desirable intervention for body focused repetitive behaviors exhibited by individuals with IDD. More research is warranted to establish the effectiveness and generality of the AED as a stand-alone procedure and as an adjunct to habit reversal for individuals with IDD.

Practice Recommendations

So far we have described five evidence-based practices that have been used to treat body-focused repetitive behaviors in individuals with intellectual disabilities: habit reversal, differential reinforcement, response interruption, redirection, or prevention, punishment, and the awareness enhancement device. These interventions have been proven to be effective to some extent in reducing or eliminating body-focused repetitive behaviors with this population. This section will review these interventions and offer recommendations for treatment selection in clinical practice.

Habit reversal is one of the most effective treatments for nervous habits and tics in individuals without disabilities (Miltenberger et al. 1998a, b; Woods and Miltenberger 1995). Habit reversal facilitates increased awareness of the undesired behavior and the use of competing responses to replace the undesired behavior (Azrin and Nunn 1973). Unfortunately, research suggests that habit reversal is not generally effective for individuals with IDD (e.g., Rapp et al. 1998). The limited effectiveness of habit reversal for people with IDD may be due to a lack of reinforcement in the natural environment for use of competing responses, a lack of motivation to decrease habit behaviors, or difficulty becoming aware of the undesired behaviors (Long et al. 1999). Habit reversal may be successful in reducing body-focused repetitive behaviors if the client is motivated to change his or her behavior and is affected by social consequences of the behavior. Motivation to change is likely a product of the inconvenience, stigma, or unpleasant social consequences of the behavior. If a client with IDD does not experience these events or is not affected by these events, the client is not likely to be motivated to change the behavior because decreasing the behavior does not function as a reinforcer. Long et al. (1999) found that habit reversal was most successful for a man diagnosed with mild intellectual disability who expressed displeasure with the appearance of his fingernails due to fingernail biting. This man also reported previous self-initiated attempts to stop biting his fingernails. Although additional contingencies were needed to eliminate his fingernail biting, habit reversal reduced the amount of time he engaged in the behavior. It may be beneficial to utilize habit reversal in a clinical setting if the client expresses motivation to stop his or her habit behavior. When appropriate, habit reversal is a desirable intervention because once the competing response is learned, the client can implement the competing response in his or her natural environment without external contingencies from therapists or caregivers. Habit reversal may promote functional independence, which is in the best interest of individuals receiving treatment. However, more research is needed to determine when habit reversal may be effective with individuals with intellectual disabilities and which adjunct procedures may enhance its effectiveness.

Differential reinforcement has been used in several studies to treat body-focused repetitive behaviors in individuals with IDD (e.g., Cavalari et al. 2013; Cowdery et al. 1990; Lang et al. 2009; Radstaake et al. 2011; Rapp et al. 2000a, b; Roscoe et al. 2013). It has been used alone and in conjunction with other interventions such as habit reversal. Differential reinforcement may take different forms including DRA, DRI, or DRO. Differential reinforcement may also be modified for specific uses related to the behavior, such as differential reinforcement of nail growth used for clients who engage in finger biting (e.g., Long et al. 1999). Differential reinforcement uses principles of positive reinforcement to increase the desired behavior and extinction to decrease the undesired behavior. Differential reinforcement is both an effective and acceptable treatment. In addition, there are opportunities to incorporate the client's preferences and choices into treatment through the selection of reinforcers for desired behaviors and through the selection of alternative or incompatible behaviors to be reinforced (Radstaake et al. 2011). Consideration of a client's preferences and choices is desirable when developing an intervention that will generalize to the client's natural environment.

Although differential reinforcement has several advantages, one disadvantage may be that it can be difficult to implement. Differential reinforcement typically requires implementation by others who are responsible for observing the client, delivering the appropriate reinforcer contingent upon occurrences of desired behavior or non-occurrence of the target behavior, and withholding the reinforcer contingent upon occurrences of the target behavior. The monitoring requirements may involve an unacceptably high level of response effort for those implementing the intervention, which is important to consider especially, when treatment must be implemented by parents, teachers, or staff. Self-monitored and self-managed differential reinforcement may be a viable alternative to traditional differential reinforcement procedures; however, more research is needed to determine if it is effective with individuals with varying levels of intellectual disabilities.

Response interruption, redirection, and prevention are interventions that involve interrupting the behavior early in the sequence, redirecting to a desired alternative behavior, and preventing undesirable behaviors through the application of physical restraints or barriers on the body. These methods have been used alone and combined with differential reinforcement to reduce body-focused repetitive behaviors such as hand mouthing, hair pulling, and hair manipulation. Although not considered functional interventions that address the reinforcing consequence for the behavior, response prevention may be functional if it masks the reinforcing stimulation arising from the behavior and response redirection may be functional if the client is directed to manipulate stimuli that are matched to the stimulation produced by the repetitive behavior (e.g., Rapp et al. 1999) Only one study directly addressed the automatic reinforcement function of body-focused repetitive behavior (hair pulling) by masking the stimulation through the use of latex gloves (Fig. 6.2) and providing stimuli for the client to manipulate that were matched to the stimulation arising from hair pulling (Rapp et al. 1999). Figure 6.2 shows the effects of providing matched stimulation on hair pulling and hair manipulation. When the client had "free hair" she no longer pulled her hair and manipulated the free hair instead of pulling hair and manipulating it.

The difficulty associated with the requirement of continuously monitoring a client's behavior when using differential reinforcement also arises with response interruption and redirection, in which the implementer must continuously observe the client in order to interrupt and redirect the behaviors when they occur. This difficulty could present a disadvantage to using response interruption and redirection with body-focused repetitive behaviors. However, response prevention in the form of applying gloves or splints to the hands of clients engaging in hand mouthing or hair pulling decreases the behaviors through simple barriers or in some cases by addressing the sensory stimulation function. Furthermore, because it does not require social mediation, it is a procedure that can be used when staff cannot be continuously present with the client or when the client is alone (Deaver et al. 2001; Rapp et al. 2000a, b). The use of response prevention devices such as gloves or hand splints should be discussed with the caregivers (as should any intervention) to establish the acceptability of the procedure. Furthermore, a treatment-fading plan should be developed with the goal of eliminating the use of the barrier devices.

Another intervention that does not require implementers to be continuously present in the environment with the client is the Awareness Enhancement Device (AED). As described previously, the AED is an electronic device that emits a tone when the wearer moves a hand towards his or her head (it could be programmed to include other body parts or locations as well). Results from the few studies that have evaluated the effectiveness of the AED indicate that it reduces body-focused repetitive behaviors including hair pulling and thumb sucking by individuals with intellectual disabilities (Rapp et al. 1998; Stricker et al. 2001). The AED promotes acquisition of a replacement behavior, which is negatively reinforced by termination of the buzzer, while decreasing the undesired behavior through positive punishment without a caregiver or staff member being present to monitor the behavior and implement an intervention (Rapp et al. 2000a, b). The AED is a promising intervention for reducing body-focused repetitive behaviors in individuals with intellectual disabilities. More research is needed that evaluates the effects of the AED across multiple types of health-threatening behaviors and individuals with varying disabilities. The AED enhances awareness of the occurrence of the behavior that produces the tone in addition to arranging automatic negative reinforcement and positive punishment contingencies. Any time punishment is used in an intervention, care must be taken to ensure the individual has access to alternative sources of reinforcement and that the treatment is acceptable to those involved.

Forms of punishment used to treat body-focused repetitive behaviors include facial screening, overcorrection, electric shock, and aromatic ammonia (e.g., Altman et al. 1978; Barmann and Vitali 1982; Barrett and Shapiro 1980; Corte et al. 1971; Gross et al. 1982). Although interventions using intense forms of punishment such as electric shock have been proven to be effective in decreasing self-injurious behavior (Corte et al. 1971; Favell et al. 1982; Linscheid et al. 1990) we do not recommend these approaches for body-focused repetitive behaviors due to their limited acceptability and the focus on functional and nonaversive approaches in contemporary practice. When possible, positive interventions should be used before interventions involving punishment (Bailey and Burch 2011). In recent years the research has moved away from punishment procedures in favor of positive interventions, but more research is needed to identify whether positive interventions are equally effective and if clinical practice follows trends in the research (Matson and LoVullo 2008).

When identifying a treatment for body-focused repetitive behaviors, several factors must be taken into consideration including the severity of the behavior and values of the consumer. If the behavior is severe or life threatening, it may be necessary to use punishment if it will yield the most efficient reduction in the behavior. Punishment may also be a necessary component of an intervention if positive practices fail to reduce a health-threatening behavior to an acceptable level. However, punishment should always be combined with reinforcement procedures such as differential reinforcement or noncontingent reinforcement (Lerman and Vorndran 2002). As in any treatment selection process, the advantages and disadvantages of punishment should be considered. For example, although contingent aromatic ammonia was effective in decreasing hair pulling and hand biting in a study by Altman et al. (1978), several issues arose during implementation including difficulty of administration due to social stigma, environmental challenges, changing topographies of behavior, and difficulty monitoring and identifying occurrences of the behavior. Ultimately, we do not recommend punishment involving the application of aversive stimulation due to current philosophies in the field, limited acceptability, and the availability of effective, less intrusive procedures. Practitioners should evaluate the needs of their specific client and determine what is best based on the behavior of concern, the values of the consumer, ethical guidelines, and empirical support from the literature.

References

Altman, K., Haavik, S., & Cook, W. (1978). Punishment of self-injurious behavior in natural settings using contingent aromatic ammonia. *Behaviour Research and Therapy, 16*, 85–96.

Azrin, N. H., & Nunn, R. G. (1973). A method of eliminating nervous habits and tics. *Behaviour Research and Therapy, 11*, 619–628.

Azrin, N. H., Nunn, R. G., & Frantz, S. E. (1980a). Habit reversal versus negative practice treatment of nailbiting. *Behaviour Research and Therapy, 18*, 281–285.

Azrin, N. H., Nunn, R. G., & Frantz-Renshaw, S. E. (1980b). Habit reversal treatment of thumbsucking. *Behaviour Research and Therapy, 18*, 195–399.

Azrin, N. H., Nunn, R. G., & Frantz-Renshaw, S. E. (1982). Habit reversal versus negative practice treatment of destructive oral habits (biting, chewing or licking of the lips, cheeks, tongue or palate). *Journal of Behavior Therapy and Experimental Psychiatry, 13*, 49–54.

Azrin, N. H., & Peterson, A. L. (1989). Reduction of an eye tic by controlled blinking. *Behavior Therapy, 20*, 467–473.

Bailey, J., & Burch, M. (2011). *Ethics for behavior analysts: Second* (expanded ed.). New York: Routledge.

Barmann, B. C., & Vitali, D. L. (1982). Facial screening to eliminate trichotillomania in developmentally disabled persons. *Behavior Therapy, 13*, 735–742.

Barrett, R. P., & Shapiro, E. S. (1980). Treatment of stereotyped hairpulling with overcorrection: A case study with long term follow-up. *Journal of Behavior Therapy and Experimental Psychiatry, 11*, 317–320.

Cavalari, R. S., DuBard, M., & Luiselli, J. K. (2013). Simplified habit reversal and treatment fading for chronic skin picking in an adolescent with autism. *Clinical Case Studies, 13*, 190–198.

Conelea, C. A., & Klein-Tasman, B. P. (2013). Habit reversal therapy for body-focused repetitive behaviors in Williams syndrome: A case study. *Journal of Developmental and Physical Disabilities, 25*, 597–611.

Corte, H. E., Wolf, M. M., & Locke, B. J. (1971). A comparison of procedures for eliminating self-injurious behavior of retarded adolescents. *Journal of Applied Behavior Analysis, 4*, 201–213.

Cowdery, G. E., Iwata, B. A., & Pace, G. M. (1990). Effects and side effects of DRO as treatment for self-injurious behavior. *Journal of Applied Behavior Analysis, 23*, 497–506.

Deaver, C. M., Miltenberger, R. G., & Stricker, J. M. (2001). Functional analysis and treatment of hair twirling in a young child. *Journal of Applied Behavior Analysis, 34*, 535–538.

Didden, R., Korzilius, H., & Curfs, M. G. (2007). Skin-picking in individuals with Prader-Willi syndrome: prevalence, functional assessment, and its comorbidity with compulsive and self-injurious behaviours. *Journal of Applied Research in Intellectual Disabilities, 20*, 409–419.

Ellingson, S. A., Miltenberger, R. G., Stricker, J. M., Garlinghouse, M. A., Roberts, J., Galensky, T. L., & Rapp, J. T. (2000). Analysis and treatment of finger sucking. *Journal of Applied Behavior Analysis, 33*, 41–52.

Favell, J. E., Azrin, N. H., Baumeister, A. A., Carr, E. G., Dorsey, M. F., Forehand, R., & Solnick, J. V. (1982). The treatment of self-injurious behavior. *Behavior Therapy, 13*, 529–554.

Foxx, R. M., & Azrin, N. H. (1973). The elimination of autistic self-stimulatory behavior by overcorrection. *Journal of Applied Behavior Analysis, 6*, 1–14.

Gross, A. M., Farrar, M. J., & Liner, D. (1982). Reduction of trichotillomania in a retarded cerebral palsied child using overcorrection, facial screening, and differential reinforcement of other behavior. *Education and Treatment of Children, 5*, 133–140.

Himle, J. A., Perlman, D. M., & Lokers, L. M. (2008). Prototype awareness enhancing and monitoring device for trichotillomania. *Behaviour Research and Therapy, 46*, 1187–1191.

Joubert, C. E. (1993). Relationship of self-esteem, manifest anxiety, and obsessive- compulsiveness to personal habits. *Psychological Reports, 73*, 579–583.

Kurtz, P. F., Chin, M. D., Huete, J. M., Tarbox, R. S. F., O'Connor, J. T., Paclawskyi, T. R., & Rush, K. S. (2003). Functional analysis and treatment of self-injurious behavior in young children: A summary of 30 cases. *Journal of Applied Behavior Analysis, 36*, 205–219.

Ladd, M. V., Luiselli, J. K., & Baker, L. (2009). Continuous access to competing stimulation as intervention for self-injurious skin picking in a child with autism. *Child & Family Behavior Therapy, 31*, 54–60.

Lang, R., Didden, R., Sigafoos, J., Rispoli, M., Regester, A., & Lancioni, G. E. (2009). Treatment of chronic skin-picking in an adolescent with Asperger syndrome and borderline intellectual disability. *Clinical Case Studies, 8*, 317–325.

Lerman, D. C., & Vorndran, C. M. (2002). On the status of knowledge for using punishment: Implications for treating behavior disorders. *Journal of Applied Behavior Analysis, 35*, 431–464.

Linscheid, T. R., Iwata, B. A., Ricketts, R. W., Williams, D. E., & Griffin, J. C. (1990). Clinical evaluation of the self-injurious behavior inhibiting system (SIBIS). *Journal of Applied Behavior Analysis, 23*, 53–78.

Long, E. S., Miltenberger, R. G., Ellingson, S. A., & Ott, S. M. (1999). Augmenting simplified habit reversal in the treatment of oral-digital habits exhibited by individuals with mental retardation. *Journal of Applied Behavior Analysis, 32*, 353–365.

Long, E. S., Miltenberger, R. G., & Rapp, J. T. (1998). A survey of habit behaviors exhibited by individuals with mental retardation. *Behavioral Interventions, 13*, 79–89.

Lydon, S., Healy, O., O'Reilly, M., & McCoy, A. (2013). A systematic review and evaluation of response redirection as a treatment for challenging behavior in individuals with developmental disabilities. *Research in Developmental Disabilities, 34*, 3148–3158.

Maguire, K., Piersel, W., & Hauser, B. (1995). A long-term treatment of trichotillomania: A case study of a woman with profound mental retardation living in an applied setting. *Journal of Developmental and Physical Disabilities, 7*, 185–202.

Matson, J. L., & LoVullo, S. V. (2008). A review of behavioral treatments for self-injurious behaviors of persons with autism spectrum disorders. *Behavior Modification, 32*, 61–76.

McEntee, J. E., Parker, E. H., Brown, M. B., & Poulson, R. L. (1996). The effects of response interruption, DRO, and positive reinforcement on the reduction of hand-mouthing behavior. *Behavioral Interventions, 11*, 163–170.

Miltenberger, R. G. (2016). *Behavior modification: Principles and procedures* (6th ed.). Pacific Grove, CA: Wadsworth.

Miltenberger, R. G., & Fuqua, R. W. (1985). A comparison of contingent versus noncontingent competing response practice in the treatment of nervous habits. *Journal of Behavior Therapy and Experimental Psychiatry, 16*, 195–200.

Miltenberger, R., Fuqua, W., & McKinley, T. (1985). Habit reversal with muscle tics: Replication and component analysis. *Behavior Therapy, 16*, 39–50.

Miltenberger, R., Fuqua, R., & Woods, D. (1998a). Applying behavior analysis with clinical problems: Review and analysis of habit reversal. *Journal of Applied Behavior Analysis, 31*, 447–461.

Miltenberger, R. G., Long, E. S., Rapp, J. T., Lumley, V. A., & Elliot, A. J. (1998b). Evaluating the function of hair pulling: A preliminary investigation. *Behavior Therapy, 29*, 211–219.

Miltenberger, R. G., Lennox, D. B., & Erfanian, N. (1989). Acceptability of alternative treatments for persons with mental retardation: Ratings from institutional and community based staff. *American Journal of Mental Retardation, 93*, 388–395.

Neef, N. A., & Iwata, B. A. (1994). Current research on functional analysis methodologies: An introduction. *Journal of Applied Behavior Analysis, 27*, 211–214.

Ollendick, T. H. (1981). Self-monitoring and self-administered overcorrection: The modification of nervous tics in children. *Behavior Modification, 5*, 75–84.

Odlaug, B. l., & Grant, J. E. (2008). Clinical characteristics and medical complications of pathologic skin picking. *General Hospital Psychiatry, 30*, 61–66.

Pelios, L., Morren, J., Tesch, D., & Axelrod, S. (1999). The impact of functional analysis methodology on treatment choice for self-injurious and aggressive behavior. *Journal of Applied Behavior Analysis, 32*, 185–195.

Piazza, C. C., Adelinis, J. D., Hanley, G. P., Goh, H. L., & Delia, M. D. (2000). An evaluation of the effects of matched stimuli on behaviors maintained by automatic reinforcement. *Journal of Applied Behavior Analysis, 33*, 13–27.

Radstaake, M., Didden, R., Bolio, M., Lang, R., Lancioni, G. E., & Curfs, L. M. G. (2011). Functional assessment and behavioral treatment of skin picking in a teenage girl with Prader-Willi syndrome. *Clinical Case Studies, 10*, 67–68.

Rapp, J. T., Miltenberger, R. G., & Long, E. S. (1998). Augmenting simplified habit reversal with an awareness enhancement device: Preliminary findings. *Journal of Applied Behavior Analysis, 31*, 665–668.

Rapp, J. T., Miltenberger, R. G., Galensky, T. L., Ellingson, S. A., & Long, E. S. (1999). A functional analysis of hair pulling. *Journal of Applied Behavior Analysis, 32*, 329–337.

Rapp, J. T., Dozier, C. L., Carr, J. E., Patel, M. R., & Enloe, K. A. (2000a). Functional analysis of hair manipulation: A replication and extension. *Behavioral Interventions, 15*, 121–133.

Rapp, J. T., Miltenberger, R. G., Galensky, T. L., Ellingson, S. A., Sricker, J., Garlinghouse, M., et al. (2000b). Treatment of hair pulling and hair manipulation maintained by digital-tactile stimulation. *Behavior Therapy, 31*, 381–393.

Realon, R. E., Favell, J. E., & Cacace, S. (1995). An economical, humane, and effective method for short-term suppression of hand mouthing. *Behavioral Interventions, 10*, 141–147.

Roscoe, E. M., Iwata, B. A., & Zhou, L. (2013). Assessment and treatment of chronic hand mouthing. *Journal of Applied Behavior Analysis, 46*, 181–198.

Snorrason, I., & Woods, D. W. (2014). Hair pulling, skin picking, and other body-focused repetitive behaviors. In E. A. Storch & D. McKay (Eds.), *Obsessive-compulsive disorder and its spectrum: A life-span approach* (pp. 163–184). Washington, DC: American Psychological Association.

Stricker, J. M., Miltenberger, R. G., Garlinghouse, M. A., Deaver, C. M., & Anderson, C. A. (2001). Evaluation of an awareness enhancement device for the treatment of thumb sucking in children. *Journal of Applied Behavior Analysis, 34*, 77–80.

Stricker, J. M., Miltenberger, R. G., Garlinghouse, M., & Tulloch, H. E. (2003). Augmenting stimulus intensity with an awareness enhancement device in the treatment of finger sucking. *Education and Treatment of Children, 26*, 22–29.

Teng, E. J., Woods, D. W., Twohig, M. P., & Marcks, B. A. (2002). Body-focused repetitive behavior problems: Prevalence in a nonreferred population and differences in perceived somatic activity. *Behavior Modification, 26*, 340–360.

Tiger, J. H., Fisher, W. W., & Bouxsein, K. J. (2009). Therapist- and self-monitored DRO contingencies as a treatment for the self-injurious skin picking of a young man with Asperger syndrome. *Journal of Applied Behavior Analysis, 42*, 315–319.

Turner, W. D., Realon, R. E., Irvin, D., & Robinson, E. (1996). The effects of implementing program consequences with a group of individuals who engaged in sensory maintained hand mouthing. *Research in Developmental Disabilities, 17*, 311–330.

Van Houton, R., & Rolider, A. (1984). The use of response prevention to eliminate nocturnal thumb sucking. *Journal of Applied Behavior Analysis, 17*, 509–520.

Woods, D. W., Flessner, C. A., Franklin, M. E., Keuthen, N. J., Goodwin, R. D., Stein, D. J., et al. (2006). The trichotillomania impact project (TiP): Exploring phenomenology, functional impairment, and treatment utilization. *The Journal of Clinical Psychiatry, 67*, 1877–1888.

Woods, D. W., Friman, P. C., & Teng, E. (2001). Physical and social functioning in persons with repetitive behavior disorders. In D. W. Woods & R. G. Miltenberger (Eds.), *Tic disorders, trichotillomania, and other repetitive behavior disorders: Behavioral approaches to analysis and treatment* (pp. 33–52). Norwell, MA: Kluwer Academic.

Woods, D. W., & Miltenberger, R. G. (1995). Habit reversal: A review of applications and variations. *Journal of Behavior Therapy and Experimental Psychiatry, 26*, 123–131.

Chapter 7
Food Refusal and Selective Eating

Valerie M. Volkert, Meeta R. Patel and Kathryn M. Peterson

Introduction

Food refusal can be characterized as a severe feeding problem wherein an individual fails to eat sufficient quantity and/or variety of foods/liquids to maintain his or her weight and height (e.g., Babbitt et al. 1994). In addition, food refusal may encompass selective eating by type where weight and growth are not of concern but where nutritional status may be compromised. Food selectivity by texture can be another form of a feeding problem where oral- motor skill deficits (e.g., dysphagia, inability to chew) may be evident.

Feeding problems can occur in about 25–45 % of typically developing children and up to 80 % of children with intellectual and developmental disabilities (Gouge and Ekvall 1975; Manikam and Perman 2000; Palmer and Horn 1978; Perske et al. 1977). Certain medical diagnoses can increase the risk of feeding problems, for example, gastroesophageal reflux [GER], aspiration, bronchopulmonary dysplasia, congenital heart disease, short-gut syndrome, prematurity, and childhood cancer (Lincheid et al. 1995). Feeding difficulties also occur in up to 49 % of children diagnosed with prematurity (Kerwin 1999). In addition, feeding problems are common in children with specific genetic disorders such as Autism Spectrum Disorder [ASD], Angelman syndrome, Down syndrome, Cystic Fibrosis, Celiac

V.M. Volkert (✉) · K.M. Peterson
Munroe-Meyer Institute, University of Nebraska Medical Center, Omaha, USA
e-mail: valerie.volkert@choa.org; vvolkert@unmc.edu

M.R. Patel
Clinic 4 Kidz, Sausalito, USA

V.M. Volkert
Marcus Autism Center, Emory University School of Medicine, Atlanta, GA, USA

J.K. Luiselli (ed.), *Behavioral Health Promotion and Intervention in Intellectual and Developmental Disabilities*, Evidence-Based Practices in Behavioral Health,
DOI 10.1007/978-3-319-27297-9_7

Disease, Pierre Robin syndrome, and Treacher Collins syndrome. Notably, Field et al. (2003) reported that 62 % of children diagnosed with ASD were likely to be food selective by type and/or texture and were less likely to display oral-motor skill deficits such as dysphagia. On the other hand, 80 % of children with Down syndrome and 68 % of children with CP were identified as having oral-motor skill deficits. Similarly, Schreck et al. (2004) found that 72 % of children with ASD experienced feeding problems and ate significantly fewer foods from all food groups, consuming approximately half the number of dairy, fruits, proteins, and vegetables consumed by children without ASD.

Feeding problems can be classified into the categories of eating nothing to minimal by mouth, liquid dependency, and food selectivity. Children who eat minimal or nothing by mouth typically receive nutrition through enteral support. Liquid dependency refers to children who rely primarily on a high calorie drink supplement (e.g., Pediasure) as the main source of nutrition with minimal consumption of solid foods. As noted previously, children who display food selectivity may be selective by type (only eating a limited number of foods), texture (only eating specific textures such as crunchy or pureed foods), brand (only eating specific brands of food), temperature (only eating food of one temperature regardless of the food type), and/or, color (only eating a specific color of food; Williams and Seiverling 2010). Some children may also be selective with regards to presentation format. For example, a child may only drink from a baby bottle and refuse all other drinking vessels at inappropriate ages. Children with developmental disabilities, especially ASD, often times have peculiar eating habits which may seem ritualistic in nature. For example, a child may only eat a perfectly round pepperoni pizza from a Pizza Hut box and refuse any other presentation format or brand of pizza.

The etiology of feeding problems is not well understood. Commonly, feeding problems may develop as a result of medical issues, anatomical abnormalities and/or oral-motor skill deficits, and behavioral/environmental factors (Rommel et al. 2003; Volkert and Piazza 2012). Medical conditions in which eating has been paired with pain or discomfort may result in food refusal. For example, if a child is experiencing pain during eating due to GER (Hyman 1994) or severe food allergies, he or she may be more likely to refuse food to avoid experiencing pain. In addition, children with other medical problems such as pulmonary or cardiac issues may have to exert more energy when eating; therefore, these children may refuse to eat simply because it is too effortful. Children with other medical conditions (e.g., childhood cancers, seizure disorders) that require noxious tasting medications by mouth may develop an oral aversion by not allowing anything near the mouth including food/liquids due to previous negative experiences, resulting in food refusal. Indeed, data from animal studies have provided support for this hypothesis (Garcia and Koelling 1966; Green and Garcia 1971; Green et al. 1974; Revusky and Bedarf 1967). Certain medications may also decrease the natural hunger and satiety signals which can lead to feeding problems, specifically medications commonly prescribed to treat symptoms of attention deficit hyperactivity disorder, such as Adderall or Ritalin.

Anatomical abnormalities can also lead to feeding problems (Palmer and Horn 1978). If a child was not born with the necessary structures to eat such as a cleft lip/palate, this condition may cause eating to be more effortful or not possible at all until a surgical procedure has been completed. Children also sometimes experience feeding difficulties because they lack the oral-motor skills needed to swallow food or liquid or are diagnosed with dysphagia. For instance, problems could occur with (a) forming the bolus, (b) elevating the tongue at the posterior, (c) contacting the tongue to the hard and soft palate sequentially, or (d) propelling the bolus into the pharynx (Vaz et al. 2012).

Feeding problems may be a result of negative experiences such as choking, gagging, or vomiting while eating. Due to these negative experiences, children learn to avoid eating. In the case of food selectivity it may be likely that the sensory properties of certain foods, textures, brands, temperatures, and/or colors are more appealing than others. Overtime these children may learn to refuse the foods that are less desirable (nonpreferred) or aversive. Lastly, children with feeding problems may engage in a variety of inappropriate mealtime behaviors such as turning their head away from food, pushing the food away, and/or crying at the presentation of food to avoid eating. If these behaviors do not produce the desired outcome, which is the removal of the food, children may learn to engage in expulsion, packing (holding food in the mouth for extended periods of time), throwing, aggression, and even gagging and vomiting. These behaviors that produce escape from eating become strengthened in the child's repertoire so eventually the child learns that consumption is not required.

Some children's feeding problems may be less severe in that they miss a small percentage of meals and refuse food occasionally. However, other children may display more serious feeding problems in which they refuse food/liquid routinely which can eventually lead to malnutrition, depleted fat stores, dehydration, imbalances in electrolytes, impaired cognitive and emotional development, impaired academic functioning, failure to thrive (FTT; deceleration of weight), hospitalization, recurrent infections, a compromised immune system, and high medical costs (Christophersen and Hall 1978; Volkert and Piazza 2012). In these cases, the majority of children require nasogastric or gastrostomy tube feedings for nutritional support. Although enteral support may be a good short-term solution, tube dependency can lead to delayed chewing and swallowing, vomiting, infection around the tube site, and continued surgeries to resize the tube. Children who are liquid dependent are also at risk for health problems. Eventually these children may not be able to meet their caloric goal via liquid only as their needs increase. In some cases, being dependent on liquids could lead to deficiencies and excesses in certain vitamins and minerals because a home-concocted liquid may not be balanced in terms of macro- and micronutrients or the parent may unknowingly use a harmful supplement.

For children who display food selectivity, immediate health risks may not be apparent if lack of weight gain/growth is not typically evident. However, children who display food selectivity are still at risk for health problems. Selective diets of children with ASD are often high in fat and/or sodium (e.g., French fries) and/or low in nutritional content (e.g., candy). For example, children that consume meals predominantly composed of high glycemic-index foods (e.g., complex carbohydrates), foods that are high in fat (e.g., fast foods), or foods that are high in sugar (e.g., candy, soda) are at greater risk for developing severe health problems such as obesity, Type-2 diabetes, and hypertension (Freedman et al. 1999; Ludwig et al. 1999). Moreover, not eating a well-balanced diet may result in iron deficiency and anemia (Latif et al. 2002). The diets of children diagnosed with intellectual and developmental disabilities are deficient in micronutrients such as iron, zinc, and vitamin C because these children often refuse to consume meat, fruits, and vegetables (Sullivan et al. 2002). Sullivan et al. also stated that iron deficiency impairs brain function which cannot be reversed if left untreated and a restricted diet has resulted in scurvy in a child with ASD (Rumsey and Rosenburg 2013).

Caregivers of children with feeding problems may also experience high levels of anxiety, stress, depression, or social stigmatization (Auslander et al. 2003; Graves and Ware 1990) due to unconventional feeding routines. Drinking a baby bottle, eating pureed foods at an inappropriate age, and frequent contact with medical providers are some of the circumstances that can provoke discomfort (Volkert and Piazza 2012). Feeding problems may also prevent families from attending routine activities, thus making it critical to assess and treat feeding problems at an early age.

Assessment of Feeding Problems

Given the complex etiology and high prevalence of feeding problems in children with intellectual and developmental disabilities, multiple strategies are often necessary to assess their origin and maintaining factors (Cohen et al. 2006). Even though many children with intellectual and developmental disabilities may not present with comorbid medical conditions, it is still crucial to evaluate whether there are any relevant medical concerns prior to initiating a feeding intervention. Thus the assessment and treatment of feeding problems should be conducted by an interdisciplinary treatment team of professionals involving speech and language pathologists, registered dieticians, and physicians (Laud et al. 2009; Silverman 2010). This team is especially important during the initial stages of the evaluation process to determine the child's safety and readiness for oral feeding. For example, trained professionals such as a speech and language pathologist should evaluate a child's skill relative to chewing, mastication, swallowing, and motor dexterity. In addition, speech and language pathologists can determine whether there is risk for aspiration or choking and whether a modified barium swallow study should be performed to rule out associated risks. Speech and language pathologists also should assess the child's ability to consume various textures and bolus sizes (Milnes and Piazza 2013a, b). Physicians, including gastroenterologists, pediatricians, or other medical specialists should evaluate the child's physical health, ruling out risks associated with eating (e.g., food allergies, GER) during the initial assessment phase. Registered dieticians also play a large role in the assessment and continued evaluation of the child by monitoring the child's growth and nutritional status. The registered dietician is able to assess and provide recommendations about the child's estimated caloric and nutritional needs. Finally, the registered dietician could recommend foods or liquids that may be beneficial for the child's growth and overall nutrition (Milnes and Piazza 2013a, b; Silverman 2010).

Once all medical conditions have been treated and once the child is declared safe and appropriate for oral feeding by the interdisciplinary team, feeding therapists who are trained in behavior analysis can begin to assess the environmental variables that impact the child's feeding behavior. Therefore, the next step of the assessment process often involves structured interviews with the child's caregivers to acquire more information about the child's feeding history. For example, Matson and Kuhn (2001) developed a standardized interview and screening tool (STEP) to identify feeding difficulties in individuals with developmental or intellectual disabilities by separating feeding difficulties into food selectivity and oral-motor skill deficits. This tool was originally developed and tested among a wide age range of individuals with developmental disabilities (ages 10–87); therefore, the extent to which it could be applied to younger children with or without developmental disabilities is unknown. Seiverling et al. (2011) recently created a modification to the STEP (STEP-CHILD) to target a wider range of children with developmental disabilities. This revised tool also included more questions to determine the extent to which parent mealtime actions impacted child feeding behavior. The STEP-CHILD is a psychometrically sound tool that may reveal useful information regarding the child's history of feeding problems and parent behavior that may influence the child's behavior. Others have developed similar tools to specifically address feeding problems in children with intellectual and developmental disabilities (e.g., Hendy et al. 2009; Lukens and Linscheid 2008), including an assessment of mastication skills (Remijn et al. 2014) and swallow functioning (Sheppard et al. 2014). These types of screening tools, while informative and easy to administer, should only be used as an initial step in the evaluative process and should never replace direct observation and measurement as the primary components of assessment. In general, there is a need to develop and/or refine assessment tools to evaluate feeding problems in children with developmental disabilities (Sharp et al. 2013). However, due to the inaccuracy of secondhand reports and the correlational nature of questionnaires in general, we cannot determine much about the underlying causes of the feeding problem or the course of treatment following this initial form of assessment.

Direct observation is often the next step of the assessment process to evaluate child behavior during meals. Given that treatments based on principles of applied behavior analysis have the most empirical support for feeding difficulties in children with and without intellectual and developmental disabilities (Kerwin 1999; Sharp et al. 2010; Volkert and Piazza 2012), assessments should be behavior analytic in nature and tailored to identify the conditions under which inappropriate mealtime behavior is likely to occur. Ahearn et al. (2001) were one of the first to use a direct observational tool to measure food acceptance in children with ASD.

More specific, Ahearn et al. measured acceptance in 30 children during a repeated observations assessment of 12 different foods from four food groups that were either a pureed or "regular table" texture. Using this strategy, Ahearn et al. were able to categorize the child's feeding difficulties as either selectivity by food type, selectivity by food texture, or food refusal (i.e., failing to accept any bites), based on the percentage of acceptance across foods and textures. Although this assessment provided useful information regarding the type of feeding problem, it did not identify putative reinforcers for inappropriate mealtime behavior.

Caregivers often try to motivate their child to eat by providing attention or frequent breaks and delivering highly preferred toys or snacks. These and similar consequences could result in the child's behavior worsening over time if those parent responses serve as reinforcers for the child's behavior (Piazza et al. 2003). One way to assess problem behavior during mealtimes is to observe parents conducting meals as they normally would at home. Through this type of direct observation, behavior analysts can assess mealtime interactions between parent and child and identify common parent responses or other environmental changes that frequently follow child behavior during meals that are either appropriate (e.g., descriptive praise) or inappropriate (e.g., reprimands, coaxing, termination of the meal following inappropriate mealtime behavior). For example, Borrero et al. (2010) used descriptive analyses to determine which type of events most often followed child inappropriate behavior during parent-fed meals. Results of the study demonstrated that escape through removal of the spoon or termination of the meal most frequently followed child inappropriate mealtime behavior, in addition to parent attention (e.g., coaxing) and delivery of preferred foods and objects.

Although Borrero et al. (2010) discovered useful information about parent behavior during mealtimes, they did not conduct additional analyses to determine the effects of those parent consequences on child behavior. Functional analyses are structured assessments which are conducted to identify the variables that influence the occurrence of problem behavior (Hanley et al. 2003). Piazza et al. (2003) were the first to conduct functional analyses of inappropriate mealtime behavior for 15 children, with and without developmental disabilities, who had feeding difficulties. More specific, they assessed child responding under the standard functional analysis conditions of escape, attention, and access to tangibles to determine how common caregiver consequences such as removal of the spoon or cup, attention, or delivery of tangible items affected child feeding behavior. Results demonstrated that parent consequences functioned as reinforcement for 10 of the 15 children's problematic mealtime behavior. Of those 10 children, 90 % of inappropriate mealtime behavior was sensitive to escape as reinforcement, suggesting that negative reinforcement may play a large role in the development and maintenance of problematic feeding behavior for many children. Bachmeyer et al. (2009) also conducted functional analyses of inappropriate mealtime behavior with four children during which, they determined all four children's behavior to be multiply controlled by escape and adult attention. Subsequent function-based treatment evaluations demonstrated that attention extinction alone was not sufficient to reduce inappropriate mealtime behavior or increase acceptance. Ultimately, a combined escape and attention extinction intervention resulted in the greatest reduction in inappropriate mealtime behavior and increase in acceptance (Bachmeyer et al. 2009).

Treatment of Feeding Problems

Given the findings from Piazza et al. (2003) and Bachmeyer et al. (2009), it appears that negative reinforcement plays a critical role in the development and/or maintenance of inappropriate mealtime behavior. Therefore, escape extinction procedures that no longer allow escape are often a necessary treatment component (Patel et al. 2002; Piazza et al. 2003; Reed et al. 2004). In fact, escape extinction is the treatment with the most empirical support for pediatric feeding disorders (Ahearn et al. 1996; Borrero et al. 2013; Cooper et al. 1987; Hoch et al. 1994; Kerwin 1999; LaRue et al. 2011; Patel et al. 2002; Piazza et al. 2003; Reed et al. 2004; Volkert and Piazza 2012).

One of the most commonly used escape-extinction procedures to treat feeding problems is nonremoval of the spoon, in which the feeder holds the spoon at the child's lips until the child opens his or her mouth and allows the feeder to deposit the bite into the mouth (Hoch et al. 1994). In general, feeders re-present bites or drinks using nonremoval of the spoon following food or drink expulsion. That is, if the child (a) spits the food or liquid, (b) removes the food or liquid from the mouth with a finger or another object, or (c) allows the food or liquid to fall or run out of the mouth, the feeder immediately scoops up the bite or drink and deposits it back inside the child's mouth to minimize escape (e.g., Wilkins et al. 2011). Research has consistently shown that acceptance of bites increased and inappropriate mealtime behavior decreased when therapists used nonremoval of the spoon as treatment for feeding problems (Patel et al. 2002; Piazza et al. 2003; Reed et al. 2004).

Physical guidance is another form of escape extinction which involves the feeder applying gentle pressure to the child's mandibular joint of the jaw (i.e., jaw prompt) until the child's mouth opens and the feeder is able to deposit the bite inside his or her mouth (Ahearn et al. 1996; Borrero et al. 2013; Kozlowski et al. 2011). Physical guidance may be most effective when children clench their teeth upon presentation of the spoon or cup to the lips, which could result in longer meal durations if the feeder is unable to deposit the bite or drink. Some have questioned the use of procedures involving physical guidance in terms of safety and social validity given the more intrusive nature of the procedure. However, Ahearn et al. (1996) and Piazza et al. (2003) both noted that some caregivers actually preferred physical guidance to nonremoval of the spoon, given that it resulted in shorter meal durations. Others have criticized the physical guidance procedure in terms of treatment fidelity (Kadey et al. 2013). More specific, "the application of gentle pressure" is a subjective description which may make it difficult to assess whether all feeders are implementing the procedure in the same manner and with the correct amount of pressure.

An alternative to physical guidance involves use of a Nuk, which is a plastic utensil that is approximately 12.5 cm long with soft rubbery bristles at one end. Kadey et al. (2013) evaluated a Nuk prompt as an alternative physical guidance strategy with two children with food selectivity and ASD. Feeders inserted the Nuk between the child's lips, alongside the child's cheek and teeth, just past the last molar. Once at this position, feeders turned the Nuk approximately 10° from the teeth while keeping it positioned against the gums to open the mouth and then deposited the bite or drink with a spoon or cup. The Nuk prompt effectively increased acceptance of previously refused foods and drinks for both children. In addition, the authors concluded that the Nuk prompt was superior to nonremoval of the spoon implemented with and without noncontingent reinforcement. The treatment involving the Nuk prompt also resulted in much shorter meal durations, given that the feeder was able to deposit the bites more quickly.

There is preliminary support for yet another variation of escape extinction that involves the feeder inserting his or her finger into the child's mouth alongside the cheek and gums to prompt the child to open. Borrero et al. (2013) compared the jaw prompt with the finger prompt in the treatment of feeding problems in four children, one of which was diagnosed with ASD. Results demonstrated that both procedures were equally effective in increasing food acceptance and reducing inappropriate mealtime behavior. Given that there is limited research, caution should be taken when using these variations of escape extinction. More research is needed to further evaluate the safety, efficacy, treatment integrity, and social validity of this form of escape extinction in the treatment of feeding problems in children with intellectual and developmental disabilities.

Although escape extinction is often a necessary treatment component, results from a series of studies conducted by Patel et al. (2002), Piazza et al. (2003), and Reed et al. (2004), have shown that differential and/or noncontingent reinforcement was not sufficient to increase acceptance alone, but when combined with escape extinction, was associated with lower levels of inappropriate mealtime behavior and/or negative vocalizations for some children. Kadey et al. (2013) also demonstrated that the addition of noncontingent reinforcement to escape extinction resulted in lower levels of inappropriate mealtime behavior and negative vocalizations for two children with ASD and food selectivity. Although these reinforcement strategies may not be sufficient to compete with negatively-reinforced behavior alone, including them in a treatment package with escape extinction could enhance the effects of extinction by mitigating undesirable side effects such as crying and inappropriate mealtime behavior. Additional research is needed to continue evaluating the effects of positive-reinforcement-based strategies alone and in combination with escape extinction on inappropriate mealtime behavior in children with intellectual and developmental disabilities.

Antecedent-based interventions. An abundance of research has focused on consequence-based procedures such as positive reinforcement and escape extinction. Escape extinction has been shown to be the most effective consequence-based procedure (e.g., Sharp et al. 2010); however, with escape extinction, extinction bursts and emotional responding may be more evident, which may result in poor social acceptability of the treatment. It is likely that escape extinction is inevitable because food refusal has typically been maintained by negative reinforcement in the form of escape. If that is the case, manipulating antecedent variables in addition to escape extinction may help ameliorate the negative side effects associated with escape extinction. Conversely, in some cases escape extinction may not even be necessary if antecedent variables are manipulated. Antecedent-based interventions that have shown to be effective in treating food refusal include simultaneous presentation, stimulus fading, and high-probability (high-p) instructional sequence.

Simultaneous presentation. Simultaneous presentation is when a non-preferred food is presented together with a highly preferred food. It is likely that the feeder presents these two foods together on a utensil or blended together. The non-preferred foods also can be covered with the preferred food or the nonpreferred food can be imbedded in the preferred food. Ahearn (2003) showed an increase in consumption of vegetables in a child with ASD when they were presented with preferred condiments in the absence of escape extinction. Similarly Buckley and Newchok (2005) evaluated simultaneous presentation of a ground cookie behind the nonpreferred food, praise for swallowing, and paused video contingent on packing. The authors showed that packing initially decreased with differential reinforcement and response cost but further decreases in packing were observed with the addition of simultaneous presentation. When packing was evaluated with simultaneous presentation only, levels of packing remained low.

Piazza et al. (2002) found similar results in that simultaneous presentation (e.g., a chip presented on top of a piece of broccoli) resulted in increases in consumption for two of the three participants diagnosed with intellectual and developmental disabilities and food selectivity when compared to sequential presentation of preferred food delivered after consumption of the nonpreferred food in the absence of escape extinction. However, for the third participant, consumption only increased in the sequential condition and not the simultaneous condition when the feeder implemented physical guidance with gentle pressure to the mandibular joint if acceptance did not occur within 30 s of the presentation and re-presentation of expelled bites. In addition, Mueller et al. (2004) showed increases in acceptance of nonpreferred foods for two children with feeding disorders when the foods were blended systematically with preferred foods. These results also generalized to other foods that were not blended. However, the authors did not evaluate simultaneous presentation in the absence of escape extinction and reinforcement; therefore, the effectiveness of simultaneous presentation alone is unknown in this study. Regardless, the authors were able to increase consumption of 16 different nonpreferred foods by eventually fading out the preferred food.

Stimulus fading. Stimulus fading in the treatment of feeding problems may involve gradually changing the concentration of preferred and nonpreferred foods, similar to the Mueller et al. (2004) study. It may also involve the gradual change in other stimulus conditions that may be aversive such as texture, presence of the food, and the number of bites required for consumption. Similar to the Mueller et al. (2004) study, Patel et al. (2001) showed that differential reinforcement and escape extinction were not effective at increasing consumption of milk mixed with Carnation Instant Breakfast (CIB; high calorie drink) for a child diagnosed with pervasive developmental disorder and gastrostomy-tube dependence. Because consumption of water was at 100 %, the authors initially faded in the CIB in 5–10 % increments to the water. Once the child was consuming 100 % of the concentration of water mixed with CIB, the authors faded out the water and milk was faded in 10 % increments. Consumption increased to 100 % for milk + CIB when the authors implemented this gradual fading procedure. Both, Mueller et al. (2004) and Patel et al. (2001) evaluated stimulus fading procedures after reinforcement and escape extinction were not effective. The authors did not evaluate stimulus fading in these studies in the absence of the treatment package. Conversely, Luiselli et al. (2005) used stimulus fading in the absence of escape extinction to increase milk consumption in a child with ASD. Similar to the Patel et al. (2001) study, the authors gradually increased the amount of milk to Pediasure, a high calorie supplemental drink that the child readily consumed. The starting point for treatment was 50 % whole milk and 50 % Pediasure because that was a concentration the child readily consumed. The authors systematically decreased the concentration of Pediasure while they increased the concentration of milk until the child was eventually consuming 100 % whole milk. These results are noteworthy because escape extinction was not necessary.

As mentioned previously, texture selectivity is also a common feeding problem in children with ASD or other intellectual or developmental delays. Shore et al. (1998) demonstrated the effectiveness of texture fading in the treatment of food selectivity by texture. The authors identified a texture that the participants would consume consistently and over time they faded in higher textures while they faded out lower texture foods. Although stimulus fading was shown to be effective, it was combined with reinforcement and escape extinction; therefore, the individual contribution of stimulus fading is unknown. In addition, the authors did not assess oral-motor skills so it was unclear whether a skill deficit with regards to chewing was evident. Regardless, the author did show that all four participants consumed age-appropriate textures by the end of treatment. As for texture selectivity, it may be important to assess oral-motor skills before proceeding with texture fading because certain skills (e.g., mashing, chewing, tongue lateralization) may be necessary to move to the next texture successfully. A child may consume a particular higher-textured food through treatments such as stimulus fading but it is critical to understand if the child is consuming the food in the correct manner (i.e., chewing and not just swallowing the food).

Najdowski et al. (2003) evaluated the effects of stimulus fading, more specifically bite fading, magnitude of reinforcement, and escape extinction in the treatment of food selectivity in a child with ASD. Initially the authors provided an entire plate of a highly preferred food contingent on taking one bite of a nonpreferred food. Over time, the authors increased the number of nonpreferred bites and decreased magnitude of reinforcement, eventually fading out the highly preferred food. As a result of this treatment package, consumption of nonpreferred foods increased. Although this treatment package was effective, it is unclear if stimulus fading would have been effective alone.

In the previous studies on stimulus fading, there was some baseline responding so a fading agent (i.e., preferred food/drink, preferred texture) could be identified. However, in some cases where a child exhibits total food refusal it may be difficult to identify a highly preferred fading agent. In those situations, it may be more appropriate to evaluate characteristics of eating that can serve as motivating operations (MOs) for behavior maintained by negative reinforcement in the form of escape. Rivas et al. (2010) evaluated the effects of distance of the spoon both with and without escape extinction on acceptance and inappropriate mealtime behavior. The authors did not describe the participants' cognitive abilities. These authors ascertained that the distance of the spoon served as the MO for escape. For example, more inappropriate mealtime behavior was observed when the spoon was at the lips compared to other distances from the lips. The authors systematically faded the spoon so that it was closer to the lips. Results indicated that initially, inappropriate behavior was lower during fading compared to when the spoon was at the lips but as fading progressed closer to the lips, inappropriate behavior increased. Because fading did not result in continued lower levels of inappropriate behavior, the authors added escape extinction to the fading procedure. Fading plus escape extinction resulted in eventual decreases in inappropriate mealtime behavior and increases in acceptance as opposed to escape extinction alone. In addition, when the authors compared fading plus escape extinction to escape extinction alone, inappropriate mealtime behavior was initially lower in the fading plus escape extinction condition relative to escape extinction alone. However, after seven sessions, inappropriate mealtime behavior was at near zero levels in both conditions. In contrast, acceptance increased more rapidly with escape extinction alone as opposed to the fading plus escape extinction treatment. Although acceptance occurred more rapidly with escape extinction alone, caregivers may opt for stimulus fading plus escape extinction because it was associated with lower levels of inappropriate behavior.

High-p instructional sequence. The high-p instructional sequence has been shown to be an effective antecedent-based treatment for feeding problems. However, some of these treatment evaluations involved the use of escape extinction. In the high-p sequence, an instruction with a low probability of compliance (low-p instruction) is preceded by instructions with a high probability of compliance (high-p instruction). McComas et al. (2000) compared a treatment package, which included escape extinction, with and without the high-p sequence for one participant diagnosed with a feeding disorder and developmental delays. Acceptance of a bite of food (low-p response) increased more rapidly when the authors implemented the high-p procedure. However, levels of acceptance also increased in the absence of the high-p procedure after five sessions. Dawson et al. (2003) also evaluated the effectiveness of the high-p sequence with and without escape extinction with one child diagnosed with developmental delays, G-tube dependence, and total food refusal. Acceptance of food did not increase when the authors implemented the high-p sequence while inappropriate mealtime behavior (e.g., head turning, batting at the spoon) produced escape from eating. By contrast, acceptance increased when they implemented escape extinction independent of the presence or absence of the high-p sequence. Although the aforementioned studies showed that the high-p sequence can be an effective intervention, the results were not achieved without escape extinction. In addition, topographically similar responses were not used as the high-p response. For example, Dawson et al. used simple motor movements as the high-p response, which were topographically dissimilar to the low-p response, which was acceptance of the spoon.

In contrast Patel et al. (2006, 2007) used acceptance of a preferred stimulus in the mouth as a high-p response (i.e., presentation of an empty Nuk, liquid from a preferred cup, preferred liquid on a spoon, and presentation of an empty spoon). In the Patel et al. (2007) study, the authors conducted a compliance assessment to determine what response would function as the high-p response. These data indicated that three presentations of an empty spoon preceding a bite of food was effective at increasing acceptance of food in the absence of escape extinction. However, in the Patel et al. (2006) study, the high-p sequence plus escape extinction resulted in increases in acceptance as opposed to high-p alone. In addition, inappropriate mealtime behavior were lower during sessions with the high-p sequence plus escape extinction compared to escape extinction alone, suggesting that the high-p sequence enhanced the effects of escape extinction and potentially made escape extinction less aversive.

The high-p sequence also has been used to treat food selectivity. Meier et al. (2012) evaluated a high-p sequence with one child with ASD who displayed food selectivity. The data indicated an increase in acceptance of the low probability food when it was preceded by three bites of a highly preferred food. These data were replicated across three different nonpreferred foods. Over time, the authors were able to fade the bites of the preferred food for two of the three foods targeted. Similarly, Penrod et al. (2012) showed the efficacy of using a high-p sequence without escape extinction in the treatment of food selectivity with two children with ASD. They combined the high-p sequence with demand fading by starting with a step the child would tolerate such as kissing the food and then eventually working up to swallowing the food. The demand fading step served as the high-p response while consumption served as the low-p response. Each child's starting point for treatment was different and was based on the behavior the child was exhibiting in baseline. The step closest to consumption was the starting point selected for treatment. Consumption of novel foods did increase to acceptable levels for both participants, but it was likely that demand fading was responsible for the behavior change and not the high-p sequence because consumption of novel foods only increased when consumption was reinforced.

Antecedent-based interventions have been proven to be successful; however, more research is necessary to determine what other antecedent variables can be manipulated so that escape extinction can be avoided. As mentioned previously, escape extinction may not be avoidable but combining it with an antecedent-based procedure may ameliorate the negative side effects sometimes associated with escape extinction. In some cases, escape extinction alone may not be effective at increasing consumption and in those cases, antecedent-based procedures may be necessary for behavior change to occur. Future research may want to evaluate the role of pretreatment assessments to determine systematically the starting point for treatment. Moreover, the role of hunger and satiety as antecedents should also be explored further.

Treatment of packing and expulsion. Although escape extinction is a well-established treatment to address food refusal by reducing inappropriate mealtime behavior and increasing acceptance (Volkert and Piazza 2012), this treatment is not always sufficient due to collateral increases in packing or expulsion. In fact, Wilkins et al. (2014) reported program data that suggested 55 % of patients in an intensive day-treatment program required additional treatment components to address packing or expulsion. Packing involves the child pocketing or holding liquids or solids in the oral cavity without swallowing (Vaz et al. 2012) and expulsion can comprise the child spitting the food or liquid out of the mouth, removing the food or liquid from the mouth with the finger or another object, or allowing the food or liquid to fall or run out of the mouth. All of the studies described below incorporated escape extinction through nonremoval of the spoon and in one case physical guidance (see Vaz et al. 2012) and re-presentation for expulsions unless otherwise stated. In addition, nearly 60 % of these studies incorporated a positive-reinforcement-based procedure such as noncontingent reinforcement.

Redistribution and/or swallow facilitation have been shown to be effective to reduce packing (Gulotta et al. 2005; Lamm and Greer 1988; Sevin et al. 2002; Volkert et al. 2011). Redistribution comprises using a utensil (e.g., flipped spoon or a Nuk) to first gather the packed food and then deposit the food on the middle of the tongue. Sevin et al. (2002) and Gulotta et al. (2005) found that redistribution of pocketed food with a Nuk either immediately, 15 s, or 30 s after the bite entered the mouth reduced packing for children with feeding problems, including those with developmental disabilities. Several of the children in the Sevin et al. and Gulotta et al. studies also had diagnoses such as Pierre Robin sequence, vocal cord paralysis, low facial muscle tone, delayed oral-motor skills, or dysphagia.

Swallow facilitation involves touching the posterior of the tongue or using a utensil to apply slight pressure to the posterior of the tongue while the bite is deposited to promote or "elicit" swallowing. Lamm and Greer (1988) increased swallowing of three infants with feeding problems, developmental delays, and dysphagia who packed food and liquid by lightly touching the left, posterior of the tongue with a finger. Volkert et al. (2011) combined redistribution and swallow facilitation using a flipped spoon to decrease packing in one child with a history of food refusal and failure-to-thrive and one child with ASD and food selectivity. The feeder used a rubber-coated baby spoon to collect the pocketed food on the spoon 15 or 20 s after the bite entered the mouth, then inserted the spoon, rotated the spoon 180°, and then deposited the food on the posterior of the tongue by applying slight pressure and dragging the spoon toward the front of mouth.

Two studies have evaluated the use of a chaser to reduce packing, that is, a liquid or solid the child readily accepts and swallows. Vaz et al. (2012) provided a chaser immediately after the bite entered the child's mouth or following 15 s to allow for chewing to reduce packing of solid food for three participants, two of which were diagnosed with developmental delays or ASD. With two children diagnosed with feeding problems and ASD, Levin et al. (2014) combined a liquid chaser with redistribution and swallow facilitation (using a Nuk with one child and a flipped spoon with the other) to reduce packing of solid food. One child was also diagnosed with dysphagia.

Several studies have examined bite presentation methods to increase mouth clean, which is a product measure of swallowing and converse of packing, and/or decrease expulsions (e.g., Girolami et al. 2007; Hoch et al. 1995; Rivas et al. 2011; Sharp et al. 2010, 2012; Wilkins et al. 2014). With one child with severe intellectual disabilities, Hoch et al. (1995) presented bites by depressing the food on the posterior of the tongue with a Nuk and then pulled the Nuk toward the front of the tongue to decrease expulsions and increase mouth clean. Girolami et al. (2007) compared the effectiveness of presenting and re-presenting bites with an upright spoon versus a Nuk on reduction of expulsions with one child with food refusal, tracheomalacia, and bronchopulmonary dysplagia who was at risk for swallowing dysfunction. When using the Nuk, the feeder deposited the bite as described in Hoch et al. but on the middle of the tongue and using a clockwise motion. Results suggested that expulsions were lowest when the feeder presented and re-presented bites with the Nuk. With one child with food refusal, developmental delays, and limited oral-motor skills, Sharp et al. (2010) compared upright-spoon, flipped-spoon, and Nuk presentations in the absence of re-presentation for expulsions. The feeder placed the bites on the center of the tongue during flipped spoon and Nuk presentations. Compared to upright-spoon presentations, mouth clean increased and expulsions decreased slightly with both flipped-spoon and Nuk presentations. However, mouth clean was a mean of 30 and 18 % for flipped-spoon and Nuk, respectively, which was not clinically meaningful (Milnes and Piazza 2013a). Sharp et al. (2012) then compared the effects of upright and flipped spoon presentations on mouth clean and expulsions and included re-presentation for expulsions with three children diagnosed with feeding problems, developmental disabilities, and oral-motor deficits. Results indicated decreased expulsions and increased mouth clean for all participants when the feeder presented bites using a flipped spoon.

Wilkins et al. (2014) sought to compare presenting and re-presenting bites on an upright spoon and a Nuk during the initial stages of treatment rather than sequentially or after expulsion or packing emerged after treatment with escape extinction or nonremoval procedures (e.g., Sevin et al. 2002; Sharp et al. 2012). The feeder gently rolled the bite of food on the middle of the child's tongue when using the Nuk. Five of eight children, four of which were diagnosed with developmental delays, had lower levels of expulsions and four of eight children had higher levels of mouth clean when bites were presented and re-presented with the Nuk.

Although in many of the studies using Nuk and flipped spoon presentations and re-presentations the feeder placed the bite on the middle of the tongue as opposed to the posterior portion of the tongue, these bite presentation methods may still be conceptualized as swallow facilitation. Bolus formation is one of the first behaviors in the chain of swallowing and placement of the food directly on the tongue serves this role and facilitates swallowing because the child only needs to elevate the tongue and propel the food into the pharynx (Wilkins et al. 2014).

Two studies have evaluated a chin prompt to decrease expulsions or increase mouth clean. Wilkins et al. (2011) found that applying gentle upward pressure on the child's chin and lower lip for 5 s after a bite or drink entered the child's mouth during bite presentations and re-presentations decreased expulsions for four children with feeding problems, two of which were diagnosed with developmental delays and other medical complications (e.g., bronchopulmonary dysplagia, tracheostomy, prematurity). For one child with feeding problems who displayed an open-mouth posture, Dempsey et al. (2011) combined a flipped spoon presentation by depositing thickened liquid behind the middle of the child's tongue using slight downward pressure with a chin prompt to increase mouth clean. The authors did not describe the cognitive ability of the participant.

Chewing. Interventions to increase chewing have been understudied in the literature to address feeding problems. In typically eating children, chewing behavior emerges in a predictable sequence without intervention (Volkert et al. 2013). With a child who displays feeding problems, this is often not the case. Many of these children are not exposed to oral nutrition early in life due to medical complications such as prematurity or aspiration and/or refusal behavior, including but not limited to head turns, expulsions, or vomiting. Illingworth and Lister (1964) have postulated that children may not develop chewing skills if they are not exposed to solid foods at 6–7 months of age. Thus although initial food refusal is treated, there is no guarantee that the child will then learn to chew table food if treatment occurs once the child is over one year of age. The child may instead expel the food, pack the food, swallow the food without chewing, or attempt to mash the food with the tongue and roof of the mouth.

Only a handful of studies have examined chewing behavior in children with feeding problems (Butterfield and Parson 1973; Eckman et al. 2008; Volkert et al. 2013, 2014). To teach one child with Down syndrome to chew solid foods, Butterfield and Parson (1973) combined modeling, prompting and praise, reinforcement with preferred food, and shaping. Eckman et al. (2008) combined nonremoval procedures, shaping, fading, oral-motor techniques (e.g., placed yogurt or pudding in corner of mouth and instructed child to "lick the food," provision of a drink to promote lip closure), and praise and reinforcement with a preferred item to increase chewing for one child with Down syndrome and one child with history of kidney transplant, seizure, stroke, and neuromotor dysfunction. Volkert et al. (2013) sought to examine the efficacy of a reduced treatment package to increase chewing and incorporated a measure of mastication to determine if the child's chew resulted in food safe to swallow. For one child with a history of failure-to-thrive, reflux, and vomiting, the authors increased chewing using nonremoval of the spoon, least-to-most prompting which included counting chews aloud, and praise. For the second child diagnosed with developmental delays, bronchopulmonary dysplagia, G-tube dependence, and fundoplication, the authors used nonremoval of the spoon and descriptive prompting and praise to increase chewing and mastication.

As previously mentioned, some children with a history of feeding problems who do not chew may swallow whole bites prematurely prior to chewing. This early swallowing makes it difficult to teach a child to chew because the child will not or cannot keep the food between the teeth. This condition may also be a safety concern because the child is at risk for choking. Volkert et al. (2014) evaluated a treatment to decrease early swallowing, assess mastication, and increase chewing in three children with normal cognitive abilities and feeding problems. They combined nonremoval procedures, least-to-most prompting with count aloud, and a fading procedure in which they required chewing first on an empty chew tube, then a 0.6-cm by 0.6-cm piece embedded at the end of the chew tube, then a strip of food on a chew tube cut in half length wise and/or strip of food, and finally the 0.6-cm by 0.6-cm piece independent of the chew tube. One participant began to display an inappropriate chew (pulled lower jaw forward while chewing), and the authors added differential reinforcement for appropriate chewing and interrupted inappropriate chewing.

Self-feeding. For individuals with intellectual and developmental disabilities who also have feeding problems it is unclear if self-feeding emerges in the absence of treatment. In most of the studies we have summarized thus far, the feeder presented the utensil to the participant's mouth. Several studies have demonstrated physical guidance combined with reinforcement to be effective to increase self-feeding behavior of individuals with intellectual or developmental disabilities (e.g., Luiselli 1993, 1988a; Piazza et al. 1993; Reidy 1979; Sisson and Dixon 1986a, b). Physical guidance involved the feeder using hand-over-hand prompting to help the participant complete the self-feeding behavior. Although children with feeding disorders may not self-feed because of a skill deficit, it is also possible that their motivation to self-feed is affected by their historical avoidance of eating or refusal to self-feed may be the function of a motivational deficit (Rivas et al. 2014). Recently investigators have evaluated response effort manipulations or altered the contingencies related to being fed to increase self-feeding (i.e., Rivas et al. 2014; Vaz et al. 2011). Rivas et al. (2014) increased self-feeding of three children with feeding problems, G-tube or bottle dependence, by allowing the child the choice to self-feed one bite or be fed multiple bites of the same food (two children) or a less preferred food (one child). One of the children was diagnosed with pervasive developmental disorder not otherwise specified and the authors did not describe the development of the remaining participants.

Guidelines for Practitioners

For those children with feeding problems and intellectual or developmental disabilities, we cannot overstate that practitioners take an interdisciplinary approach to the assessment and treatment of the feeding problem due to its multifaceted etiology (Silverman 2010). As previously outlined in this chapter, the etiology of a feeding disorder is often a combination of medical/physiological, oral-motor, and behavioral factors. Before beginning treatment of the feeding problems, a practitioner should consult with the child's primary care physician and/or other physicians involved in the child's care (e.g., gastroenterologist, cardiologist, pulmonologist, allergist) to determine that there are no ongoing medical concerns that would preclude the child from participating in treatment (Milnes and Piazza 2013a, b). For example, if a child has unmanaged eosinophilic esophagitis (inflammation of the esophagus which is a reaction to foods, acid reflux, or allergens) which is contributing to a child's refusal to eat, the problem may be exacerbated during treatment. It is possible that a child with food selectivity is refusing to eat certain foods because of untreated esophagitis. When possible, having the consultation of a gastroenterologist or physician during the course of treatment is also recommended (Milnes and Piazza 2013a).

Due to the medical conditions associated with feeding problems, a child may be at risk for aspiration. A speech and language pathologist may determine that a modified barium swallow study is warranted to rule out aspiration or to determine the best method to reduce the risk, for example, presenting thickened liquid on a spoon rather than thin liquids from a cup while the child undergoes treatment (Silverman 2010). Thus, practitioners are cautioned to rule out swallowing concerns before beginning treatment of the feeding problem. In addition, if a child has very limited experience consuming liquids and solids, swallowing concerns may arise during the course of treatment. Although coughing and gagging may occur initially because this behavior previously resulted in escape from the drink or bite, this type of behavior should decrease. If coughing and gagging persist and are paired with abnormal or wet vocal quality, the child may be aspirating and this would necessitate consultation with a speech and language pathologist to assess this possibility.

During treatment of feeding problems, practitioners should work or consult with a registered dietician to monitor intake, growth, and other parameters of nutritional status. A registered dietician is needed to provide an estimate of energy requirements (estimated amount of calories), including fluid needs for hydration, to ensure continued growth or to maintain a child's weight and height. The registered dietician can prescribe the nutritionally appropriate formula for the child to consume so that the child's diet is balanced in terms of macro- and micronutrients. The registered dietician can inform the practitioner if the child's growth is adequate. Although weight gain is often a goal of treatment, overnutrition may become a problem (Dahl et al. 1996) and if the weight or body mass index of a child with a history of growth failure begins to accelerate too quickly, this may put the child at risk for health problems (e.g., hypertension) later in life (Adair et al. 2009).

When proceeding to treatment of total food refusal, liquid dependence, or food selectivity in a child with intellectual or developmental disabilities, there is a wealth of empirically-supported interventions based on principles of behavior analysis for practitioners to select from and implement. Therefore, practitioners should not attempt these procedures unless they are board certified behavior analysts (BCBA) or licensed psychologists with behavioral training, or are supervised by an individual with one of these credentials. Given the role negative reinforcement plays in maintaining feeding problems, it is not surprising that escape extinction has become a well-established intervention to increase acceptance and consumption of liquids and solids (Volkert and Piazza 2012). However, the literature suggests that practitioners should combine escape extinction with reinforcement-based procedures, such as noncontingent or differential reinforcement, to ameliorate inappropriate mealtime behavior and negative vocalizations (Patel et al. 2002; Piazza et al. 2003; Reed et al. 2004). Nonremoval procedures; physical guidance, which involves the feeder applying slight pressure to the mandibular joint (Ahearn et al. 1996); or using a Nuk to guide the child's mouth open (Kadey et al. 2013); or a finger prompt procedure (Borrero et al. 2013) where the feeder inserts the index finger along the upper gum line, have been used by investigators to increase acceptance.

Children with intellectual or developmental disabilities may exhibit more passive forms of food refusal (Borrero et al. 2013). For example, the child may not turn his or her head or bat at the cup or spoon, but instead, clinch the teeth so that the feeder cannot deposit the liquid or bite. Thus, the Nuk and finger prompts are viable treatments to increase acceptance when teeth clinching is the topography of refusal behavior the child exhibits. However, we caution practitioners to attempt antecedent- or reinforcement-based procedures first because limited research has been conducted regarding the safety and social validity of these procedures. For instance, when the feeder uses the Nuk prompt, the bristles of the brush may scrape the gums and cause bleeding and the feeder may be at risk of the child biting his or her finger when implementing the finger prompt. Practitioners should assess social validity of these procedures by requesting that the caregivers complete an acceptability questionnaire during or following implementation of the treatment.

Research has shown that various antecedent-based interventions, such as simultaneous presentation, the high-p instructional sequence, and stimulus fading are worthwhile strategies when used alone or in conjunction with escape extinction. Given that only a few studies have shown that antecedent manipulations are effective independent of escape extinction or other forms of treatment (e.g., demand fading), more research is necessary to determine whether these and other antecedent-based strategies are effective in isolation. In addition, future researchers should examine possible assessments that may guide practitioners in the use of antecedent-based interventions and the starting point for these strategies. More specific, assessments should identify the conditions under which antecedent manipulations may be most effective and useful in clinical settings. For example, the high-p sequence may be effective for children with ASD who have less severe inappropriate mealtime behavior and more mild forms of food selectivity (Meier et al. 2012). Manipulating antecedent variables may be especially optimal when the practitioner wishes to avoid or reduce the negative side effects often associated with escape extinction (e.g., screaming or crying, inappropriate mealtime behavior). For example, children with cardiac issues could be at greater risk for medical complications if his or her heart rate is elevated for prolonged periods of time. However, as we highlighted earlier in the chapter, before using an antecedent-based intervention such as texture fading to progress the texture of the food a child consumes, it is critical that practitioners understand if the child is or is capable of consuming the food in the correct manner.

After initial food refusal behavior is treated, many children continue to have difficulty consuming a drink or bite due to the emergence of packing or expulsion. This may not be unexpected given that oral-motor skill deficits commonly contribute to feeding problems and the child may lack the skills to actually swallow the bite. Research has demonstrated that redistribution and/or swallow facilitation procedures with the Nuk or flipped spoon are effective to reduce packing for children with intellectual and developmental disabilities (e.g., Gulotta et al. 2005; Sevin et al. 2002; Volkert et al. 2011). Investigators have hypothesized that in the case of redistribution, bolus formation is aided when the feeder collects the packed food and places it back on the child's tongue as now the child only has to propel the bolus into the pharynx by elevating the tongue. Swallow facilitation when combined with redistribution may take this one step further because this procedure involves the feeder stimulating the rear portion of the tongue with a utensil, which results in arching of the tongue (Lamm and Greer 1988), and improves or aides the child's ability to propel the bolus into the pharynx. Research has also lent support to the use of a chaser to reduce packing and investigators have speculated that this procedure may also compensate for poor oral-motor skills and facilitate a swallow by aiding bolus propulsion (Vaz et al. 2012).

Research has demonstrated the usefulness of the feeder presenting bites using a Nuk or flipped spoon rather than an upright spoon to increase mouth clean or reduce expulsions (e.g., Sharp et al. 2010, 2012; Wilkins et al. 2014). We postulate that these bite presentation methods also compensate for poor oral-motor skills because swallowing is facilitated by how the feeder deposits the bite directly on the child's tongue and this aides bolus propulsion. Two studies have also found the use of a chin prompt to either decrease expulsions or increase mouth clean (Dempsey et al. 2011; Wilkins et al. 2011) and described the participants as having an open-mouth posture (i.e., the mouth hung open). The authors in these studies also suspected that the chin prompt compensated for oral-motor skill deficits because facilitating a closed mouth allowed the child to more easily complete the remainder of the swallowing sequence.

Thus, if escape-extinction procedures combined with re-presentation do not treat packing and expulsion, it is possible that the child has oral-motor skill deficits and the literature suggests that practitioners could alter the way that the bite is presented by using a Nuk or flipped spoon or add redistribution- and/or swallow facilitation- or chin-prompt component(s) to the intervention. As we previously stated, most investigators combined these treatment components with re-presentation, thus, it is not clear if they would be effective in isolation.

Although we are hypothesizing that redistribution, swallow facilitation, and chin prompts may compensate for a child's limited oral-motor skills, it may be that positive punishment or negative reinforcement contributed to the decreases in packing or expulsions. For example, the child may have learned to swallow the bite or drink to avoid redistribution and/or swallow facilitation if these procedures were more aversive than swallowing (Volkert et al. 2011). Given this possibility, practitioners should also assess social validity or caregiver acceptability of these treatment components given their potential intrusive or aversive properties.

Although a lot is known about the assessment and treatment of feeding problems in children with intellectual and developmental disabilities and there is an abundance of literature for practitioners to reference, we feel that research efforts should begin to develop more prescriptive models to treat feeding problems such as packing and expulsion (Levin et al. 2014). It is likely that these behaviors are also maintained by avoidance or escape in many cases, however, some children may exhibit packing or expulsion even after treatment involving escape extinction. Packing and expulsion may appear in many forms. That is, a child may pack by holding food or liquid, or in some cases allowing the food or liquid to pool, between the cheek and gums, under the tongue, or between the lower lip and front teeth. Some children may have small particles of food dispersed across the entire tongue and/or on top of the teeth. Similarly, a child may expel by forcefully pushing or spraying the food or liquid from the mouth, use the hand or an object to wipe or remove the food from the mouth, or allow the food to fall out of the mouth due to an open-mouth posture. It will be important for researchers to determine what treatments are best suited or prescribed to reduce different topographies of packing or expulsion to better aid practitioners.

References

Adair, L. S., Martorell, R., Stein, A. D., Hallal, P. C., Sachdev, H. S., Prabhakaran, D., et al. (2009). Size at birth, weight gain in infancy and childhood, and adult blood pressure in 5 low- and middle-income-country cohorts: when does weight gain matter? *American Journal of Clinical Nutrition, 89*, 1383–1392.

Ahearn, W. H. (2003). Using simultaneous presentation to increase vegetable consumption in a mildly selective child with autism. *Journal of Applied Behavior Analysis, 36*, 361–365.

Ahearn, W. H., Castine, T., Nault, K., & Green, G. (2001). An assessment of food acceptance in children with autism or pervasive developmental disorder-not otherwise specified. *Journal of Autism and Developmental Disabilities, 31*, 505–511.

Ahearn, W. H., Kerwin, M. E., Eicher, P. S., Shantz, J., & Swearingin, W. (1996). An alternating treatments comparison of two intensive interventions for food refusal. *Journal of Applied Behavior Analysis, 29*, 321–332.

Auslander, G., Netzer, D., & Arad, I. (2003). Parental anxiety following discharge from hospital of their very low birth weight infants. *Family Relations, 52*, 12–21.

Babbitt, R. L., Hoch, T. A., & Coe, D. A. (1994). Behavioral feeding disorders. In D. Tuchman & R. Walters (Eds.), *Pediatric feeding and swallowing disorders: Pathology, diagnosis, and treatment*. San Diego, CA: Singular Publishing Group.

Bachmeyer, M. H., Piazza, C. C., Fredrick, L. D., Reed, G. K., Rivas, K. D., & Kadey, H. J. (2009). Functional analysis and treatment of multiply controlled inappropriate mealtime behavior. *Journal of Applied Behavior Analysis, 42*, 641–658.

Borrero, C. S., Schlereth, G. J., Rubio, E. K., & Taylor, T. (2013). A comparison of two physical guidance procedures in the treatment of pediatric food refusal. *Behavioral Interventions, 28*, 261–280.

Borrero, C. S., Woods, J. N., Borrero, J. C., Masler, E. A., & Lesser, A. D. (2010). Descriptive analyses of pediatric food refusal and acceptance. *Journal of Applied Behavior Analysis, 43*, 71–88.
Buckley, S. D., & Newchok, D. K. (2005). An evaluation of simultaneous presentation and differential reinforcement with response cost to reduce packing. *Journal of Applied Behavior Analysis, 20*, 155–163.
Butterfield, W. H., & Parson, R. (1973). Modeling and shaping by parents to develop chewing behavior in their retarded child. *Journal of Behavior Therapy and Experimental Psychiatry, 4*, 285–287.
Christophersen, E. R., & Hall, C. L. (1978). Eating patterns and associated problems encountered in normal children. *Issues in Comprehensive Pediatric Nursing, 3*, 1–16.
Cohen, S. A., Piazza, C. C., & Navathe, A. (2006). Feeding and nutrition. In I. L. Rubin & A. C. Cooper, L. J., Wacker, D. P., McComas, J. J., Peck, S. M., Richman, D., Drew, J.,…Brown, K. (1995). Use of component analyses to identify active variables in treatment packages for children with feeding disorders. *Journal of Applied Behavior Analysis, 28*, 139–154.
Cooper, J. O., Heron, T. E., & Heward, W. L. (1987). *Applied Behavior Analysis*. New Jersey: Prentice Hall, Inc.
Dahl, M., Thommessen, M., Rasmussen, M., & Selberg, T. (1996). Feeding and nutritional characteristics in children with moderate or severe cerebral palsy. *Acta Paediatrics, 85*, 697–701.
Dawson, J. E., Piazza, C. C., Sevin, B. M., Gulotta, C. S., Lerman, D., & Kelley, M. (2003). Use of the high-probability instructional sequence and escape extinction in a child with a feeding disorder. *Journal of Applied Behavior Analysis, 36*, 105–108.
Dempsey, J., Piazza, C. C., Groff, R. A., & Kozisek, J. M. (2011). A flipped spoon and chin prompt to increase mouth clean. *Journal of Applied Behavior Analysis, 44*, 961–965.
Eckman, N., Williams, K. E., Riegel, K., & Paul, C. (2008). Teaching chewing: A structured approach. *American Journal of Occupational Therapy, 62*, 514–521.
Field, P., Garland, M., & Williams, K. (2003). Correlates of specific childhood feeding problems. *Journal of Pediatric Child Health, 39*, 299–304.
Freedman, D. S., Dietz, W. H., Srinivasan, S. R., & Berenson, G. S. (1999). The relation of overweight to cardiovascular risk factors among children and adolescents: The Bogalusa Heart Study. *Pediatrics, 103*, 1175–1182.
Garcia, J., & Koelling, R. A. (1966). Relation of cue to consequence in avoidance learning. *Psychonomic Science, 6*, 123–124.
Girolami, P. A., Boscoe, J. H., & Roscoe, N. (2007). Decreasing expulsions by a child with a feeding disorder: Using a brush to present and re-present food. *Journal of Applied Behavior Analysis, 40*, 749–753.
Gouge, A. L., & Ekvall, S. W. (1975). Diets of handicapped children: Physical, psychological and socioeconomic correlations. *American Journal of Mental Deficiency, 80,* 149–157.
Graves, J. K., & Ware, M. E. (1990). Parents and health professionals' perceptions concerning parental stress during a child's hospitalization. *Child Health Care, 19*, 37–42.
Green, K.F., & Garcia, J. (1971). Recuperation from illness flavor enhancement for rats. *Science, 173,* 749–751.
Green, K. F., Holmstrom, L. S., & Wollman, M. A. (1974). Relation of cue to consequence in rats: effect of recuperation from illness. *Behavioral Biology, 10*, 491–503.
Gulotta, C. S., Piazza, C. C., Patel, M. R., & Layer, S. A. (2005). Using food redistribution to reduce packing in children with severe food refusal. *Journal of Applied Behavior Analysis, 38*, 39–50.
Hanley, G. P., Iwata, B. A., & McCord, B. E. (2003). Functional analysis of problem behavior: A review. *Journal of Applied Behavior Analysis, 36*, 147–185.
Hendy, H. M., Williams, K. E., Camise, T. S., Eckman, N., & Hedemann, A. (2009). The parent mealtime action scale (PMAS). Development and association with children's diet and weight. *Appetite, 52*, 328–339.
Hoch, T. A., Babbitt, R. L., Coe, D. A., Duncan, A., & Trusty, E. M. (1995). A swallow induction avoidance procedure to establish eating. *Journal of Behavior Therapy and Experimental Psychiatry, 26*, 41–50.

Hoch, T. A., Babbitt, R. L., Coe, D. A., Krell, D. M., & Hackbert, L. (1994). Contingency contacting: Combining positive reinforcement and escape extinction procedures to treat persistent food refusal. *Behavior Modification, 18*, 106–128.

Hyman, P. E. (1994). Gastroesophageal reflux: One reason why baby won't eat. *The Journal of Pediatrics, 125*, 103–109.

Illingworth, R. S., & Lister, J. (1964). The critical or sensitive period, with special reference to certain feeding problems in infants and children. *Journal of Pediatrics, 65*, 839–848.

Kadey, H. J., Roane, H. S., Diaz, J. C., & McCarthy, J. M. (2013). An evaluation of chewing and swallowing for a child diagnosed with autism. *Journal of Developmental and Physical Disabilities, 25*, 343–354.

Kerwin, M. E. (1999). Empirically supported treatments in pediatric psychology: Severe feeding problems. *Journal of Pediatric Psychology, 24*, 193–214.

Kozlowski, K. M., Matson, J. L., Fodstad, J. C., & Moree, B. N. (2011). Feeding therapy in a child with autistic disorder. *Clinical Case Studies, 20*, 1–11.

Lamm, N., & Greer, D. (1988). Induction and maintenance of swallowing responses in infants with dysphasia. *Journal of Applied Behavior Analysis, 21*, 143–156.

LaRue, R. H., Stewart, V., Piazza, C. C., Volkert, V. M., Patel, M. R., & Zeleny, J. (2011). Escape as reinforcement and escape extinction in the treatment of feeding problems. *Journal of Applied Behavior Analysis, 44*, 719–735.

Latif, A. H., Heinz, P., & Cook, R. (2002). Iron deficiency in autism and Asperger Syndrome. *Autism, 6*, 103–114.

Laud, R. B., Girolami, P. A., Boscoe, J. H., & Gulotta, C. S. (2009). Treatment outcomes for severe feeding problems in children with autism spectrum disorder. *Behavior Modification, 33*, 520–536.

Levin, D., Volkert, V. M., & Piazza, C. C. (2014). A multicomponent treatment package to reduce packing in children with feeding and autism spectrum disorders. *Behavior Modification, 38*, 940–963.

Linscheid, T. R., Budd, K. S., & Rasnake, L. K. (1995). Pediatric feeding disorders. In M. C. Roberts (Ed.), *Handbook of pediatric psychology* (pp. 501–515). New York: Guilford.

Ludwig, D. S., Majzoub, J. A., Al-Zahrani, A., Dallal, G. E., Blanco, I., & Roberts, S. B. (1999). High glycemic index foods, overeating, and obesity. *Pediatrics, 103*, e26.

Luiselli, J. K. (1988a). Behavioral feeding intervention with deaf-blind, multihandicapped children. *Child and Family Behavior Therapy, 10*, 49–62.

Luiselli, J. K. (1993). Training self-feeding in children who are deaf and blind. *Behavior Modification, 17*, 457–473.

Luiselli, J. K., Ricciardi, J. N., & Gilligan, K. (2005). Liquid fading to establish milk consumption by a child with autism. *Behavioral Interventions, 20*, 155–163.

Lukens, C. T., & Linscheid, T. R. (2008). Development and validation of an inventory to assess mealtime behavior problems in children with autism. *Journal of Autism and Developmental Disorders, 38*, 342–352.

Manikam, R., & Perman, J. A. (2000). Pediatric feeding disorders. *Journal of Clinical Gastroenterology, 30*, 34–46.

Matson, J. L., & Kuhn, D. E. (2001). Identifying feeding problems in mentally retarded persons: development and reliability of the screening tool for feeding problems (STEP). *Research in Developmental Disabilities, 21*, 165–172.

McComas, J. J., Wacker, D. P., Cooper, L. J., Peck, S., Golonka, Z., Millard, T., et al. (2000). Effects of the high-probability request procedure: Patterns of responding to low-probability requests. *Journal of Developmental and Physical Disabilities, 12*, 157–171.

Meier, A. E., Fryling, M. J., & Wallace, M. D. (2012). Using high-probability foods to increase acceptance of low-probability foods. *Journal of Applied Behavior Analysis, 45*, 149–153.

Milnes, S. M., & Piazza, C. C. (2013a). Feeding disorders. In R. Hastings & J. Rojahn (Eds.), *International review of research in developmental disabilities* (pp. 143–166). London: Academic Press.

Milnes, S. M., & Piazza, C. C. (2013b). Intensive treatment of pediatric feeding disorders. In. D. D. Reed, F. D. Digennaro Reed, & J. K. Luiselli (Eds.), *Handbook of crisis intervention and developmental disabilities* (pp. 393–408). New York: Springer.

Mueller, M. M., Piazza, C. C., Patel, M. R., Kelley, M. E., & Pruett, A. (2004). Increasing variety of foods consumed by blending nonpreferred foods into preferred foods. *Journal of Applied Behavior Analysis, 37*, 159–170.

Najdowski, A. C., Wallace, M. D., Doney, J. K., & Ghezzi, P. M. (2003). Parental assessment and treatment of food selectivity in the natural settings. *Journal of Applied Behavior Analysis, 36*, 383–386.

Palmer, S., & Horn, S. (1978). Feeding problems in children. In S. Palmer & S. Ekvall (Eds.), *Pediatric nutrition in developmental disorders* (pp. 107–129). Springfield, Ill: Charles C. Thomas.

Patel, M. R., Piazza, C. C., Kelly, M. L., Ochsner, C. A., & Santana, C. M. (2001). Using a fading procedure to increase fluid consumption in a child with feeding problems. *Journal of Applied Behavior Analysis, 34*, 357–360.

Patel, M. R., Piazza, C. C., Martinez, C. J., Volkert, V. M., & Santana, C. M. (2002). An evaluation of two differential reinforcement procedures with escape extinction to treat food refusal. *Journal of Applied Behavior Analysis, 35*, 363–374.

Patel, M. R., Reed, G. K., Piazza, C. C., Bachmeyer, M. H., Layer, S. A., & Pabico, R. S. (2006). An evaluation of a high-probability instructional sequence to increase acceptance of food and decrease inappropriate behavior in children with pediatric feeding disorders. *Research in Developmental Disabilities, 27*, 430–442.

Patel, M., Reed, G. K., Piazza, C. C., Mueller, M., Bachmeyer, M. H., & Layer, S. A. (2007). Use of a high-probability instructional sequence to increase compliance to feeding demands in the absence of escape extinction. *Behavioral Interventions, 22*, 305–310.

Penrod, B., Gardella, L., & Fernand, J. (2012). An evaluation of a high-probability instructional sequence combined with low-probability demand fading in the treatment of food selectivity. *Journal of Applied Behavior Analysis, 45*, 527–537.

Perske, R., Clifton, A., McClean, B. M., & Stein, J. I. (1977). *Mealtimes for severely and profoundly handicapped persons: New concepts and attitudes*. Baltimore: University Park Press.

Piazza, C. C., Anderson, C., & Fisher, W. W. (1993). Teaching self-feeding skills to children with Rett syndrome. *Developmental Medicine and Child Psychology, 35*, 991–996.

Piazza, C. C., Fisher, W. W., Brown, K. A., Shore, B. A., Patel, M. R., Katz, R. M., et al. (2003a). Functional analysis of inappropriate mealtime behaviors. *Journal of Applied Behavior Analysis, 36*, 187–204.

Piazza, C. C., Patel, M. R., Gulotta, C. S., Sevin, B. M., & Layer, S. A. (2003b). On the relative contributions of positive reinforcement and escape extinction in the treatment of food refusal. *Journal of Applied Behavior Analysis, 36*, 309–324.

Piazza, C. C., Patel, M. R., Santana, C. M., Goh, H. L., Delia, M. D., & Lancaster, B. M. (2002). An evaluation of simultaneous and sequential presentation of preferred and nonpreferred foods to treat food selectivity. *Journal of Applied Behavior Analysis, 35*, 259–270.

Remijn, L., Speyer, R., Groen, B. E., van Limbeek, J., & Nijhuis-van der Sanden, M. W. G. (2014). Validity and reliability of the mastication observation and evaluation (MOE) instrument. *Research in Developmental Disabilities, 35*, 1551–1561.

Reed, G. K., Piazza, C. C., Patel, M. R., Layer, S. A., Bachmeyer, M. H., Bethke, S. D., et al. (2004). On the relative contributions of noncontingent reinforcement and escape extinction in the treatment of food refusal. *Journal of Applied Behavior Analysis, 37*, 24–42.

Reidy, T.J. (1979). Training appropriate eating behaviour in a pediatric rehabilitation setting: a case study. *Archives of Physical Medicine and Rehabilitation, 60*, 226–230.

Revusky, S. H., & Bedarf, E. W. (1967). Association of illness with prior ingestion of novel foods. *Science, 155*, 219–220.

Rivas, K. D., Piazza, C. C., Patel, M. R., & Bachmeyer, M. H. (2010). Spoon distance fading with and without escape extinction as treatment for food refusal. *Journal of Applied Behavior Analysis, 43*, 673–683.

Rivas, K. D., Piazza, C. C., Kadey, H. J., Volkert, V. M., & Stewart, V. (2011). Sequential treatment of a feeding problem using a pacifier and flipped spoon. *Journal of Applied Behavior Analysis, 44*, 387–391.

Rivas, K. M., Piazza, C. C., Roane, H. S., Volkert, V. M., Stewart, V., Kadey, H. J., Groff, R. A. (2014). Analysis of self-feeding in children with feeding disorders. *Journal of Applied Behavior Analysis, 47*, 1–14.

Rommel, N., De Meyer, A. M., Feenstra, L., & Veereman-Wauters, G. (2003). The complexity of feeding problems in 700 infants and young children presenting to a tertiary care institution. *Journal of Pediatric Gastroenterology and Nutrition, 37*, 75–84.

Rumsey, D. G., & Rosenberg, A. M. (2013). Childhood scurvy: A pediatric rheumatology perspective. *Journal of Rheumatology, 40*, 201–202.

Schreck, K. M., Williams, K. E., & Smith, A. F. (2004). A comparison of eating behaviors between children with and without autism. *Journal of Autism and Developmental Disorders, 34*, 433–438.

Seiverling, L., Hendy, H. M., & Williams, K. E. (2011). The screening tool of feeding problems applied to children (STEP-CHILD): Psychometric characteristics and associations with child and parent variables. *Research in Developmental Disabilities, 32*, 1122–1129.

Sevin, B. M., Gulotta, C. S., Sierp, B. J., Rosica, L. A., & Miller, L. J. (2002). Analysis of response covariation among multiple topographies of food refusal. *Journal of Applied Behavior Analysis, 35*, 65–68.

Sharp, W. G., Harker, S., & Jaquess, D. L. (2010a). Comparison of bite-presentation methods in the treatment of food refusal. *Journal of Applied Behavior Analysis, 43*, 739–743.

Sharp, W. G., Jaquess, D. L., & Lukens, C. T. (2013). Multi-method assessment of feeding problems among children with autism spectrum disorders. *Research in Autism Spectrum Disorders, 7*, 56–65.

Sharp, W. G., Jaquess, D. L., Morton, J. F., & Herzinger, C. V. (2010b). Pediatric feedind disorders: A quantitative synthesis of treatment outcomes. *Clinical Child and Family Psychological Review, 13*, 348–365.

Sharp, W. G., Odom, A., & Jaquess, D. L. (2012). Comparison of upright and flipped spoon presentations to guide treatment of food refusal. *Journal of Applied Behavior Analysis, 45*, 83–96.

Sheppard, J. J., Hochman, R., & Baer, C. (2014). The dysphagia disorder survey: Validation of an assessment for swallowing and feeding function in developmental disability. *Research in Developmental Disabilities, 25*, 929–942.

Shore, B. A., Babbitt, R. L., Williams, K. E., Coe, D. A., & Snyder, A. (1998). Use of texture fading in the treatment of food selectivity. *Journal of Applied Behavior Analysis, 31*, 621–633.

Silverman, A. H. (2010). Interdisciplinary care for feeding problems in children. *Nutrition in Clinical Practices, 25*, 160–165.

Sisson, L. A., & Dixon, M. J. (1986a). A behavioral approach to the training and assessment of feeding skills in multihandicapped children. *Applied Research in Mental Retardation, 7*, 149–163.

Sisson, L. A., & Dixon, M. J. (1986b). Improving mealtime behaviors through token reinforcement. A study with mentally retarded behaviorally disordered children. *Behavior Modification, 10*, 333–354.

Sullivan, P. B., Juszczak, E., Lambert, B. R., Rose, M., Ford-Adams, M. E., & Johnson, A. (2002). Impact of feeding problems on nutritional intake and growth: Oxford feeding study II. *Developmental Medicine and Child Neurology, 44*, 461–467.

Vaz, P. M., Piazza, C. C., Stewart, V., Volkert, V. M., Groff, R. A., & Patel, M. R. (2012). Using a chaser to decrease packing in children with feeding disorders. *Journal of Applied Behavior Analysis, 45*, 97–105.

Vaz, P. M., Volkert, V. M., & Piazza, C. C. (2011). Using negative reinforcement to increase self-feeding in a child with food selectivity. *Journal of Applied Behavior Analysis, 44*, 915–920.
Volkert, V. M., & Piazza, C. C. (2012). Empirically supported treatments for pediatric feeding disorders. In P. Sturmey & M. Herson (Eds.), *Handbook of evidence based practice in clinical psychology*. Hoboken, NJ: Wiley, USA.
Volkert, V. M., Peterson, K. M., Zeleny, J., & Piazza, C. C. (2014). A clinical protocol to increase chewing and assess mastication in children with feeding disorders. *Behavior Modification, 38*, 705–729.
Volkert, V. M., Piazza, C. C., Vaz, P. M., & Frese, J. (2013). A pilot study to increase chewing in children with feeding disorders. *Behavior Modification, 37*, 391–408.
Volkert, V. M., Vaz, P. M., Piazza, C. C., Frese, J., & Barnett, L. (2011). Using a flipped spoon to decrease packing in children with feeding disorders. *Journal of Applied Behavior Analysis, 44*, 617–621.
Wilkins, J. W., Piazza, C. C., Groff, R. A., & Vaz, P. M. (2011). Chin prompt plus re-presentation as treatment for expulsion in children with feeding disorders. *Journal of Applied Behavior Analysis, 44*, 513–522.
Williams, K. E., & Seiverling, L. (2010). Eating problems in children with autism spectrum disorders. *Topics in Clinical Nutrition, 25*, 27–37.
Wilkins, J. W., Piazza, C. C., Groff, R. A., Volkert, V. M., Koziesk, J. M., & Milnes, S. M. (2014). Utensil manipulation during initial treatment of pediatric feeding disorders. *Journal of Applied Behavior Analysis, 47*, 694–709.

Chapter 8
Sleep and Sleep-Related Problems

James K. Luiselli

Many children and adults with intellectual and developmental disabilities (IDD) also have serious, persistent, and sometimes treatment-resistant sleep problems (Durand 2014a; Lancioni et al. 1999; Luiselli 1995). Summarizing a large body of sleep research in IDD, Richdale and Baker (2014) reported poor sleep habits and sleep disorders in a range of 24–86 %. Notably, certain clinical populations within IDD have a high prevalence of sleep problems, for example, Angelman's syndrome, Down syndrome, and Prader-Willi syndrome (Cotton and Richdale 2010; Stores and Stores 2013). As well, impaired sleep occurs in 33–80 % of individuals with autism spectrum disorder (ASD) (Goldman et al. 2011; Mannion and Leader 2013; Rzepecka et al. 2011). Population statistics notwithstanding, Richdale and Baker (2014) cautioned that sleep research in IDD features heterogeneous samples, variable definitions of sleep problems, and different sleep assessment instruments with inconsistent psychometric properties. Furthermore, many sleep problems among people with IDD do not conform to the diagnostic criteria contained in formal classification nosology such as the *Diagnostic and Statistical Manual of Mental Disorders—Fifth Edition* (*DSM-V*) (American Psychiatric Association 2013) and the *International Classification of Sleep Disorders* (*ICSD*-2).

More specifically, *disruptive bedtime routines* are frequently displayed by children and adults who have IDD. This problem occurs as a person actively resisting a parent or care-provider request to "get ready for bed." A child, for example, may simply refuse to stop playing or watching television when his mother or father

J.K. Luiselli (✉)
Clinical Solutions, Inc., North East Educational and Developmental Support Center, 1120 Main Street, Tewksbury, MA 018776, USA
e-mail: jluiselli@needsctr.org

J.K. Luiselli (ed.), *Behavioral Health Promotion and Intervention in Intellectual and Developmental Disabilities*, Evidence-Based Practices in Behavioral Health,
DOI 10.1007/978-3-319-27297-9_8

initiate the bedtime instruction. Similarly, an adult in a residential group-home might walk away from a care-provider and engage in a competing activity at bedtime. Some children and adults exhibit noncompliance with co-occurring challenging behavior such as throwing objects, loud vocalizing, self-injury, and aggression.

Delayed sleep onset is a second sleep problem among people with IDD. Certainly, a child or adult with bedtime resistance will not be in bed and fall asleep at a desired time. However, delayed sleep onset can present in other ways. One example is a parent or care-provider who allows a later bedtime to avoid compliance conflicts. Children, in particular, may be permitted to play with toys and other preferred objects in bed because "it keeps them quiet." Unfortunately, this strategy only delays sleep and over time, contributes to poor sleep hygiene (Ferber 2006).

A third problem, *sleep-wake cycle disturbance*, manifests as erratic and typically short-bout sleeping episodes during the evening and early morning hours. In some cases a child or adult may go to bed, fall asleep at an acceptable time, but then wake-up prematurely and remain awake. The person may be relatively quiet or more commonly, get out of bed, become disruptive, and distract other people in the living environment. Among children in particular this situation can lead to a further problem of co-sleeping in the parent's bed.

Finally, a difficulty initiating and maintaining sleep can result in *hypersomnia*, a condition of excessive daytime sleep (Alik et al. 2006; Liu et al. 2006). Some parents and care-providers are reluctant to interrupt a person sleeping during the day because their actions provoke agitation and oppositional behavior. Unfortunately, prolonged periods of diurnal sleep compromise instructional and habilitation activities with a child or adult, as well as promote sleep-wake cycle disturbance previously described.

This chapter reviews the research base and practice applications of behavioral sleep intervention for people with IDD. I describe several studies which illustrate well established procedures within the discipline of applied behavior analysis (ABA), the results of systematic intervention, and several research-to-practice considerations.

Negative Effects of Sleep Problems in IDD

Regardless of behavior topography, there are similar detrimental effects when a person sleeps poorly. One set of concerns is an increased risk for medical conditions, possibly cardiovascular abnormalities, obesity, and diabetes (Colton and Altevogt 2006; Doran et al. 2006). Additionally, sleep disturbance negatively influences mood, affect, energy level, and executive function (Stores 2002). Within families of children with IDD, mothers report increased stress, anxiety, and depression (Chu and Richdale 2009; Gallagher et al. 2010; Meltzer and Mindell 2007). A child with a sleep problem may also disrupt the sleeping of family members (Cotton and Richdale 2010), producing further distress that exacerbates an already tension-filled home. The same concern is apparent with adults who have IDD and reside with peers in a staff-supervised group-home or congregate living arrangement (Harvey et al. 2003).

Several applied behavior analytic studies have confirmed functional relationships between impaired sleep and daytime performance of people with IDD. O'Reilly (1995) described a 31-year-old man with IDD who had sleep deprivation, typically waking up between 2:00–3:00 a.m., and not returning to bed. During an experimental functional analysis, the man either received attention from a therapist or removal of task demands contingent on his aggression. Results showed that aggression was demonstrably higher in the demand condition when the man had less than 5 h sleep the night before compared to preceding evenings when he slept more than 5 h. In summary, the man was better able to tolerate therapist-presented demands when he slept more soundly.

Kennedy and Meyers (1996) reported a similar finding with a 15-year old boy and an 18-year old girl who had IDD. Both individuals participated in functional analysis sessions in which attention, demand termination, and no attention were contingent on their destructive behavior. In each case, sleep deprivation the day before functional analysis sessions was associated with higher behavior frequencies in the demand termination condition as opposed to when the boy and girl were not sleep-deprived.

Reed et al. (2005) evaluated the effects of sleep disruption on mealtime behavior of a 4-year old boy who had developmental delays and a complex medical profile consisting of broncho-pulmonary dysplasia, gastroesophageal reflux, and immune deficiency. Disrupted sleep was defined as having to awake the boy from periods of daytime sleeping 15 min preceding meals at a pediatric inpatient unit. Under baseline conditions he had zero-to-low percentages of food consumption when his sleep was disrupted. These findings were similar during an initial intervention phase with consumption-contingent positive reinforcement. Adding escape extinction to intervention improved bite acceptance under both sleep-disrupted and sleep-not disrupted conditions. The implication from these findings is that certain mediating conditions might attenuate the behavior-compromising effects of sleep deprivation.

In a clinical example, Eshbaugh et al. (2004) reported the case of a 32-year old man who had IDD, autism, late sleep onset, frequent night awakenings, and hypersomnia. During the day he displayed aggression and self-injury, many times in response to instructional and sleep-interruption interactions from care-providers. After being prescribed a sleep-facilitating medication at bedtime, the man had fewer instances of daytime challenging behavior and sleeping episodes. Eshbaugh et al. (2004) suggested that this outcome was likely the result of him better tolerating care-provider demands because he slept more hours the night before. Although this case study was not planned as an experimental evaluation, the results once again illustrate how problem behavior during waking hours can be linked to nocturnal sleep disturbance.

Sleep Assessment and Measurement

Pre-intervention screening is necessary to precisely identify and define a person's sleep problem. Instruments such as the *Pediatric Sleep Questionnaire* (Chervin et al. 2000), *Children's Sleep Habits Questionnaire* (*CSHQ*) (Owens et al. 2000), and *Behavioral Evaluation of Disorders of Sleep* (*BEDS*) (Schreck et al. 2003) are used clinically and in research protocols (Malow et al. 2014; Taylor et al. 2012). However, many of these questionnaires are not designed for people who have IDD. It is also worth noting that most standardized screening instruments applied in IDD, as well as sleep assessment methods in general, have focused on children and youth but not adults. Another qualification is that questionnaires and survey-like formats document the subjective impressions of respondents—ideally, these reports should be validated through objective measurement.

A second facet of pre-intervention screening is ruling out medical conditions that possibly contribute to a sleep problem (e.g., obstructive sleep apnea). Physician evaluation would be the first step in this regard. Assessment can also be performed with an instrument such as the 24-h *Sleep History Questionnaire* (*SHQ*) (Garcia and Wills 2000). And as discussed below, functional behavioral assessment done by a qualified professional can isolate potential non-social precursors to sleep problems and recommendation for more extensive review from a medical specialist.

Once pre-intervention screening is completed, it is customary to have parents, care-providers, and research staff record sleep problems through *direct measurement*. The different methods for gathering data include frequency counts, cumulative duration, interval recording, or some combination of procedures. For example, Luiselli et al. (2005) described a data recording methodology that care-providers implemented to document sleep patterns of 59 adults with IDD (M age = 42.5 years) living in 16 community-based group homes. A recording form designated consecutive, 30-min intervals starting at 7:00 p.m. in the evening and concluding at 7:00 a.m. the next day. Three sleep behaviors were included on the form: (a) *awake*: adult's eyes are open while she/he is in or out of bed, (b) *asleep*: adult's eyes are closed while she/he is in bed, and (c) *awake and disruptive*: adult's eyes are open while she/he is in or out of bed and displaying specified disruptive behavior. An assigned care-provider began each 30-min interval by circulating through the group-home, locating each adult, observing for approximately 10-s, and recording which of the three sleep behaviors were occurring at that time. These data were subsequently converted for each adult by summing the respective 30-min intervals per behavior. This measurement method is similar to a *sleep diary* that parents often complete and Durand (2014a) noted "yields useful information that can assist with assessing the sleep problem and designing an intervention plan" (p. 178).

Actigraphy is an automated objective measurement method that can be combined with parent and care-provider reports (Meltzer et al. 2012; Wiggs and Stores 2004). A person wears an actigraph on the wrist to monitor and record limb movements in bed. The actigraphy data provide an estimate of time sleeping but in some cases may not reliably represent actual sleep duration (Sadeh 2011). An additional complication with actigraphy is a child or adult who will not tolerate wearing a wrist device. Positioning an actigraph on another part of the body or in a pajama pocket may be an alternative arrangement (Souders et al. 2009). Measuring sleep through portable time-lapse video recording, known as *videosomnography*, also eliminates the need for direct observational measurement and has been shown to correlate well with actigraphy (Sitnick et al. 2008).

As a point of emphasis, direct measurement should serve the purpose of clarifying antecedent and consequence variables which set the occasion for and maintain a sleep problem. Functional behavioral assessment is performed using indirect methods such as the *Motivation Assessment Scale* (*MAS*) (Durand and Crimmins 1992), *Functional Analysis Interview* (*FAI*) (O'Neill et al. 1997), and *Questions About Behavior Function* (*QABF*) (Paclawskyi et al. 2000). Another approach to functional behavioral assessment is descriptive methods consisting of antecedent-behavior-consequence (A-B-C) data recording and analysis (Reed and Azuly 2011). In a study with 6 children who had developmental disabilities and sleep problems, Didden et al. (1998) first interviewed parents "during which information was obtained on medical history, emergence of sleeping problems, and antecedents and consequences of nighttime disruptive behaviors" (p. 88). The next phase of assessment was having parents keep a 6-night record of their child's sleeping problems and associated conditions. The hypotheses derived from these functional behavioral assessments were that four of the children were disruptive at bedtime as the consequence of parental attention, one child was fearful of falling asleep, and one child reacted to nighttime seizures and attention contingencies. Function-based intervention plans were subsequently introduced with each child.

Behavioral Sleep Intervention

Most behavioral intervention research for sleep and sleep-related problems in IDD has combined antecedent and consequence procedures. The goal of antecedent intervention is to prevent problem behavior from occurring by manipulating (a) the presence and absence of discriminative stimuli, and (b) the motivating operations (MOs) that influence response-environmental relationships (Luiselli 2008). Consequence procedures include positive reinforcement of alternative behavior, compliance, periods of time without disruption, and less frequently, contingent negative events (punishment). Sleep intervention behavior plans are optimally effective when they are function-based and implemented in a person's natural environment by familiar care-providers. This section of the chapter describes several intervention studies that addressed problems of delayed sleep onset, disruptive bedtime routines, early morning and night awakenings, daytime sleeping, and sleep terrors.

Delayed Sleep Onset-Disruptive Bedtime Routines-Night Awakenings. In a study with children who has developmental disabilities, Didden et al. (1998) defined a conventional *extinction* approach to disruptive behavior evident at bedtime: "Parents were asked to put the child in bed and to carry out a bedtime routine. After bidding the child 'good night' they had to leave the room and were instructed not to re-enter the room until the morning" (p. 89). To be effective, the stimuli that reinforce problem behavior must be accurately identified and continuously withheld when extinction is applied. Unfortunately, extinction is usually accompanied by intensive "bursts" of behavior that can be prolonged and not easily tolerated by parents and care-providers. As such, standard extinction programming is generally not recommended as sleep intervention in IDD (Durand 2014b). An alternative method, *graduated extinction*, has some empirical support with typically developing infants and children (Adams and Rickert 1989; Kuhn and Eliot 2003; Meltzer and Mindell 2004). This procedure entails a parent or care-provider immediately attending to the person when she/he is disruptive but then withholding attention for gradually increasing periods of time until problem behavior ceases.

Piazza and Fisher (1991) evaluated an antecedent and consequence control intervention for delayed sleep onset and sleep-wake cycle disturbance in four children with IDD. Conducted on a specialized inpatient unit, the dependent measures in this study were the percentage of recording intervals the children were either awake or asleep while in or out of bed. During baseline phases of a multiple baseline design, care-providers prompted each child to go to bed according to a consistent bedtime routine. They repeated prompting if the children did not go to bed when requested or if they had early or night awakenings. From baseline data the research staff determined the average time of rapid sleep onset for each child. With a *faded bedtime* protocol in effect, an initial bedtime was set by adding 30 min to the baseline average, then "adjusting the child's bedtime by 30 min each night based on the latency to sleep onset for the previous night" (p. 132). A child's success or failure each evening made time-to-bed 30 min earlier or later the next night respectively. A *response cost* component of intervention removed the children from their rooms for 60 min if they were not asleep within 15 min of the scheduled bedtime—they were then returned to bed and the procedures were re-implemented if necessary. This faded bedtime + response cost intervention successfully increased durations of appropriate sleep and decreased frequency of night awakenings for all of the children.

A study by O'Reilly et al. (2004) exemplifies the process of assessment-derived sleep intervention. The participant was a 5-year old girl who had IDD and difficulty falling asleep when put to bed. During a pre-intervention choice assessment the girl was allowed to play with favorite toys, watch videos, and interact with her mother following her getting out of bed and leaving the bedroom. This assessment revealed that she preferred being with her mother most of the time. Next, the researchers evaluated the effects of systematic sleep scheduling on delayed sleep onset. They requested mother to put the girl to bed at 8:00 p.m. each evening, eliminate access to books and toys, and return her to bed when she exited the bedroom. This intervention plan was ineffective until it was augmented with mother delivering fixed-time (FT) social attention to the girl every 5 min until she fell asleep. An ABAB reversal design verified that sleep scheduling + FT attention improved sleep onset and reduced frequency of leaving the bedroom. The success of this intervention can be attributed to documenting the girl's preference for her mother's attention and programming social reinforcement accordingly.

Knight and Johnson (2014) designed a four-component intervention plan to treat bedtime resistance and night awakenings of three children (4–5 years old) with ASD. Parents were trained to implement procedures in their homes during the children's natural bedtime routines. They applied *circadian rhythm management* (Ferber 2006) by establishing fixed bedtime and wake times for their children and not allowing the children to lie in the dark or watch television after awakening. The second component of intervention was presenting *white noise* in the children's bedrooms, set at 50–75 dB, throughout the overnight hours. Prior to going to bed the parents instructed their child to complete a *pre-bedtime calming routine* of 4–6 quiet activities such as reading a story or taking a bath. Finally, the parents responded with *graduated extinction* if the children exhibited disruptive behavior at bedtime or any other time before waking up in the morning. A multiple baseline design across children revealed that the intervention plan reduced sleep awakenings and sleep latency. Social validation assessment showed that parents were generally satisfied with the intervention procedures and sleep outcomes.

One other approach to bedtime resistance, as yet only evaluated with typically developing children, is the Bedtime Pass Program (BPP) piloted by Friman and colleagues (Friman et al. 1999; Moore et al. 2007). To implement the BPP, parents put their child to bed according to schedule and give the child a card (pass) exchangeable for one "free trip" out of the bedroom or one parent visit before returning to bed. Parents subsequently "ignore" the child's attention-generating behavior. The BPP is an extinction-based procedure that was shown to be effective in reducing bedtime crying and leaving the bedroom in two, single-case studies (Friman et al. 1999) and a randomized control trial (Moore et al. 2007). Further endorsement of the program was realized by parental reports of high satisfaction and intervention acceptability. Future research may find that the BPP is equally beneficial with children who have IDD.

Large-scale parent training programs have been an effective modality for sleep problems. To illustrate, Malow et al. (2014) included 80 children (2–10 years old) with ASD and sleep onset difficulties. A parent sleep education program was evaluated within individual and group formats featuring a comprehensive curriculum that covered (a) the factors contributing to normative and disruptive sleep, (b) appropriate sleep hygiene, (c) specific sleep problems, and (d) intervention methods with empirical support. The children's sleep was monitored with actigraphy and parents completed several questionnaires at baseline and one-month following program implementation. This study found improved sleep latency and sleep duration via parent report but less confirmatory evidence from actigraphy measurement. These outcomes were similar for both individual and group education formats.

Morning Sleep Awakening Disruption. Thiele et al. (2001) intervened with a 17-year old male who had IDD and lived at a specialized residential school. Upon wakening up in the morning between 6:30 and 7:00 a.m., he regularly cried, screamed, and engaged in self-injury during interactions with care-providers. This combination of behaviors was defined as a tantrum. Tantrum frequency was recorded each morning, first under baseline conditions and then during sequentially introduced intervention within a multiple baseline design. In baseline care-providers assisted the boy after he woke up, guiding him through a self-care routine before preparing for breakfast. They delivered physical touch (pats on the shoulder) and praise approximately every 30-s that he did not display a tantrum. When a tantrum was encountered, the care-providers tried prompting the boy to complete his self-care activities. If prompting was unsuccessful after 30-s, they stopped interacting with him, waited until he was not agitated for 60-s, and resumed the earlier routine.

Before intervening with the boy, clinical supervisors at the residential school conducted functional behavioral assessment that constituted (a) reviewing previously recorded A-B-C data, (b) interviewing the care-providers who supported the boy, and (c) observing the boy and care-providers several times during morning wake-up. The conclusion from functional behavioral assessment was that tantrum behavior was reinforced by care-provider attention and the physical prompting they provided. Accordingly, an intervention plan was designed to pre-empt tantrums by having one of several care-providers that the boy preferred greet him immediately upon awakening. The attending care-provider conversed with the boy about pleasurable topics for several minutes, ensured that he was "calm," and initiated the self-care routine. These antecedent procedures essentially eliminated morning sleep awakening disruption though a 9-month follow-up period.

Daytime Sleeping. Targeting a 13-year old boy with autism, Freidman and Luiselli (2008) addressed his daytime sleeping at school. Classroom teachers reported that he frequently fell asleep during the class-day and was difficult to wake up. At home the boy napped occasionally and slept soundly at night. He was in good health and did not take medication. Preceding the study classroom teachers completed the *MAS* (Durand and Crimmins 1992) and the *Functional Analysis Screening Tool* (*FAST*) (Iwata et al. 2013) as indirect methods of functional behavioral assessment. The results suggested that the boy's daytime sleeping was maintained by automatic reinforcement. A second type of functional behavioral assessment was a detailed recording checklist on which classroom teachers documented the time, location, and context of daytime sleeping. The checklist information indicated that the boy slept most often during breaks from instruction, under conditions of reduced teacher supervision, and when he was not engaged in purposeful activities. The usual consequence for daytime sleeping was classroom teachers not attending to the boy until he was awake.

Freidman and Luiselli (2008) introduced baseline and intervention phases in an ABAB reversal design. The baseline conditions allowed the boy to sleep without interruption or formal attempts to prevent his sleeping. Intervention has three components:

Stimulus change. The boy typically slept on a soft floor mat or a large "bean-bag" chair in one area of the classroom. The mat and chair were removed to eliminate sleep-associated stimuli.

Response interruption-redirection. Whenever the boy put his head down or appeared sleepy (closing eyes), one of the classroom teachers guided him to a location that contained stimulating objects and motor tasks. The redirected activity lasted 5–10 min with teacher prompting to sustain engagement as necessary.

Positive interactions. Classroom teachers praised the boy and patted his back during their daily interactions with him. This procedure had the dual objective of preventing sleep attempts and positively reinforcing non-sleep behavior throughout the day.

Within the initial baseline phase the boy slept an average of 46 min each day. Daytime sleeping did not occur when intervention was first implemented, increased to an average of 22 min per day in the reversal-to-baseline phase, and was absent again with intervention. At a 6-month follow-up, the boy continued to be awake all day.

Sleep Terrors. Few studies have treated sleep terrors in people with IDD. One exception is Durand (2002) in which parents of three children with autism applied *scheduled awakenings* as a solitary behavioral intervention. Scheduled awakening consisted of arousing a child 15–30 min before the time(s) that night terrors were usually experienced. The three children had fewer night terrors with intervention in effect and 12 months later. Clearly, more research is needed to replicate these findings and to study other potentially effective procedures.

Summary and Practice Recommendations

There are several reasons to recommend behavioral intervention for improving sleep of people who have IDD. Notably, clinicians have several procedures at their disposal with good evidence support in treating particular sleep problems. Various methods of functional behavioral assessment can provide vital information for tailoring a sleep intervention to the unique presentation of children and adults. The research reviewed in this chapter further supports parents and care-providers implementing behavioral intervention within different applied settings such as homes, schools, and hospital units. Many of these intervention procedures also appeal to parents and care-providers because of high satisfaction and treatment acceptability.

Equally important are some relative limitations with the extant behavioral intervention sleep research. For example, the vast majority of studies evaluated multicomponent intervention plans that may or may not have required the full complement of procedures (Freidman and Luiselli 2008; Knight and Johnson 2014; O'Reilly et al. 2004). This matter has practical significance for parents and care-providers who generally prefer methods that are easy to understand and institute (Knight and Johnson 2014). A second concern is that most research has not included assessment of intervention integrity—do parents and care-providers implement intervention procedures as they were trained and presented in a written plan? Intervention integrity assessment cannot be overlooked as an integral feature of outcome evaluation (Sanetti and Kratochwill 2014). Lastly, although there is some evidence that the salutary effects of behavioral intervention for sleep problems in IDD are maintained long-term (Durand 2002; Piazza and Fisher 1991; Thiele et al. 2001), research has not consistently reported follow up measures months and years post-intervention.

Establishing appropriate sleep hygiene is recognized as a prerequisite to behavioral intervention (Durand 2014a; Knight and Johnson 2014; Malow et al. 2014). Minimally, a sleep hygiene protocol should emphasize regular evening bedtimes and morning wake up times. Parents and care-providers are advised to plan relaxing activities with children and adults at least 30 min before going to bed. It is desirable to eliminate sleep-interfering and distracting ambient stimulation in the bedroom, namely noise, light, and uncomfortable temperatures. Often overlooked, parents and care-providers should restrict ingestion of caffeine-laden liquids and foods (e.g., coffee, tea, cola soft drinks, chocolate). A sleep hygiene orientation can further include sleep facilitating stimulation, for example, continuous white noise (Forquer and Johnson 2005). Attention to sleep hygiene is a relatively low-demand approach to improving sleep, can be accommodated within most living environments, and may preclude the need for more intensive behavioral intervention.

When behavioral intervention is indicated, clinicians should be cognizant of the unique circumstances facing parents and care-providers. By definition, sleep problems occur at inconvenient times, either at the end of the day, the middle of the night, and early morning before the day begins. The already existing fatigue that parents and care-providers experience in dealing with a sleep problem is further intensified by having to intervene in such contexts. Furthermore, many sleep intervention plans can be difficult to implement because the procedures themselves are time-consuming, not always possible to apply with fidelity, and may provoke other challenging behavior from the child or adult. Using an instrument such as the *Selecting Sleep Interventions Questionnaire* (*SSIQ*) described by Durand (2014a) can help clinicians choose intervention procedures that parents and care-providers judge most palatable. The *SSIQ* solicits people's attitudes about the disruption-distress they are able to tolerate in dealing with sleep problems as well as other beliefs that could compromise a potentially effective intervention plan. Such pre-intervention assessment is strongly recommended.

Designing sleep intervention plans to be implemented by parents and care-providers also means that behavioral specialists will have to interact with other professionals. Multidisciplinary collaboration can be expected among physicians, nurses, nutritionists, and related health practitioners. In such circumstances, it is necessary for clinicians to be "consultation savvy" and prepared to assist with evaluating complimentary treatment protocols, most likely pharmacology-medication regimens (Cortesi et al. 2012; Richdale 2013).

Behavioral intervention for sleep and sleep-related problems has focused primarily on people who have ASD (Mannion and Leader 2013) but less so with other developmental disabilities. Clinical practice will be enhanced through more widespread application and evaluation within the larger IDD population. Allen et al. (2013) as an example reported promising findings from behavioral sleep intervention with children who had Angelman syndrome. Similarly, and as noted previously, studies have been dominated by children and youth. It would be valuable to concentrate efforts on adults and the types of sleep problems that differentiate them from pediatric samples (van de Wouw et al. 2012).

Another suggestion for clinicians is to combine multiple methods when conducting sleep intervention assessment and measurement (Hodge et al. 2012). Integrated measures would include direct observational coding, informant questionnaires, rating scales, and actigraphy. Social validity assessment also serves a critical evaluative function (Knight and Johnson 2014; Moore et al. 2007). Of course, various assessment and measurement modalities will have to be adjusted to the behaviors of concern, setting resources, ease of documentation, and treatment objectives that apply to each case. Multi-method evaluation will best represent the often multiple facets of a sleep problem and the total impact from a comprehensively formulated and implemented behavioral intervention plan.

References

Adams, L. A., & Rickert, V. I. (1989). Reducing bedtime tantrums: Comparison between positive routines and graduated extinction. *Pediatrics, 84*, 756–761.

Allen, K. D., Kuhn, B. R., DeHaai, K. A., & Wallace, D. P. (2013). Evaluation of a behavioral treatment package to reduce sleep problems in children with Angelman syndrome. *Research in Developmental Disabilities, 34*, 676–686.

Allik, H., Larsson, J., & Smedje, H. (2006). Insomnia in school-age children with Asperger syndrome or high-functioning autism. *BMC Psychiatry, 6*, 6–18.

American Psychiatric Association. (2013). *Diagnostic and statistical manual of mental disorders* (5th ed.). Washington, DC: Author.

Chevrin, R. D., Hedger, K., Dillon, J. E., & Pituch, K. J. (2000). Pediatric sleep questionnaire (PSQ): Validity and reliability of scales for sleep-disordered breathing, snoring, sleepiness, and behavioral problems. *Sleep Medicine, 1*, 21–32.

Chu, J., & Richdale, A. L. (2009). Sleep quality and psychological wellbeing in mothers of children with developmental disabilities. *Research in Developmental Disabilities, 30*, 1512–1522.

Colton, H. R., & Altevogt, V. M. (Eds.). (2006). *Sleep disorders and sleep deprivation: An unmet health problem*. Washington, DC: National Academics Press.

Cortesi, F., Giannotti, F., Sebastiani, T., Panunzi, S., & Valente, D. (2012). Controlled-release melatonin, singly and combined with cognitive behavioral therapy, for persistent insomnia in children with autism spectrum disorders: A placebo-controlled trial. *Journal of Sleep Research, 21*, 700–709.

Cotton, S., & Richdale, A. (2010). Brief report: Parental descriptions of sleep problems in children with autism, Down syndrome, and Prader-Willi syndrome. *Research in Developmental Disabilities, 27*, 151–161.

Didden, R., Curfs, L. M. G., Sikkema, S. P. E., & de Moor, J. (1998). Functional assessment and treatment of sleeping problems with developmentally disabled children: Six case studies. *Journal of Behavior Therapy and Experimental Psychiatry, 29*, 85–97.

Doran, S. M., Harvey, M. T., & Horner, R. H. (2006). Sleep and developmental disabilities: Assessment, treatment, and outcome measures. *Mental Retardation, 44*, 13–27.

Durand, V. M. (2002). Treating sleep terrors in children with autism. *Journal of Positive Behavioral Interventions, 4*, 66–72.

Durand, V. M. (2014a). Sleep problems. In J. K. Luiselli (Ed.), *Children and youth with autism spectrum disorder (ASD): Recent advances and innovations in assessment, education, and intervention* (pp. 174–192). New York: Oxford University Press.

Durand, V. M. (2014b). *Sleep better! A guide to improving sleep for children with special needs* (revised ed.). Baltimore, MD: Paul H. Brookes.

Durand, V. M., & Crimmins, D. (1992). *The motivation assessment scale administrative guide*. Topeka, KS: Monaco & Associates.

Eshbaugh, B., Martin, W., Cunningham, K., & Luiselli, J. K. (2004). Evaluation of bedtime medication regimen on daytime sleep and challenging behaviors of an adult with intellectual disabilities. *Mental Health Aspects of Developmental Disabilities, 7*, 21–25.

Ferber, R. (2006). *Solve your child's sleep problems* (2nd ed.). New York: Fireside Books.

Forquer, L. M., & Johnson, C. M. (2005). Continuous white noise to reduce resistance going to sleep and night wakings in toddlers. *Child & Family Behavior Therapy, 27*, 1–10.

Freidman, A., & Luiselli, J. K. (2008). Excessive daytime sleep: Behavioral assessment and intervention in a child with autism. *Behavior Modification, 32*, 548–555.

Friman, P. C., Hoff, K. E., Schnoes, C., Freeman, K. A., Woods, D. W., & Blum, N. (1999). The bedtime pass: An approach to bedtime crying and leaving the room. *Archives of Pediatric and Adolescent Medicine, 153*, 1027–1029.

Gallagher, S., Phillips, A. C., & Carroll, D. (2010). Parental stress is associated with poor sleep quality in parents caring for children with developmental disabilities. *Journal of Pediatric Psychology, 35*, 728–737.

Garcia, J., & Wills, L. (2000). Sleep disorders in children and teens: Helping patients and their families get some rest. *Postgraduate Medicine, 107*, 161–178.

Goldman, S. E., Mcgraw, S., Johnson, K. P., Richdale, A. L., Clemons, T., & Malow, A. (2011). Sleep is associated with problem behaviors in children and adolescents with autism spectrum disorders. *Research in Autism Spectrum Disorders, 5*, 1223–1229.

Harvey, M. T., Baker, D. J., Horner, R. H., & Blackford, J. U. (2003). A brief report on the prevalence of sleep problems in individuals with mental retardation living in the community. *Journal of Positive Behavioral Interventions, 5*, 195–200.

Hodge, D., Parnell, A. M. N., Hoffman, C. D., & Sweeney, D. P. (2012). Methods for assessing sleep in children with autism spectrum disorders: A review. *Research in Autism Spectrum Disorders, 6*, 1337–1344.

Iwata, B. A., DeLeon, I. G., & Roscoe, E. M. (2013). Reliability and validity of the functional analysis screening tool. *Journal of Applied Behavior Analysis, 46*, 271–284.

Kennedy, C. H., & Meyer, K. A. (1996). Sleep deprivation, allergy symptoms, and negatively reinforced problem behavior. *Journal of Applied Behavior Analysis, 29*, 133–135.

Knight, R. M., & Johnson, C. M. (2014). Using a behavioral treatment package for sleep problems in children with autism spectrum disorders. *Child & Family Behavior Therapy, 36*, 204–221.

Kuhn, B. R., & Eliot, A. J. (2003). Treatment efficacy in behavioral pediatric sleep medicine. *Journal of Psychosomatic Research, 54*, 587–597.

Lancioni, G. E., O'Reilly, M. F., & Basili, G. (1999). Review of strategies for treating sleep problems in persons with severe and profound mental retardation or multiple handicaps. *American Journal of Mental Deficiency, 104*, 170–186.

Liu, X., Hubbard, J. A., Fabes, R. A., & Adam, J. B. (2006). Sleep disturbances and correlates of children with autism spectrum disorders. *Child Psychiatry and Human Development, 37*, 179–191.

Luiselli, J. K. (1995). Behavioral assessment and treatment of sleep disorders in persons with developmental disabilities. *Habilitative Mental Healthcare Newsletter, 14*, 68–73.

Luiselli, J. K. (2008). Antecedent (preventive) intervention. In J. K. Luiselli, S. Wilczynski, D. C. Russo, & W. P. Christian (Eds.), *Effective practices for children with autism: Educational and behavior support interventions that work* (pp. 393–412). New York, NY: Oxford University Press.

Luiselli, J. K., MaGee, C., Sperry, J. M., & Parker, S. (2005). Descriptive assessment of sleep patterns among community-living adults with mental retardation. *Mental Retardation, 43*, 416–420.

Malow, B. A., Adkins, K. W., Reynolds, A., Weiss, S. K., Loh, A., & Fawkes, D. et al. (2014). Parent-based sleep education for children with autism spectrum disorders. *Journal of Autism and Developmental Disorders, 44*, 216–228.

Mannion, A., & Leader, G. (2013). Sleep problems in autism spectrum disorder: A literature review. *Review Journal of Autism and Developmental Disorders, 1*, 101–109.

Meltzer, L. J., & Mindell, J. A. (2004). Non-pharmacologic treatments for pediatric sleeplessness. *Pediatric Clinics of North America, 51*, 135–151.

Meltzer, L. J., & Mindell, J. A. (2007). Relationship between child sleep disturbances and maternal sleep, mood, and parenting stress: A pilot study. *Journal of Family Psychology, 21*, 67–73.

Meltzer, L. J., Montgomery-Downs, H. E., Insana, S. P., & Walsh, C. M. (2012). Use of actigraphy for assessment in pediatric sleep research. *Sleep Medicine Reviews, 16*, 463–475.

Moore, B. A., Friman, P. C., Fruzzetti, A. E., & MacAleese, K. (2007). Brief report: Evaluating the bedtime pass program for child resistance to bedtime—a randomized, controlled trial. *Journal of Pediatric Psychology, 32*, 283–287.

O'Neill, R. E., Horner, R. H., Albin, R. W., Sprague, J. R., Storey, K., & Newton, J. S. (1997). *Functional assessment and program development for problem behavior: A practical handbook*. Pacific Grove, CA: Brookes/Cole.

O'Reilly, M. F. (1995). Functional analysis and treatment of escape-maintained aggression correlated with sleep deprivation. *Journal of Applied Behavior Analysis, 28*, 225–226.

O'Reilly, M. F., Lancioni, G. E., & Sigafoos, J. (2004). Using paired-choice assessment to identify variables maintaining sleep problems in a child with severe disabilities. *Journal of Applied Behavior Analysis, 37*, 209–212.

Owens, J. A., Spirito, A., & Mcguinn, M. (2000). The children's sleep habits questionnaire (CSHQ): Psychometric properties of a survey instrument for school-age children. *Sleep, 23*, 1043–1052.

Paclawskyi, T. R., Matson, J. L., Rush, K. S., Smalls, Y., & Vollmer, T. R. (2000). Questions about behavior function (QABF): A behavioral checklist for functional assessment of aberrant behavior. *Research in Developmental Disabilities, 21*, 223–229.

Piazza, C. C., & Fisher, W. (1991). A faded bedtime with response cost protocol for treatment of multiple sleep problems in children. *Journal of Applied Behavior Analysis, 24*, 129–140.

Reed, D. D., & Azulay, R. (2011). Functional behavioral assessment. In J. K. Luiselli (Ed.), *Teaching and behavior support for children and adults with autism spectrum disorder: A practitioner's guide* (pp. 13–21). New York: Oxford University Press.

Reed, G. K., Dolezal, D. N., Cooper-Brown, L. J., & Wacker, D. P. (2005). The effects of sleep disruption on the treatment of a feeding disorder. *Journal of Applied Behavior Analysis, 38*, 243–245.

Richdale, A. L. (2013). Autism and other developmental disabilities. In A. R. Wofson & H. Montgomery-Downs (Eds.), *The oxford handbook of infant, child, and adolescent sleep* (pp. 471–494). New York: Oxford University Press.

Richdale, A. L., & Baker, E. K. (2014). Sleep in individuals with an intellectual or developmental disability: Recent research reports. *Current Developmental Disorders Reports, 1*, 74–85.

Rzepecka, H., McKenzie, K., McClure, I., & Murphy, S. (2011). Sleep, anxiety, and challenging behavior in children with intellectual disability and/or autism spectrum disorder. *Research in Developmental Disabilities, 16*, 2758–2766.

Sadeh, A. (2011). The role and validity of actigraphy in sleep medicine: An update. *Sleep Medicine Reviews, 15*, 259–267.
Sanetti, L. M. H., & Kratochwill, T. R. (2014). *Treatment integrity: A foundation for evidence-based practice in applied psychology*. Washington, DC: American Psychological Press.
Schreck, K. A., Mulick, J. A., & Rojahn, J. (2003). Development of the behavioral evaluation of disorders of sleep scale. *Journal of Child and Family Studies, 12*, 349–359.
Sitnick, S. L., Goodline-Jones, B. L., & Anders, T. F. (2008). The use of actigraphy to study sleep disorders in preschoolers: Some concerns about detection of nighttime awakenings. *Sleep, 31*, 395–401.
Souders, M. C., Mason, T. B. A., Valladares, O., Bucan, M., Levy, S. E., & Mandell, D. S. (2009). Sleep behaviors and sleep quality in children with autism spectrum disorders. *Sleep, 32*, 1566–1578.
Stores, G. (2002). Annotation: Children's sleep disorders: Modern approaches, developmental effects, and children at special risk. *Developmental Medicine and Child Neurology, 41*, 568–573.
Stores, G., & Stores, R. (2013). Sleep disorders and their clinical significance in children with Down syndrome. *Developmental Medicine and Child Neurology, 30*, 126–130.
Taylor, M. A., Schreck, K. A., & Mulick, J. A. (2012). Sleep disruption as a correlate to cognitive and adaptive behavior problems in autism spectrum disorders. *Research in Developmental Disabilities, 33*, 1408–1417.
Thiele, T., Blew, P., & Luiselli, J. K. (2001). Antecedent control of sleep awakening disruption. *Research in Developmental Disabilities, 22*, 399–406.
Van de Wouw, E., Evenhuis, H. M., & Echtld, M. A. (2012). Prevalence, associated factors, and sleep problems in adults with intellectual disability: A systematic review. *Research in Developmental Disabilities, 33*, 1310–1332.
Wiggs, L., & Stores, G. (2004). Sleep patterns and sleep disorders in children with autistic spectrum disorders: Insights using parent report and actigraphy. *Developmental Medicine and Child Neurology, 46*, 372–380.

Chapter 9
Rumination Disorders

David A. Wilder and Joshua L. Lipschultz

Rumination is the deliberate regurgitation, chewing, and swallowing of stomach contents, and operant vomiting is the purposeful expulsion of regurgitated stomach contents from the mouth (Fredericks et al. 1998; Lang et al. 2011; Starin and Fuqua 1987). Operant vomiting is frequently caused by placing fingers in the mouth or by engaging in tongue thrusting (Winton and Singh 1983). Rumination has been reported across a wide range of ages (0–89 years; Parry-Jones 1994) and in both typically developing individuals and individuals with intellectual and developmental disabilities, but is much more common among the latter (Winton and Singh 1983). The mean age of onset for typically developing children ranges from 3 weeks to 12 months, while onset among children with intellectual and developmental disabilities may not occur until years later (Winton and Singh 1983). Rumination in typically developing children is often transient, while rumination in children with intellectual and developmental disabilities may persist for many years. Although no formal data on the prevalence of rumination exist, the prevalence of rumination among individuals with intellectual disabilities is estimated to range from 6 to 10 % (Lang et al. 2011; Starin and Fuqua 1987; Winton and Singh 1983). A recent review of the current state of feeding and eating disorders, under which rumination disorder is categorized in the *Diagnostic and Statistical Manual of Mental Disorders* (DSM-5; American Psychiatric Association 2013), states that there are insufficient data to determine lifetime prevalence (Kelly et al. 2014).

D.A. Wilder (✉)
School of Behavior Analysis, Florida Institute of Technology,
150 W University Blvd, Melbourne, FL 32901, USA
e-mail: dawilder@fit.edu

D.A. Wilder · J.L. Lipschultz
Florida Institute of Technology, Melbourne, FL, USA

J.K. Luiselli (ed.), *Behavioral Health Promotion and Intervention in Intellectual and Developmental Disabilities*, Evidence-Based Practices in Behavioral Health,
DOI 10.1007/978-3-319-27297-9_9

There are many negative medical side effects associated with rumination disorder. The chronic vomiting associated with rumination can lead to many serious health problems such as irritation of the mouth, throat, and esophagus, dehydration, malnutrition, lowered resistance to diseases, weight loss, tooth decay, choking, gastrointestinal bleeding, and possibly death (Fredericks et al. 1998; Kelly et al. 2014; Lang et al. 2011; Tierney and Jackson 1984; Winton and Singh 1983). Furthermore, individuals who do not take in a sufficient amount of food (which is associated with chronic rumination) may have to be placed on feeding tubes (Kuhn and Matson 2004). Feeding tubes may be associated with other health risks and can further inhibit the development of appropriate and effective eating behavior. Cited mortality rates associated with rumination disorder range from 12.5 to 50 % (Tierney and Jackson 1984), and rumination is the primary cause of death in 5–10 % of people who ruminate (Fredericks et al. 1998).

In addition to medical side effects, there are many negative social side effects associated with rumination. Chronic vomiting and rumination may have a damaging effect on the individual's overall appearance and lead to halitosis and foul body odor (Starin and Fuqua 1987), possibly resulting in social isolation and reduced educational or vocational opportunities. Poor social and family functioning are also commonly associated with rumination disorder (Kelly et al. 2014).

A complication in identifying, diagnosing, and measuring rumination disorder is that it can be difficult to detect. In some individuals, subtle throat movements are the only indication that rumination is occurring. In addition, some individuals may only ruminate when alone due to a history of punishment for rumination. In some cases, rumination may not occur in discrete movements; clinicians may have to measure duration instead of, or in addition to, frequency.

A distinction between rumination and vomiting is often made; vomiting involves the expulsion of food from the mouth whereas rumination involves bringing up vomitus into the mouth without expulsion. Vomiting when sick or after eating dangerous food is largely a respondent behavior (i.e., a reflex). However, some individuals engage in operant vomiting, or vomiting with a purpose (i.e., it produces or terminates something for the individual). It has been suggested that some individuals may ruminate because they are physically unable to recruit other sources of stimulation due to physical limitations (e.g., non-ambulatory individuals; Kuhn and Matson 2004). Some individuals who ruminate also engage in operant vomiting, although the extent to which these two are co-morbid is unknown. Interestingly, Amarnath et al. (1986) found that many individuals who engage in rumination exhibit increased movements in the abdomen without compressions of other gastrointestinal areas typically exhibited during vomiting. This type of responding may contribute to the difficulty in identifying rumination and may help explain why it appears so easy for people who engage in rumination to bring food up into the mouth (Fredericks et al. 1998). Some researchers have noted that vomiting may reliably precede rumination in some individuals (Singh 1981). In other cases, vomiting becomes more common after a history of rumination, which may indicate more serious gastrointestinal abnormalities (Kuruvilla and Trewby 1989).

A comprehensive medical evaluation should be conducted to assess the presence of abnormalities in cases such as this.

History of Rumination

Rumination was first described clinically in 1618 by Italian anatomist Fabricious ab Aquapendente. Interestingly, there is speculation that rumination occurred prior to this, but that it was not considered a disorder or problem. Instead, it may have been a common, accepted cultural practice. That is, typically developing people may have ruminated because they found it pleasurable, and good-tasting food may have been in shorter supply than in modern times. Rumination may have become a clinical problem or disorder only after it was linked with the behavior of cattle (Parry-Jones 1994). Throughout history, comparisons between rumination and other eating disorders have been made. While evidence for symptom overlap with anorexia nervosa is limited, more evidence for symptom overlap with bulimia exists. Due to this symptomology overlap with rumination, both disorders have been perceived as degenerate behaviors, leading to the social embarrassment and impairment associated with these disorders in the present (Parry-Jones and Parry-Jones 1994).

In the 1700s and early 1800s, as rumination became an oddity, individuals who ruminated were often highlighted in circuses along with other unusual human physical characteristics and activities such as bearded women and leather-skinned children. The use of rumination as an exhibitionist oddity offers another interesting parallel with bulimia, as individuals with both disorders used their eating abnormalities to earn their living in fairs, circuses, or side-shows (Parry-Jones and Parry-Jones 1994). As it became less common among the general population, medical and scientific interest in rumination turned to individuals with disabilities. Later, in the 20th century, attention turned toward rumination among infants (Parry-Jones 1994).

Treatment of rumination first emerged in the 1950s. The psychoanalytic conceptualization of abnormal behavior, popular at the time, described problematic mother-child relationships as the culprit. These problematic relationships were said to cause the individual to seek internal gratification, sometimes in the form of rumination. Treatments consisted of a "mother substitute" who interacted with the individual in a warm manner. Parents were trained to implement the new approach to interaction at home. Another important factor related to psychiatric treatments was the dependent variables used to demonstrate clinical progress in patients. The dependent variables commonly used were weight of the ruminator, apparent emotional state of the patient (inferred from facial expressions), and therapy progress by the ruminator and/or parents (Starin and Fuqua 1987). Anecdotal reports suggest that these interventions could be effective in some cases (Winton and Singh 1983), but these conclusions were limited in that most research in the psychiatric literature consists of uncontrolled case studies (Starin and Fuqua 1987).

Once attention turned toward viewing rumination as a learned behavior, behavior analytic treatments became more common. As opposed to the dependent variables typically used in psychoanalytic/psychiatric treatments, behavior analytic treatments often used discrete, observable response measures such as frequency or duration of rumination (Starin and Fuqua 1987). These types of interventions have remained the most commonly used class of intervention for rumination to this day. Early behavior analytic interventions often focused on punishment-based procedures. However, more recent interventions have focused on interventions informed by a functional assessment. Thus, behavioral interventions for rumination can be classified into two types: interventions informed by a functional assessment, and non-assessment-based interventions. Rumination has also been treated medically in some cases.

Rumination Due to Medical Issues

The possibility that rumination is due to a medical cause should be examined before proceeding to other forms of assessment and intervention. If medical causes are implicated, a medical intervention may be most appropriate. Rogers et al. (1992) found that over 90 % of participants evaluated for rumination had gastroesophageal abnormalities, although it is not clear if the rumination was a cause or result of the abnormalities. Kuruvilla and Trewby (1989) found that 50 % of individuals with rumination had reflux and esophagitis (inflammation of the esophagus), although again, it is not clear if rumination was the cause or an effect of this condition. Some medications (neuroleptics in particular) may make swallowing difficult and should be ruled out as causes or contributors to rumination.

In terms of specific diagnostic procedures, a barium esophogram, an endoscopy, and radiological studies can be conducted to evaluate physical causes of rumination (Rogers et al. 1992). In addition, Kuruvilla and Trewby (1989) recommend H2 blockers (acid reducers) or antacids to rule out physical causes of rumination. Although these procedures may be invasive, they can save time by identifying problems which may be relevant for treatment.

Medical interventions consist of surgery, which may target repair of hiatal hernia and has been shown to reduce rumination secondary to a hernia or other gastroesophageal abnormality. Some medications have also been used, although reports of these medications consist of uncontrolled case studies. In particular, the opioid agonist, paregoric inhibited rumination in two participants (Blinder et al. 1986). Surprisingly, little data on the use of antacid medications to treat rumination has been published (although see Luiselli et al. 1993, 1994, for exceptions). In general, although medical etiologies are important to rule out, medical interventions, and particularly surgery, might best be considered after less invasive behavioral interventions have failed.

Non-assessment-Based Behavioral Interventions for Rumination

Non-assessment-based interventions for rumination can be classified into three types: differential reinforcement-based procedures, dietary interventions, and punishment-basedprocedures.

Differential Reinforcement Procedures. Differential reinforcement (DR) procedures have been used to treat rumination in a number of studies. Of course, in the absence of a functional assessment identifying and targeting the function of rumination, the effectiveness of DR procedures depends entirely on the extent to which the reinforcer employed as part of the DR procedure can "overpower" the reinforcer maintaining rumination. Given that rumination is often maintained by automatic reinforcement and that the reinforcer is therefore always available to the participant, clinicians may have difficulty maintaining the effects of DR procedures. In other words, the long term effects of DR procedures may be questionable, and few studies have employed long-term follow-up measures of DR procedures. Clinicians might enhance the likelihood of treatment efficacy by using highly preferred items, formally identified via a stimulus preference assessment, as part of the DR procedure and by restricting access to the items used in the DR procedure.

Kelly and Heffner (1988) evaluated a differential reinforcement of alternative behavior contingency with a 24-year-old male who engaged in operant vomiting. Specifically, they removed all attention for 2 min contingent upon each instance of vomiting. In addition, they provided attention on a dense fixed time schedule. The results showed that the DR procedure was effective; vomiting was reduced and the participant's weight increased from a dangerously low level to average for his height and age. In addition, the effects were maintained for 2 months.

Sanders-Dewey and Larson (2006) evaluated a differential reinforcement of other behavior (DRO) schedule with a 20-year-old man who engaged in rumination. The authors provided verbal attention contingent upon the absence of rumination for various periods of time. In addition, they also delivered a small taste of a sour drink contingent upon rumination or pre-rumination behaviors. The results show that rumination decreased upon introduction of the procedure. In addition, the authors were able to gradually remove the sour drink from the treatment package; the treatment was evaluated 8 days later and remained effective.

Dietary Interventions. Jackson et al. (1975) were the first to evaluate a food satiation procedure, in which participants were provided with large quantities of food as a treatment for rumination. The procedure used in the study allowed the participant to eat all of the food that he or she could consume. Although the results of the study showed that satiation was an effective procedure to decrease rumination/vomiting in two participants, the procedure involved both participants eating at least twice the amount of food typically consumed during meals, so weight gain was a concern. However, as with many individuals who ruminate, these participants were underweight. Other researchers (Libby and Phillips 1979; Rast et al.

1984, 1981) have replicated and added to this procedure. While Jackson et al. (1975) and Libby and Phillips (1979) allowed access to at least twice the amount of food typically given during meals along with snacks to maintain satiation, Rast et al. (1981, 1984) evaluated the exact relation between food quantity and rumination behavior by conducting a parametric analysis of varying amounts of food and rumination frequency and duration. These two studies identified an inverse relation between caloric density of diet and frequency of rumination. Overall, the results of these studies have shown that food satiation procedures produce robust and sustaining reductions in rumination (Starin and Fuqua 1987), although the procedure has the potential to result in excessive weight gain. Despite the potential negative side effects of food satiation, manipulation of dietary variables has become one of the most common interventions for rumination (Sharp et al. 2012).

Rast et al. (1988) evaluated a novel intervention for three women with intellectual disabilities who engaged in rumination. The authors provided access to sugarless chewing gum before meals, which was intended to act as an abolishing operation by decreasing the value of chewing, and therefore decreasing the frequency of rumination. The intervention was effective; rumination decreased when the pre-meal chewing program was in place. The authors also ruled out increased caloric intake as a possible mechanism for the reduction of rumination by using zero-calorie gum (some researchers have speculated that satiation procedures may be effective due to increased caloric intake). Years later, Rhine and Tarbox (2009) replicated the gum chewing intervention to decrease rumination in a young boy with autism. The replication was equally effective. One notable feature of these studies is that rumination decreased without increased caloric intake, circumventing the potential for excessive weight gain.

Yang (1988) evaluated a food satiation procedure with an adolescent with an intellectual disability who lived in a residential treatment facility. The satiation procedure included access to typical meals *in addition to* 20 slices of white bread at each meal. Once an effect was obtained, the author systematically decreased the number of white bread slices available, until, after 10 weeks, no additional bread was available at meals. Rumination remained at low levels during the fading process. At a 12-week follow-up, the participant remained rumination free and had gained weight. Clauser and Scibak (1990) used a similar procedure with three adults with intellectual disabilities who engaged in rumination; the procedure was effective to reduce the target behavior. Interestingly, the authors also noted a decrease in other forms of self-injurious behavior when the satiation procedure was in place.

Greene et al. (1991) evaluated the delivery of various amounts and types of peanut butter on rumination exhibited by five individuals with intellectual disabilities. Some researchers have hypothesized that the thick, sticky consistency of peanut butter makes rumination more difficult. The peanut butter was given during meals. Ingeniously, the authors evaluated lower calorie as well as higher calorie peanut butter in order to separate any effects due to increased caloric intake from effects due to the consistency of peanut butter. The authors also varied peanut butter texture, as thick textured peanut butter could be more effective than thin textured peanut butter to decrease rumination. The results showed that as the amount of peanut butter consumed increased, rumination decreased. Calories appeared to be more important than texture; the texture of the peanut butter had little effect on rumination.

Johnston et al. (1991) evaluated increased caloric intake with three adults with intellectual disabilities. The authors increased the participants' caloric intake from 700 to 900 calories per meal to 2800 to 3000 calories per meal. The increased caloric intake reduced rumination during lunch. This study was particularly informative because all other variables (e.g., attention delivered to participants) remained the same during baseline and intervention.

Luiselli et al. (1993) evaluated a package intervention to decrease rumination and operant vomiting in an adolescent with an intellectual disability. The dietary components of the intervention consisted of paced access to food during meals and limited access to liquids, dairy products and spicy foods. The treatment package also included medication (i.e., an antacid, as well as two additional medications used to treat heartburn) and behavioral components (i.e., delivery of attention during meals and a reprimand contingent upon rumination or vomiting). The food pacing and liquid restriction components were gradually reduced. Both rumination and vomiting decreased to low levels; these results were maintained at a two year follow-up.

Luiselli et al. (1994) evaluated another multi-component treatment to reduce rumination and operant vomiting in an adolescent male with an intellectual disability. Their intervention included dietary components (i.e., bite pacing, reductions of fatty foods and lactose, and an increase in healthier foods), behavioral components (i.e., delivery of attention when not ruminating, required assistance in cleaning up vomitus), and an antacid. Both rumination and vomiting decreased to low levels; these results were maintained for four months.

Dunn et al. (1997) provided free access to foods high in starch (e.g., potatoes, pasta) and then later to fruits and vegetables in addition to regular meals. The amount of food delivered was reduced to control weight gain. Unfortunately, rumination returned after two years; free access to food was again provided. The satiation procedure was effective to reduce rumination up to 7 years later. Dudley et al. (2002) evaluated a similar procedure with a young boy and found it to be effective. Follow-up data four years later suggested the intervention remained effective.

Wilder et al. (1997) compared three interventions to reduce rumination in an adult with an intellectual disability. They evaluated noncontingent delivery of bites of preferred food every 20 s for 30 min immediately following meals, competing stimulation (they required the participant to take a shower during which the participant would sing), and reduced liquid intake. The noncontingent delivery of food produced the greatest reductions in rumination. The reduced liquid intake produced moderate levels of reduction, and competing stimulation was the least effective intervention.

Thibadeau et al. (1999) evaluated an intervention to decrease rumination and vomiting by an 18-year-old male with an intellectual disability. Their procedure included access to white bread upon request for one hour following meals.

This is similar to the procedure described by Yang (1988), but Thibadeau incorporated participant choice into the intervention. The procedure was effective; even after 15 months rumination remained low. In addition, bread consumption was reduced but not eliminated. Masalsky and Luiselli (1998) replicated this procedure with a 44-year-old male with an intellectual disability and visual impairment. Participant choice was still utilized in this study; however, instead of giving full slices of white bread, only a small piece of white bread was available for up to 30 min following the last bite of a meal. Follow-up data showed that rumination remained below original levels. Darling et al. (2011) replicated Thibadeau et al.'s procedure with a 27-year-old man with an intellectual disability and found similar results. In this study, the participant did not gain any additional weight.

Heering et al. (2003) conducted a pre-intervention dietary assessment with a 19-year-old male who engaged in rumination. The assessment suggested that rumination was less likely when the participant did not consume liquids during meals and when he did consume peanut butter before meals. The authors then implemented an intervention in which they withheld liquid until 1.5 h after mealtime. The results suggest that the liquid rescheduling reduced rumination during both breakfast and lunch, although the design employed to assess the effects during lunch was pre-experimental.

Recently, Sharp et al. (2012) compared four dietary modification-based interventions to treat rumination among two individuals with autism. The interventions were increased meal size, supplemental feedings, fixed-time provision of peanut butter, and liquid rescheduling. During the increased meal size condition, participants received double their usual portion size at meals. The supplemental feedings condition consisted of splitting a meal in two halves and providing half of the meal in small bites on a fixed time 1 min schedule for 30 min after the first half of the meal was consumed. The fixed-time provision of peanut butter condition consisted of the delivery of half a teaspoon of peanut butter on a fixed-time 1 min schedule for 30 min after a meal. The liquid rescheduling condition consisted of withholding drinks for 60 min after a meal. Of these, liquid rescheduling was the most effective. In addition, the authors also found that the most effective schedule upon which the liquid was administered varied by participant.

The mechanism(s) responsible for the effects of dietary interventions probably varies by procedure. For procedures in which large quantities of food are provided, the increased caloric intake may produce satiation, which may be responsible for treatment effects. For procedures in which food is delivered on fixed-time schedules after meals, chewing the food may compete with rumination. For procedures in which a thick food such as peanut butter or bread is delivered before, during, or after meals and procedures in which liquid is withheld during meals, the mechanism of action might be prevention. That is, rumination might be prevented from occurring due to the participant's inability to bring food up into the mouth. Other possible explanations for the efficacy of access to peanut butter and bread include the increased consumption of concentrated starches (which are high in caloric content), and the possibility that eating these foods provides a sensory consequence that competes with rumination behavior. Of course, this is just speculation;

additional research is needed to determine the mechanism of action for these and many other interventions for rumination. In addition to varying by procedure, the mechanism of action may vary by individual. As a result, more research on an individual basis is needed. Since the literature on the treatment of rumination largely consists of within subject experimental designs with a small number of participants, large-scale studies employing group designs to evaluate dietary interventions (as well as other interventions) are also necessary.

Punishment-Based Procedures. A number of studies have used punishment-based procedures to treat rumination. In nearly all of these studies, positive punishment (i.e., the addition of a stimulus contingent upon a behavior which results in a decrease in that behavior) was used. Most of these studies were published early in the history of the treatment of rumination; more recent interventions have focused on dietary manipulations (reviewed above), as well as interventions based on a functional assessment (described below).

Although it is not common today, electric shock has been used to decrease rumination in a number of studies. Bright and Whaley (1968) used contingent electric shock to decrease rumination and vomiting in an 11-year-old boy with an intellectual disability. The procedure was reportedly effective; rumination was eliminated. Other early studies on the use of shock to decrease rumination reported similar results (Galbraith et al. 1970; Kohlenberg 1970; Luckey et al. 1968). Unfortunately, many of these studies employed inadequate research designs, so the extent to which the effects were due to the shock alone is difficult to determine.

In addition to problematic research methodology, a number of studies using electric shock have reported unwanted side effects. These side effects include emotional behavior, masturbation, hair pulling, and other self-injurious behaviors (Starin and Fuqua 1987). The use of electric shock is now considered to be inhumane by many and is seldom, if ever, approved by human rights committees.

Other punishment-based procedures have also been used to treat rumination. Minness (1980) used contingent pinching to decrease operant vomiting by an adolescent female with an intellectual disability. The author reported pinching the back of the participant's hand contingent upon the participant putting her hand into her mouth. A time-out period, as well as reinforcement for alternative behavior, was also used. The procedure was effective in both the original setting as well as a generalization setting; operant vomiting decreased to near-zero levels. Unfortunately, once treatment was removed, vomiting returned.

Another form of punishment procedure that has been used to treat rumination is the contingent application of unpleasant tastes. Lemon juice, hot sauce, and antiseptic have all been applied contingent upon rumination. Most often, a small amount (5–10 cc) of the substance is squirted into the participant's mouth immediately following an instance of rumination. In one case, however, Bright and Whaley (1968) sprayed hot sauce on to previously expelled vomitus in order to decrease re-ingestion of the vomitus.

Sajwaj et al. (1974) used contingent lemon juice to decease life-threatening rumination in a six-month-old infant. The procedure decreased rumination to near-zero levels and the authors reported few, if any, negative side effects. This study is unusual in that the participant was a typically developing female; the majority of studies evaluating treatments for rumination have been conducted with individuals with intellectual disabilities. Marholin et al. (1980) replicated this procedure in an adolescent with an intellectual disability; operant vomiting and vomiting-related behavior decreased to near-zero levels. In addition, the contingent lemon juice was removed after 62 days of treatment and vomiting remained at low levels.

Becker et al. (1978) used contingent lemon juice to treat rumination exhibited by a 3-year-old girl with an intellectual disability. The procedure reduced rumination and the authors were able to train the participant's mother to implement the intervention. The authors did report some negative side effects of the procedure, including other forms of self-injury.

Foxx et al. (1979) used an oral hygiene punishment procedure to treat rumination exhibited by two women with intellectual disabilities. The oral hygiene procedure consisted of cleansing the participant's teeth with an alcohol-based mouthwash for two min contingent upon rumination. Interestingly, the authors first implemented a satiation procedure with the participants; although satiation was somewhat effective, it did not decrease rumination to near-zero levels. The addition of the oral hygiene procedure reduced rumination to 1–3 % of baseline levels for both participants.

Overcorrection, another form of punishment, has also been used to treat rumination. The published studies on the use of overcorrection have used restitution, a form of overcorrection in which the participant is required to restore the environment to an improved state, to treat operant vomiting or rumination. Azrin and Wesolowski (1975) used a restitution procedure as well as positive practice, in which the participant was required to practice the correct way to vomit (i.e., over a sink or toilet) 15 times. The total duration of the overcorrection procedure was 20–60 min. The participant was a woman with an intellectual disability who engaged in operant vomiting. The procedure was effective within one week and was discontinued shortly after. At a one-year follow-up, operant vomiting was still absent. Duker and Seys (1977) replicated the procedure but used a shorter overall duration of the overcorrection procedure; they found that the briefer version of the overcorrection procedure was also effective.

Assessment-Based Behavioral Interventions for Rumination

Interventions for many forms of challenging behavior among individuals with intellectual disabilities have become increasingly non-aversive over the past 25 years (Lang et al. 2011), and interventions for rumination are no exception. The advent and use of functional assessment technology to identify the environmental variables responsible for challenging behavior has led to an increase in assessment-based interventions for rumination and a decrease in punishment-based procedures. Table 9.1 provides a succinct description of the research on assessment-based behavioral interventions for rumination.

Lockwood et al. (1997) conducted a descriptive analysis in which they recorded narrative data on rumination exhibited by a 34-year old woman with an intellectual disability. Their assessment results suggested that the participant's rumination was maintained by social negative reinforcement in the form of escape from demands. Based on these results, they instituted an intervention which included escape extinction, a correction procedure involving cleaning any expelled vomitus, and choice of foods. They found the procedure to be effective at decreasing rumination. In addition, the effects generalized across settings and maintained for 3 years. Notably, this is the only published study in which a functional assessment suggested maintenance of rumination via social variables as opposed to non-social variables (i.e., automatic reinforcement).

Kenzer and Wallace (2007) conducted a functional analysis on rumination exhibited by a 59-year old male with an intellectual disability. The analysis suggested that rumination was maintained by automatic reinforcement. During intervention, the authors compared access to larger portions of food during meals to supplemental post-meal opportunities to eat. Results showed that the supplemental feedings produced a greater reduction in the rate of rumination than the large portions treatment.

Lyons et al. (2007) conducted a functional analysis with two adolescents who engaged in rumination. The results suggest that rumination was maintained by automatic reinforcement for both participants. These researchers then evaluated a chew ring intended to match (to some extent, at least) the oral stimulation produced by rumination, as well as a supplemental feeding session that involved access to food and liquids. Their results showed that the chew ring initially reduced rumination for one of the participants, but the effects were not maintained. The supplemental feeding component reduced rumination and the intervention effects were maintained for 3 months.

Wilder et al. (2009) conducted a functional analysis on rumination exhibited by an adult with autism. They conducted a functional analysis both pre- and post-meal to verify that rumination only occurred after food consumption and to determine the variables responsible for maintenance. The authors found that rumination did only occur after meals and the results of the functional analysis suggest that rumination was maintained by automatic reinforcement. They then evaluated the use of flavor sprays (i.e., zero calorie sprays which taste like various foods) to reduce rumination. The intervention was moderately effective and the participant was also taught to self-administer the spray.

Baker et al. (2010) assessed operant vomiting in an 8-year old boy with autism. During a functional analysis, vomiting was shown to persist in the absence of social consequences. Interestingly, the behavior seemed to be maintained by the site of the vomitus once it was expelled. Interventions involving noncontingent reinforcement (NCR) and differential reinforcement of other behavior (DRO) were ineffective, but a visual screen, which prevented the boy from seeing the vomitus, reduced rumination to low levels. The effects were maintained for 4 months and generalized across settings.

Table 9.1 Rumination studies in which a functional assessment was conducted

Citation	Participant(s)	Dependent variables	Functional assessment (FA) / Intervention (INT)	Results
Baker et al. (2010)	8 YO male with autism	Mean number of vomits per week	FA: Automatic reinforcement INT: Contingent antiseptic and visual screen in which view of vomitus was blocked	Contingent antiseptic ineffective; visual screen effective
Dominguez et al. (2014)	11 YO male with autism	Rumination per min during 30 min after dinner	FA: Automatic reinforcement INT: Contingent verbal reprimand	Contingent verbal reprimand effective
Kenzer and Wallace (2007)	59 YO male with intellectual disability	Rumination per min	FA: Automatic reinforcement INT: Food satiation and 15 min, 30 min supplemental feedings	Food satiation ineffective; supplemental feedings effective (30 min more effective than 15 min)
Kliebert and Tiger (2011)	11 YO male with autism	Percentage of sessions with rumination after lunch	FA: Automatic reinforcement INT: Fixed time 15 s access to apple juice	Fixed time access to apple juice effective
Lockwood et al. (1997)	34 YO female with intellectual disability	Vomiting incidents per day	FA: Escape from demands INT: Differential reinforcement, escape extinction, food choice	Combination of differential reinforcement, escape extinction, and food choice effective
Lyons et al. (2007)	14 YO male with developmental delay and 11 YO male autism	Percentage of intervals with rumination	FA: Automatic reinforcement (both participants) INT: Fixed time 30 s access to food or liquid (14 YO); Fixed time 30 s access to food or liquid and continuous access to a chew ring (11 YO)	Fixed time access to food and liquid effective (fruit juice most effective) for 14 YO; fixed time access to food and liquid effective (pretzel most effective) for 11 YO

(continued)

Table 9.1 (continued)

Citation	Participant(s)	Dependent variables	Functional assessment (FA) / Intervention (INT)	Results
Wilder et al. (2009)	37 YO male with autism	Rumination per min	FA: Automatic reinforcement INT: Fixed time delivery of a flavor spray	Fixed time delivery of a flavor spray effective (taught self-administration of flavor spray)
Woods et al. (2013)	19 YO male with intellectual disability	Percentage of intervals with rumination	FA: Automatic reinforcement INT: Continuous access to auditory, visual and food; continuous access to foods differing in texture and taste; pre-session, access to granola bar	Pre-session and continuous access to granola bar effective
Wrigley et al. (2010)	Female with severe intellectual disability	Frequency of rumination	FA: Automatic reinforcement INT: Interruption of precursor behavior, 10 min periods of instruction and exercise, 10 min NCR with attention, DRO	Four-component intervention effective; similar effectiveness observed when DRO and instruction/exercise components were removed

Wrigley et al. (2010) evaluated a multi-component intervention to treat rumination exhibited by an adult female with intellectual disabilities. After a functional analysis demonstrated that the participant's rumination was maintained by automatic reinforcement, the researchers implemented an intervention consisting of the interruption of precursor behavior, noncontingent attention, and a 1-min DRO. The intervention reduced rumination by 82 % relative to baseline. The authors then systematically removed each component to determine its effects; interestingly, each component was found to contribute to the overall treatment effect.

Kliebert and Tiger (2011) evaluated the effects of noncontingent juice delivery on rumination exhibited by a young boy with autism. After a functional analysis showed that rumination was maintained by automatic reinforcement, the authors delivered preferred juice independent of rumination. In addition, they measured rumination during juice delivery as well as rumination that occurred well after juice delivery. The juice eliminated rumination during juice delivery, but had no effect on rumination after noncontingent juice was delivered. These results are interesting in that previous studies (e.g., Heering et al. 2003) have suggested that access to liquids might increase the likelihood of rumination; this study suggested the opposite effect (i.e., access to liquids decreased the likelihood of rumination).

Woods et al. (2013) conducted a functional analysis of rumination exhibited by a man with autism. The functional analysis suggested that rumination was maintained via automatic reinforcement. The authors then implemented an intervention in which they provided noncontingent access to supplemental food at meals. They found that noncontingent food was more effective than noncontingent inedible stimuli, certain types of food were more effective at reducing rumination than others, and that both pre-session as well as continuous access to food were more effective to reduce rumination than fixed-time access to food.

Finally, Dominguez et al. (2014) conducted a pre-treatment screening analysis to verify that rumination occurred in the absence of social consequences for an 11-year-old boy with autism. The analysis suggested a non-social function. They then implemented a verbal reprimand contingent upon rumination; the target behavior decreased to near-zero levels. The authors also collected follow-up data 18 months after the intervention; the reprimand was still effective at reducing rumination. This study is unusual in that a punishment-based procedure (which is non-function-based) was selected after the functional analysis showed maintenance via automatic reinforcement.

Practice Recommendations

Since the treatment of rumination began in the 1960s, a number of behavioral interventions have been employed. Punishment-based procedures such as contingent electric shock, contingent unpleasant taste, and overcorrection have all been shown to be effective to treat rumination. Dietary-based interventions, including food satiation, liquid rescheduling, and the response-independent delivery of food after meals have also been shown to be effective to treat rumination in a number of studies. Differential reinforcement procedures have been shown to be effective in some cases. A more recent development has been the use of functional assessment procedures to identify the function of rumination before implementing an intervention.

A decision tree depicting one possible framework for selecting behavioral interventions for rumination is provided in Fig. 9.1. This decision tree is based on the

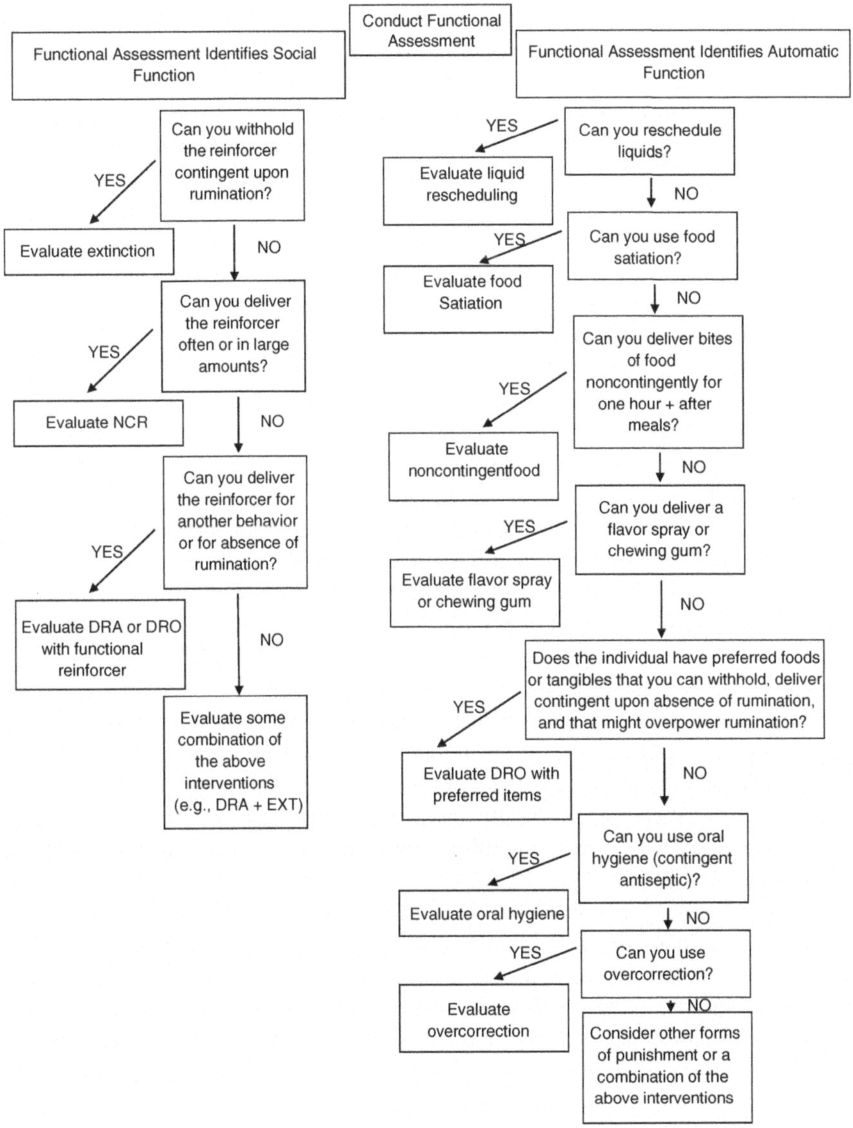

Fig. 9.1 Decision Tree for Model for Behavioral Interventions for Rumination

existing literature on the treatment of rumination and describes the least restrictive, most effective behavioral interventions published to date. Of course, individual practitioners may have constraints not considered in the development of this tree; therefore, it should only be used as a general guide to the development of an intervention.

Practitioners should first obtain a medical evaluation to determine the extent to which rumination is due to, or a by-product of, a medical problem. If medical causes and/or interventions are ruled out, the next step is to conduct a functional assessment to determine the function of rumination. Although it is likely that rumination is maintained by automatic reinforcement, it has been shown to be sensitive to social variables (i.e., escape from demands; Lockwood et al. 1997) in one case. If rumination is maintained by or sensitive to social variables, treatment will center on manipulation of those variables. For example, treatment might consist of eliminating the motivation to engage in rumination by delivering a large amount of the reinforcer on a response-independent basis (noncontingent reinforcement), withholding the reinforcer contingent upon rumination (i.e., extinction), delivering the reinforcer contingent upon a socially appropriate alternative behavior (i.e., differential reinforcement), or some combination of these.

If rumination is maintained by automatic reinforcement (i.e., it produces its own reinforcement, independent of social consequences), a different approach to treatment will be necessary. Because they are generally not very intrusive and have been shown to be effective, dietary interventions might be evaluated first. The dietary intervention that is least likely to produce side effects would be liquid rescheduling, or, if the individual is of below average or average weight, food satiation (i.e., providing large quantities of food during a meal). The response independent delivery of food on a fixed time schedule might also be an option, but this may be time-intensive, and thus, difficult to implement. If these interventions are ineffective, and if it is possible to deliver stimulation that is similar to the stimulation produced by rumination (e.g., delivery of a flavor spray, chewing gum) after meals, this is a viable approach. If delivery of a flavor spray or chewing gum cannot be done or is ineffective, a differential reinforcement procedure using a highly preferred item might be attempted. A stimulus preference assessment should be conducted first; once a high preference item has been identified, it can be delivered contingent on the absence of rumination (i.e., a DRO). Finally, if all of these procedures fail, a combination of the interventions described above might be attempted.

As a last resort, punishment-based procedures might be used. Of course, permission from a guardian and/or a human rights committee will be necessary before evaluating a punishment-based procedure. An overcorrection procedure or a verbal reprimand might be evaluated first. If these are ineffective, an oral hygiene procedure using an antiseptic might be applied. If rumination is unresponsive to all of these interventions (remember that a punishment procedure can be combined with one of the interventions described above), more intrusive punishment-based procedures might be considered, taking into account the individual's current state of health and the urgency of decreasing rumination.

To summarize, rumination and operant vomiting can have serious adverse health consequences and should be addressed as soon as they are identified. If no medical cause is apparent, behavioral interventions are the least intrusive, most effective procedures to treat rumination. A functional assessment should first be conducted to identify the variables maintaining rumination. Based on assessment results, a number of interventions might be evaluated.

References

Amarnath, R. P., Abell, T. L., & Malagelada, J. R. (1986). The rumination syndrome in adults: A characteristic manometric pattern. *Annals of Internal Medicine, 105*, 513–518. doi:10.7326/0003-4819-105-4-513

American Psychiatric Association. (2013). *Diagnostic and statistical maunal of mental disorders* (5th ed.). Washington, D.C.: Author.

Azrin, N. H., & Wesolowski, M. D. (1975). Eliminating habitual vomiting in a retarded adult by positive practice and self-correction. *Journal of Behavior Therapy and Experimental Psychiatry, 6*, 145–148. doi:10.1016/0005-7916(75)90040-3

Baker, L. M., Rapp, J. T., & Carroll, R. A. (2010). Treating operant vomiting with visual screening. *Clinical Case Studies, 9*, 218–224. doi:10.1177/1534650110372253

Becker, J. V., Turner, S. M., & Sajwaj, T. E. (1978). Multiple behavioral effects of the use of lemon juice with a ruminating toddler-age child. *Behavior Modification, 2*, 267–278. doi:10.1177/014544557822007

Blinder, B. J., Bain, N., & Simpson, R. (1986). Evidence for an opioid neurotransmission mechanism in adult rumination. *The American Journal of Psychiatry, 143*, 255.

Bright, G. O., & Whaley, D. L. (1968). Supression of regurgitation and rumination with aversive events. *Michigan Mental Health Research Bulletin, 11*, 17–20.

Clauser, B., & Scibak, J. W. (1990). Direct and generalized effects of food satiation in reducing rumination. *Research in Developmental Disabilities, 11*, 23–36. doi:10.1016/0891-4222(90)90003-Q

Darling, J. A., Otto, J. T., & Buckner, C. K. (2011). Reduction of rumination using a supplemental starch feeding procedure. *Behavioral Interventions, 26*, 204–213. doi:10.1002/bin.331

Dominguez, A., Wilder, D. A., Cheung, K., & Rey, C. (2014). The use of a verbal reprimand to decrease rumination in a child with autism. *Behavioral Interventions, 29*, 339–345. doi:10.1002/bin.1390

Dudley, L. L., Johnson, C., & Barnes, R. S. (2002). Decreasing rumination using a starchy food satiation procedure. *Behavioral Interventions, 17*, 21–29. doi:10.1002/bin.104

Duker, P. C., & Seys, D. M. (1977). Elimination of vomiting in a retarded female using restitutional overcorrection. *Behavior Therapy, 8*, 255–257. doi:10.1016/S0005-7894(77)80275-X

Dunn, J., Lockwood, K., Williams, D. E., & Peacock, S. (1997). A seven year follow-up of treating rumination with dietary satiation. *Behavioral Interventions, 12*, 163–172. doi:10.1002/(SICI)1099-078X(199710)12:4<163:AID-BRT175>3.0.CO;2-X

Foxx, R. M., Snyder, M. S., & Schroeder, F. (1979). A food satiation and oral hygiene punishment program to suppress chronic rumination by retarded persons. *Journal of Autism and Developmental Disorders, 9*, 399–412. doi:10.1007/BF01531447

Fredericks, D. W., Carr, J. E., & Williams, W. L. (1998). Overview of the treatment of rumination disorder for adults in a residential setting. *Journal of Behavior Therapy and Experimental Psychiatry, 29*, 31–40. doi:10.1016/S0005-7916(98)00002-0

Galbraith, D. A., Byrick, R. J., & Rutledge, J. T. (1970). An aversive conditioning approach to the inhibition of chronic vomiting. *Canadian Psychiatric Association Journal, 15*, 311–313.

Greene, K. S., Johnston, J. M., Rossi, M., Rawal, A., Winston, M., & Barron, S. (1991). Effects of peanut butter on ruminating. *American Journal on Mental Retardation, 95*, 631–645.

Heering, P. W., Wilder, D. A., & Ladd, C. (2003). Liquid rescheduling for the treatment of rumination. *Behavioral Interventions, 18*, 199–207. doi:10.1002/bin.137

Jackson, G. M., Johnson, C. R., Ackron, G. S., & Crowley, R. (1975). Food satiation as a procedure to decelerate vomiting. *American Journal of Mental Deficiency, 80*, 223–227.

Johnston, J. M., Greene, K. S., Rawal, A., Vazin, T., & Winston, M. (1991). Effects of caloric level on ruminating. *Journal of Applied Behavior Analysis, 24*, 597–603. doi:10.1901/jaba.1991.24-597

Kelly, M. B., & Heffner, H. E. (1988). The role of attention in the elimination of chronic, life-threatening vomiting. *Journal of Mental Deficiency Research, 32*, 425–431.

Kelly, N. R., Shank, L. M., Bakalar, J. L., & Tanofsky-Kraff, M. (2014). Pediatric feeding and eating disorders: Current state of diagnosis and treatment. *Current Psychiatry Reports, 16*, 1–12. doi:10.1007/s11920-014-0446-z

Kenzer, A. L., & Wallace, M. D. (2007). Treatment of rumination maintained by automatic reinforcement: A comparison of extra portions during a meal and supplemental post-meal feedings. *Behavioral Interventions, 22*, 297–304. doi:10.1002/bin.249

Kliebert, M. L., & Tiger, J. H. (2011). Direct and distal effects of noncontingent juice on rumination exhibited by a child with autism. *Journal of Applied Behavior Analysis, 44*, 955–959.

Kohlenberg, R. J. (1970). The punishment of persistent vomiting: A case study. *Journal of Applied Behavior Analysis, 3*, 241–245. doi:10.1901/jaba.1970.3-241

Kuhn, D. E., & Matson, J. L. (2004). Assessment of feeding and mealtime behavior problems in persons with mental retardation. *Behavior Modification, 28*, 638–648. doi:10.1177/0145445503259833

Kuruvilla, J., & Trewby, P. N. (1989). Gastro-oesophageal disorders in adults with severe mental impairment. *British Medical Journal, 299*(6691), 95–96.

Lang, R., Mulloy, A., Giesbers, S., Pfeiffer, B., Delaune, E., Didden, R., et al. (2011). Behavioral interventions for rumination and operant vomiting in individuals with intellectual disabilities: A systematic review. *Research in Developmental Disabilities, 32*, 2193–2205.

Libby, D. G., & Phillips, E. (1979). Eliminating rumination behavior in a profoundly retarded adolescent: An exploratory study. *Mental Retardation, 17*, 94–95.

Lockwood, K., Maenpaa, M., & Williams, D. E. (1997). Long-term maintenance of a behavioral alternative to surgery for severe vomiting and weight loss. *Journal of Behavior Therapy and Experimental Psychiatry, 28*, 105–112. doi:10.1016/S0005-7916(97)00009-8

Luckey, R. E., Watson, C. M., & Musick, J. K. (1968). Aversive conditioning as a means of inhibiting vomiting and rumination. *American Journal of Mental Deficiency, 73*, 139–142.

Luiselli, J. K., Haley, S., & Smith, A. (1993). Evaluation of a behavioral medicine consultative treatment for chronic, ruminative vomiting. *Journal of Behavior Therapy and Experimental Psychiatry, 24*, 27–35. doi:10.1016/0005-7916(93)90005-H

Luiselli, J. K., Medeiros, J., Jasinowski, C., Smith, A., & Cameron, M. J. (1994). Behavioral medicine treatment of ruminative vomiting and associated weight loss in an adolescent with autism. *Journal of Autism and Developmental Disorders, 24*, 619–629. doi:10.1007/BF02172142

Lyons, E. A., Rue, H. C., Luiselli, J. K., & DiGennaro, F. D. (2007). Brief functional analysis and supplemental feeding for postmeal rumination in children with developmental disabilities. *Journal of Applied Behavior Analysis, 40*, 743–747.

Marholin, D., Luiselli, J. K., Robinson, M., & Lott, I. T. (1980). Response-contingent taste-aversion in treating chronic ruminative vomiting of institutionalised profoundly retarded children. *Journal of Mental Deficiency Research, 24*, 47–56.

Masalsky, C. J., & Luiselli, J. K. (1998). Effects of supplemental feedings of white bread on chronic rumination. *Behavioral Interventions, 13*, 227–233. doi:10.1002/(SICI)1099-078X(199811)13:4<227:AID-BIN18>3.0.CO;2-C

Minness, P. M. (1980). Treatment of compulsive hand in mouth behaviour in a profoundly retarded child using a sharp pinch as the aversive stimulus. *Australian Journal of Developmental Disabilities, 6*, 5–10.

Parry-Jones, B. (1994). Merycism or rumination disorder: A historical investigation and current assessment. *The British Journal of Psychiatry, 165*, 303–314. doi:10.1192/bjp.165.3.303

Parry-Jones, W. L., & Parry-Jones, B. (1994). Implications of historical evidence for the classification of eating disorders: A dimension overlooked in DSM-III—R and ICD-10. *The British Journal of Psychiatry, 165*, 287–292. doi:10.1192/bjp.165.3.287

Rast, J., Johnston, J. M., & Drum, C. (1984). A parametric analysis of the relationship between food quantity and rumination. *Journal of the Experimental Analysis of Behavior, 41*, 125–134. doi:10.1901/jeab.1984.41-125

Rast, J., Johnston, J. M., Drum, C., & Conrin, J. (1981). The relation of food quantity to rumination behavior. *Journal of Applied Behavior Analysis, 14*, 121–130. doi:10.1901/jaba.1981.14-121

Rast, J., Johnston, J. M., Lubin, D., & Ellinger-Allen, J. (1988). Effects of premeal chewing on ruminative behavior. *American Journal on Mental Retardation, 93*, 67–74.

Rhine, D., & Tarbox, J. (2009). Chewing gum as a treatment for rumination in a child with autism. *Journal of Applied Behavior Analysis, 42*, 381–385. doi:10.1901/jaba.2009.42-381

Rogers, B., Stratton, P., Victor, J., Kennedy, B., & Andres, M. (1992). Chronic regurgitation among persons with mental retardation: A need for combined medical and interdisciplinary strategies. *American Journal on Mental Retardation, 96*, 522–527.

Sajwaj, T., Libet, J., & Agras, S. (1974). Lemon-juice therapy: The control of life-threatening rumination in a six-month-old infant. *Journal of Applied Behavior Analysis, 7*, 557–563. doi: 10.1901/jaba.1974.7-557

Sanders-Dewey, N. E. J., & Larson, M. E. (2006). Chronic rumination reduction in a severely developmentally disabled adult following combined use of positive and negative contingencies. *Journal of Behavior Therapy and Experimental Psychiatry, 37*, 140–145. doi:10.1016/j.jbtep.2005.03.001

Sharp, R. A., Phillips, K. J., & Mudford, O. C. (2012). Comparisons of interventions for rumination maintained by automatic reinforcement. *Research in Autism Spectrum Disorders, 6*, 1107–1112. doi:10.1016/j.rasd.2012.03.002

Singh, N. N. (1981). Rumination. In N. R. Ellis (Ed.), *International review of research in mental retardation* (Vol. 10, pp. 139–182). New York: Academic Press.

Starin, S. P., & Fuqua, R. W. (1987). Rumination and vomiting in the developmentally disabled: A critical review of the behavioral, medical, and psychiatric treatment research. *Research in Developmental Disabilities, 8*, 575–605. doi:10.1016/0891-4222(87)90055-2

Thibadeau, S., Blew, P., Reedy, P., & Luiselli, J. K. (1999). Access to white bread as an intervention for chronic ruminative vomiting. *Journal of Behavior Therapy and Experimental Psychiatry, 30*, 137–144. doi:10.1016/S0005-7916(99)00012-9

Tierney, D. W., & Jackson, H. J. (1984). Psychosocial treatments of rumination disorder: A review of the literature. *Australia and New Zealand Journal of Developmental Disabilities, 10*, 81–112.

Wilder, D. A., Draper, R., Williams, W. L., & Higbee, T. S. (1997). A comparison of noncontingent reinforcement, other competing stimulation, and liquid rescheduling for the treatment of rumination. *Behavioral Interventions, 12*, 55–64. doi:10.1002/(SICI)1099-078X(199704)12:2<55::AID-BIN167>3.0.CO;2-7.

Wilder, D. A., Register, M., Register, S., Bajagic, V., & Neidert, P. L. (2009). Functional analysis and treatment of rumination using fixed-time delivery of a flavor spray. *Journal of Applied Behavior Analysis, 42*, 877–882. doi:10.1901/jaba.2009.42-877

Winton, A. S. W., & Singh, N. N. (1983). Rumination in pediatric populations: A behavioral analysis. *Journal of the American Academy of Child Psychiatry, 22*, 269–275. doi:10.1016/S0002-7138(09)60376-9

Woods, K. E., Luiselli, J. K., & Tomassone, S. (2013). Functional analysis and intervention for chronic rumination. *Journal of Applied Behavior Analysis, 46*, 328–332.

Wrigley, M., Kahn, K., Winder, P., Vollmer, T. R., & Sy, J. R. (2010). A multi-component approach to the treatment of chronic rumination. *Behavioral Interventions, 25*, 295–305. doi:10.1002/bin.313

Yang, L. (1988). Elimination of habitual rumination through the strategies of food satiation and fading: A case study. *Behavioral Residential Treatment, 3*, 223–234. doi:10.1002/bin.2360030306

Chapter 10
Substance Use and Health Related Issues

Robert Didden, Joanneke VanDerNagel and Neomi van Duijvenbode

Introduction

Substance use (SU) is highly prevalent among the adult population. For example, results of the National Survey on Drug Use and Health (Substance Abuse and Mental Health Services Administration [SAMHSA] 2014) indicate that in the United States, more than 80 % of the population aged 18 and older has ever used alcohol in his or her life. In addition, roughly half of this population has ever used cannabis and other illicit drugs. While SU in itself is not necessarily problematic and is often also socially acceptable—especially in the case of tobacco and alcohol use—a number of people develop a substance use disorder (SUD).

According to the American Psychiatric Association (APA 2013), SUD is characterised by a problematic and recurrent pattern of SU that results in significant impairments in day-to-day functioning, including failures to meet responsibilities at work, school or home. It is diagnosed on a continuum from mild to severe, using 11 criteria related to impaired control over SU, social impairments as a result of SU, risky SU and symptoms of tolerance and withdrawal. Recent findings from the general United States population estimate the lifetime prevalence of alcohol use disorder around 8 % and illicit drug use disorder around 2–3 % (Swendsen et al. 2012). Similar findings have been reported in studies on the epidemiology of SUD among European countries, with prevalence rates for alcohol use disorder of roughly 6 % for males and 1 % for females (Rehm et al. 2005) and rates varying between 0.3 and 2.9 % for drug use disorder (Rehm et al. 2005).

R. Didden (✉) · J. VanDerNagel · N. van Duijvenbode
Radboud University Nijmegen, Nijmegen, The Netherlands
e-mail: r.didden@pwo.ru.nl

J.K. Luiselli (ed.), *Behavioral Health Promotion and Intervention in Intellectual and Developmental Disabilities*, Evidence-Based Practices in Behavioral Health,
DOI 10.1007/978-3-319-27297-9_10

Individuals with intellectual and developmental disabilities (IDD) seem to be at risk for developing SUD. Although reliable data on the prevalence of SU(D) in individuals with IDD are scarce (Carroll Chapman and Wu 2012), it is suggested that all substances are used by individuals with IDD. Alcohol is reported to be the main substance used and misused among this group, with prevalence rates similar or lower compared to those in the general population (To et al. 2014; VanDerNagel et al. 2011a). Prevalence rates of cannabis and other illicit drug use among individuals with IDD, on the other hand, seem higher compared to those in the general population (VanDerNagel et al. 2011a). The overall prevalence rate of SUD was estimated by Sturmey et al. (2003) around 0.5–2 % of the IDD population. However, it should be noted that these rates highly depend on sample characteristics, with relatively high prevalence rates found in referred samples (e.g., Didden et al. 2009) and forensic samples (e.g., Lindsay et al. 2013).

The consequences of SUD are often detrimental and are a major public health and economic concern (Martin et al. 2014). For example, problematic alcohol use is responsible for 2.74 million deaths annually (4 % of the worldwide total), being the fifth leading risk factor for global diseases (Scott and Kaner 2014). In addition to these somatic consequences, SUD is also related to a wide range of (neuro) psychological and behavioral problems, including aggression, violence, mental ill-health and suicide (Room et al. 2005). Research suggests that SUD also has a negative influence on the brain, especially on executive control (e.g., Loeber et al. 2009). Examples include a decreased working memory capacity, a poorer inhibitory control, slowed processing speed, impaired cognitive and behavioral flexibility and impaired emotion regulation (e.g., Bravers et al. 2014). In individuals with IDD these substance use-related somatic, psychological and social problems might be even more prevalent and more severe (Slayter 2008). SUD is also related to problems with work, housing and the social network of individuals with IDD (Slayter 2008) and is a risk factor for emotional and behavioral problems (Didden et al. 2009) and delinquency (Lindsay et al. 2013). Therefore, it has not only a large and negative impact on the wellbeing of the individual, but also on the society as a whole.

Despite these severe consequences, however, individuals often continue the use of substances. Wiers and Stacy (2006) have called this 'the paradox of addiction' and noted that "…the typical problem in addiction is not that drug abusers do not realize that the disadvantages of continued drug use outweigh the advantages. The central paradox in addictive behaviors is that people continue to use substances even though they know the harm." Dual process models of addiction (e.g., Strack and Deutsch 2004) have tried to explain this paradox, and postulate that behavior is influenced by both implicit, automatic processes and explicit, controlled processes. Implicit processes are considered to be spontaneous, fast, can sometimes occur outside of conscious awareness and cannot easily be controlled. Examples of such processes are attention selection and allocation and automatic action tendencies. Explicit processes, on the other hand, are deliberate, slow and require conscious awareness and include executive functioning and motivation. As a result of chronic and/or excessive SU, the implicit processes get stronger and the rewarding effects of substances and related stimuli become overvalued at the expense of other rewards. At the same time, the explicit or controlled processes become weaker as a result of a disrupted inhibitory control system and reduced top-down control over behavior. Together, these disruptions indicate a growing loss of control over SU. It should be noted, however, that research on these neuropsychological disruptions in individuals with IDD is still limited (e.g., Van Duijvenbode et al., submitted; Van Duijvenbode et al., under review). The same conclusion holds true for research on the relationship between SUD and mental health and psychosocial problems of individuals with IDD.

SUD is a chronic and multifaceted problem that is caused by biological, psychological and social factors and is often associated with comorbid psychiatric disorders and psychosocial problems (Van Duijvenbode et al. 2015). This complexity is first reflected in the fact that SUD cannot be explained by a single factor, but rather is a result of an interplay between biological, psychological and social risk factors (Donovan 2005). Second, SUD often co-occurs with other somatic and psychiatric problems, which increases symptom severity, complicates treatment and often causes additional psychosocial problems (Sterling et al. 2011). Third and last, SUD is a chronic disorder that often lasts for several decades and is characterized by relapse and multiple treatment episodes before reaching full recovery (Swendsen et al. 2012). Together, these factors mean that patients with SUD form a heterogeneous group, with differences in risk factors for SUD, patterns of SU(D) (e.g., number and types of substances used, severity of SUD, experienced consequences of SUD), type and degree of comorbidity with somatic and mental health problems, and individual characteristics (including motivation to enter into and adhere to treatment goals, risk and protective factors and context).

Priority Concerns

Given that SUD is a chronic and complex disorder that is associated with potentially detrimental negative consequences, it is not surprising that SU(D) among individuals with IDD has received growing attention over the past decade. However, there are still many lacunae in our knowledge base. For example, knowledge regarding prevalence and risk factors is limited and assessment tools and evidence-based treatment interventions are scarce (also see Sect. "Conclusions About Evidence-Based Practice"). Van Duijvenbode et al. (2015) have therefore proposed several directions for future research and recommendations for policy and practice that will be briefly summarised here and that will be discussed in more detail in the remainder of this chapter.

First, research should be directed at establishing the prevalence and risk factors of SU(D) among individuals with IDD. More knowledge on this topic is needed to plan treatment capacity, to develop prevention strategies and to facilitate early detection of SU(D). This research may include a variety of methods—including biomedical markers, administrative data and meta-data—and should be aimed at both the general population of individuals with IDD and specific risk groups, such as those with comorbid psychiatric disorders and forensic patients. Identifying risk groups will then also lead to more knowledge on specific risk factors for SUD, including motives for SU, client characteristics and social factors, which could subsequently be targeted in primary and secondary prevention strategies. Considering the high rates of comorbidity between SUD and other psychiatric disorders, and the influence comorbidity has on symptom severity and treatment success (Sterling et al. 2011), studies into the prevalence of a so-called 'triple diagnosis' (e.g., the co-occurrence of IDD, SUD and a psychiatric disorder) are especially needed.

Second, screening and assessment instruments of SU(D)—and co-morbid psychiatric disorders and psychosocial problems—should be developed and validated for those with IDD. The majority of IDD service providers do not systematically screen for SU(D) in clients but instead rely on the clinical judgement of staff members. However, staff members indicate that they lack the skills and knowledge to do so (McLaughlin et al. 2007; VanDerNagel et al. 2011a) and these judgements are proven to be unreliable (Wilson et al. 2004). Thus, it is likely that only the more severe cases of SU(D) are noticed and opportunities to intervene at an early stage are missed. It is therefore advised to systematically screen for SU(D) among clients with IDD and implement this screening in the routine diagnostic procedure [as opposed to limiting screening to clients at risk for developing SUD]. Examples of instruments that are now being studied are the *Substance Use and Misuse in Intellectual Disability—Questionnaire* (SumID-Q; VanDerNagel et al. 2011b) and indirect measures of substance use-induced deficiencies in information processing (e.g., cognitive biases and executive dysfunction; Van Duijvenbode et al., under review; Van Duijvenbode et al., submitted).

Third, although there are a small number of published papers on SUD interventions for individuals with IDD, the body of evidence on their effectiveness is small (see Sect. "Conclusions About Evidence-Based Practice"). One line of research is therefore to develop treatment interventions tailored to the needs of those with IDD and study their effectiveness using strong methodological designs and larger samples of participants. These treatment interventions should take into account the diverse (risk) factors for SUD, and should include biological, psychological and social interventions (Reif et al. 2014). Especially the development of treatment interventions for individuals with dual and triple diagnoses is warranted. Also, as SUD is a chronic disorder that often lasts several decades and that is characterised by multiple relapses, treatment interventions should be structured according to the chronic care approach (McLellan et al. 2005), for example, by developing a broad spectrum of less to more intensive treatment forms, the implementation of stepped care, long-term management and monitoring of patients and a focus on relapse prevention strategies, chronic care and harm reduction.

Last, the negative consequences and the complex, multifaceted nature of SUD requires specialised treatment. This calls for a close collaboration and cross-fertilisation between the different sectors of the health care system, including addiction medicine, IDD service providers and general psychiatry (also see Slayter 2010).

As noted by McLaughlin et al. (2007), professionals working in the field of IDD should be educated about the nature of SU(D) and the care for and treatment of patients with SUD. Professionals working within addiction medicine, on the other hand, should be educated about the needs of those with IDD, for example, when it comes to communication strategies and tailoring treatment interventions to those with IDD. This could initiate a joint strategy and improve SUD treatment for patients with IDD.

Efficacy of Methods

Interventions for Substance Use

Kerr et al. (2013) conducted a mixed method review of studies regarding the effectiveness of interventions for SU in individuals with IDD. They assessed feasibility, appropriateness, and meaningfulness of the interventions for tobacco smoking and alcohol drinking. A total of nine papers were included in their review covering 341 participants with mild IDD who were between 14 and 54 years of age. Four papers focused on tobacco-related interventions, three on alcohol-related interventions and two studies addressed both alcohol and tobacco.

Of the tobacco-related interventions, most were aimed at increasing knowledge levels about smoking and its financial and somatic consequences. For example, in the study by Chester et al. (2011) an educational course was combined with nicotine replacement which appeared effective in cutting down smoking rates and tobacco consumption in individuals with IDD residing in a forensic inpatient unit. Intervention consisted of 7 weekly group sessions with discussions, quizzes, and videos. Next to this, nurses provided individual health information supporting clients in the cessation of smoking. Results were positive in that there were 48 smokers on admission and 15 were successful in their attempt to stop smoking.

The alcohol-related studies were aimed at increasing knowledge and motivation to change behavior and increase client's readiness to change. In these studies, motivational interviewing techniques were used. For example, Mendel and Hipkins (2002) used motivational interviewing in 7 males (18–54 years old) who had a history of alcohol abuse from a medium secure forensic unit. Group intervention consisted of three 1-hour sessions over a 2-week period. Findings indicate that there had been a cognitive shift in that six individuals recognized more negative than positive consequences of their behavior than prior to the intervention. Also, four participants reported an increased confidence in their ability to change their level of alcohol consumption once discharged back to the community.

Lindsay et al. (1998) evaluated an education program for smoking cigarettes and drinking alcohol in a relatively large sample ($N = 48$) of individuals with IDD. Both alcohol and smoking groups were compared to age and gender matched control groups, and data on knowledge about smoking and drinking were collected in a randomized controlled group design. Intervention consisted of 8 sessions given by one trainer to groups containing 5 to 6 participants, which included group discussions, role-play, quizzes, fact sheets and team games. The intervention resulted in a significant increase in knowledge regarding smoking and alcohol drinking.

Conclusions About Evidence-Based Practice

Several conclusions may be drawn from the review. First, results of the studies suggest that—with adaptations to communication, use of pictorial stimuli, and number, format and duration of sessions—educating clients with IDD about the adverse effects and risks of SU may improve their substance-related knowledge. Educational interventions typically consist of several weekly group sessions, in which clients are provided with information (e.g., motives for drinking and/or smoking, legal issues, short-term and long-term effects and adverse consequences of smoking and drinking) about tobacco smoking and alcohol drinking and which aim to reduce SU and to prevent SU developing into SUD. It should be noted, however, that these interventions not always lead to a reduction in SU.

Second, a number of interventions aimed for behavioral change, such as cutting down or quitting SU, and improving skills related to this change such as social skills, coping skills and refusal skills. These interventions seemed effective in eliciting behavioral change and reducing SU. However, a range of problems can be identified when examining both the design and methodology of the studies as well as the interventions themselves. By far most studies were of poor to moderate methodological quality, often used small sample sizes and in most cases failed to include a control condition. Notable exception is the study by Lindsay et al. (1998). Recently, Singh et al. (2014) conducted a study that was not covered in Kerr et al.'s (2013) review. They used a mindfulness-based cessation program versus treatment as usual in a randomized controlled group design for 51 individuals with mild ID who smoked between 80 and 85 cigarettes per week. Long-term evaluation showed that individuals receiving the intervention were more successful at abstaining from smoking cigarettes at a 1-year follow-up than the controls. Singh et al.'s study is of high quality because of an internally valid design, reliability measures on dependent variables and clear description of the procedure.

And third, interventions were often fairly short (i.e., 3–12 sessions) and/or lacked a theoretical foundation. They seemed to focus on SU rather than SUD, and disregarded possible comorbid problems related to mental health and psychosocial functioning of individuals involved. Most often, treatment packages were implemented and no conclusions can be drawn on which elements contributed to the effectiveness of an intervention.

Practice Recommendations

The relative lack of evidence-based methods (see Sect. "Conclusions About Evidence-Based Practice") for individuals with IDD and SU(D) should not discourage clinicians from addressing this topic. Given the negative impact that SU(D) can have on health, psychological and social well-being, prevention, detection and screening, early intervention and treatment are of importance.

Prevention of Substance Use and Substance Use Disorder

Prevention starts with the recognition of the omnipresence of SU and individuals with IDD as a group at risk for substance-related problems. Limited cognitive abilities and impaired adaptive functioning do not preclude individuals from using substances, neither does the fact that they receive professional care or live in a sheltered environment. Awareness among staff members of the risk factors for both initial SU and progression to SUD is a centerpiece in prevention, as is implementing strategies to reduce these factors. These strategies can include: (a) identifying and influencing individual risk factors for SU, such as for instance mental health problems, inadequate coping styles, and psychological stress, (b) reducing social risks for SU, such as setting institutional rules for a smoke-free living environment, regulations that prevent professionals from using substances (including smoking) in the presence of clients, and reducing social pressure from peers, and (c) promoting a healthy lifestyle and introducing or strengthening protective factors such as having meaningful daytime activities, fulfilling social contacts, etcetera.

Restrictive policies in a facility regarding SU, such as prohibition of use, punishment after using substances, and limiting substance users' freedom of movement within and outside their place of residence may seem effective in short-term, but may also further secretive use as well as ingenious methods to continue use despite these restrictive measures. Educating clients with IDD about the risks and dangers of SU as a sole intervention has not proven effective in discouraging them to use substances (see Kerr et al. 2013). However, providing clients with adequate and factual information may be helpful in supporting them to make informed decisions and remain open to communicate about their SU with their caregivers.

Direct caregivers and family members play an essential role in the prevention of SU and SUD. A large range of actions may be taken in the case of prevention, such as increasing staff members' awareness, educating them on SU and effective preventive interventions, promoting healthy role modeling, fostering an environment in which SU can be discussed openly, and improving staff members' communication skills to address SU of their clients.

Detection of and Screening for Substance Use

Case identification is the next crucial step in reducing the risks of SU and the progression towards SUD. Promoting an open and non-confrontational manner in which SU can be discussed before problems arise contributes to timely case identification (VanDerNagel et al. 2013). Conversely, a judgemental approach may deter clients from speaking openly about their SU, hindering both early detection and intervention. In a number of clients, SU may be directly observed and/or may be discussed openly. In many other cases SU is less overt. Then, a wide variety of signs and signals indicate the possibility of SU (VanDerNagel et al. 2013). These include (a) physical signs and symptoms (e.g., weight loss, decreased level of fitness, impeded motor skills), (b) psychological signs and symptoms (e.g., increased moodiness, impulsivity, concentration problems, deviant behavior), and (c) social signs [e.g., avoiding caregivers, changing the social environment, lateness (for work, school), increased financial or legal issues].

When SU is suspected, the client should be told which signs and symptoms are seen, and—without judgement—be asked what could be their cause. If SU is not mentioned by the client, the topic could be introduced in the form of a question or hypothesis ("I wonder if…"). When the client still denies using substances, refrain from arguing and propose to discuss this topic at a later time. Only when serious adverse consequences of SU(D) are imminent, a more coercive approach and measures to protect the client's and third party's safety may be called for. Again, a non-confrontational approach generally renders the best results in the long-term. Unfortunately, because the symptoms can be subtle, it is often only with the benefit of hindsight that early signs and signals of SU or even SUD are identified as such. Therefore, a more active approach with systematic screening in high-risk groups is recommended.

Screening for SU should be preferably done regularly (e.g., during each treatment evaluation) and with the use of a standardized screening instrument. The use of mainstream instruments, such as used in general medical practices, may not be feasible or appropriate in individuals with IDD. Widely used instruments such as the AUDIT (Alcohol Use Disorder Identification Test; Babor et al. 2001) for instance contain complex sentences that require insight in own behavior, timeframes and relations between events (e.g., "How often during the last year have you needed a first drink in the morning to get yourself going after a heavy drinking session?"). Even seemingly simple terms may pose difficulties. For instance, for an individual with IDD it may not be clear that the term 'alcohol' only may refer to strong spirits but also to beer. To add to this: the straightforward focus and style of mainstream questionnaires on the topic of an individual's SU may evoke evasive responses, especially when the individual fears negative consequences of admitting to using substances.

The aforementioned *SumID-Q* (VanDerNagel et al. 2011b), a Dutch language questionnaire on SU for individuals with IDD first addresses the topic of SU in general. Using pictures of both widely used substances (such as tobacco and alcohol) and pictures of illicit drugs (cannabis, cocaine et cetera) evaluates client's familiarity with substances in general and assesses the terminology the client uses for each substance. Then the client is interviewed on knowledge of and attitude towards SU. After this, SU in the individual's social environment (e.g., family, professional caregivers, peers) is inventoried. Only after this initial phase, in which the client experiences that s/he can talk freely about SU, his or her own SU is addressed. This strategy—though time-consuming—elicits valuable information and is well appreciated by both clients and professionals (VanDerNagel et al. 2011b, 2013). Further studies into the validity and feasibility of the *SumID-Q* and its translation into other languages are underway.

Since SU may not be a problem in and of itself, not all SU must lead to active interventions. In some cases 'watchful waiting', that is monitoring SU and possible adverse consequences, may suffice. When the individual who uses substances seems unaware of (potential) risks, or when future risks are foreseen, early intervention is called for. Additional substance education may be helpful if the client is open to it. Informal education ('small talk' and inquiring on the client's views and experience) and exploring with the client educational material or the internet may be more helpful than protocolled educational interventions. The use of 'minimal interventions' (i.e., the simple advice of a general practitioner to stop smoking, leaving the decision to the patient) is sometimes effective in the general population and may be of use in individuals with IDD as well.

Treatment of Substance Use Disorder

SUD is a complex and potentially serious health problem that warrants clinical attention, intensified staff support, and possibly referral to an addiction center. If substance-related problems arise, further diagnosis and assessment is needed. This should include (a) functional analysis of the relationship between the SU in this patient and biological, social and psychological risk factors and adverse consequences, (b) assessment whether the DSM-5 criteria of SUD are met and its severity level, and (c) somatic and mental health evaluation. The possibility of poly SU (i.e., use of several substances) or co-occurrence of SU and mental health problems should always be considered.

The assessment process can be complicated by the patient's reluctance to talk about his SU or sheer denial that s/he uses or misuses substances. It can also be complicated by the effects of co-occurring mental health conditions on the presentation of symptoms. For instance, patients with ADHD may not display typical symptoms, such as agitation, disorganization, and concentration problems, from the misuse of stimulants but may, paradoxically, become more quiet and focussed. Vice versa, symptoms of SU(D) may complicate assessment of other psychiatric illness. Minimally, an assessment should include a patient interview, observation, and a full medical check at least, preferably in all cases, but certainly in the case of a triple diagnosis. A psychiatric evaluation and information from family members or professional caregivers on patient history, symptoms and changes in health or behaviour should be incorporated in the assessment.

Interventions for SUD in individuals with IDD depend on its severity and complexity. However, SUD is often a chronic, relapsing and remitting condition that warrants prolonged treatment and a multimodal approach (Van Duijvenbode et al. 2015). In more progressed cases this generally requires the involvement of addiction services, although they often are not well-equipped to meet the needs of those with IDD. Therefore, a close collaboration between IDD service providers and addiction centers is warranted (Slayter 2010; Van Duijvenbode et al. 2015).

Addiction treatment often requires motivating patients to change their behavior. Though patients, including those with IDD, are generally (at least partially) aware of the problems that arise from their use, they are unable to control or cease their substance use (also see Wiers and Stacey 2006). Motivational interviewing is a client-centered, directive approach that helps clients to reflect on how their SU (or in general: behavior) impacts their lives and values, to consider what the benefits of behavioral change can be, and to explore how positive change can be achieved. Motivational interviewing is used in a wide spectrum of problems and disorders, and various populations, including individuals with IDD. A small number of studies have been published on motivational interviewing which suggest that this type of intervention may be used in clients with IDD and that it is a promising intervention for SU(D) (see Kerr et al. 2013).

The centerpiece of most SUD treatment programs is cognitive behavioral therapy (CBT), often combined with other treatment forms such as pharmacological treatment, training of adaptive skills or motivational interviewing. Adapted versions of mainstream programs for CBT in addiction can be used in patients with IDD. However, addiction facilities may lack the experience in treating individuals with IDD and may require help from IDD services to adapt patient communication, treatment procedures (e.g., length and number of treatment sessions might need to be adapted), wording and examples in the CBT protocols, and so on. Treatment of co-occurring psychiatric disorder ('dual diagnosis') generally requires similar adaptations when protocols for integrated treatment of dual diagnosis are used in patients with triple diagnosis. In all types of interventions, professionals from addiction services might need support from IDD services in helping the patient apply newly learned skills in daily life.

Many addiction services provide outpatient and inpatient services. Inpatient services are needed when the patient requires permanent supervision or when complications within the detoxification process are expected. These problems could include medical complications (such as seizures or delusions during alcohol withdrawal), but also behavioral or psychological disturbances, or the inability of the patient to follow through with the program leading to drop out. Generally, inpatient detoxification programs have a short duration (several days to two weeks) and focus on physical recovery. For many patients, inpatient detoxification is not required and a medically supervised outpatient detoxification, together with support and supervision from IDD services, will be sufficient. Some services also provide long-term (several months) inpatient programs aiming for prolonged abstinence and reduction of risk factors. These programs often provide groupwise therapy sessions, which may not always be suitable for patients with IDD if they are placed in groups with patients without IDD. Communication and group interactions may be too complex, differences between group members in the problems they encounter and the solutions that apply may be too large, and vulnerable individuals with IDD may be exploited or negatively influenced by group members. To prevent these obstacles, in the Netherlands, for example, several clinics have developed wards that specialize in the treatment of individuals with IDD.

Even when treatment of SUD is successful, relapses are part and parcel of this disorder. A relapse prevention program might help patients and staff members to reduce the frequency and severity of relapses and to prevent further complications. Therefore, regardless of whether abstinence or reduction of use has been achieved, patients with SUD generally require prolonged aftercare. However, both patients with IDD and their caregivers may be reluctant to engage in such programs because they regard the SUD as a problem from the past. Education on the nature of SUD (as a chronic condition, just like many medical conditions) and motivational approaches may be needed to promote treatment engagement.

For some patients long-term or even short-term abstinence seems unattainable. Sometimes this is seen by service providers as a valid reason to withdraw from these patients. This in itself may contribute to an increase in SU and preclude the patient from interventions that may be beneficial, even when SU continues. This tertiary prevention, or harm reduction measures, includes prevention of detrimental physical effects (e.g., by prescribing vitamin B to prevent Korsakows amnesia in alcoholics) as well as promotion of protective factors.

Conclusion

It may be concluded that SU(D) in individuals with IDD has gained attention over the past decade. It is generally assumed that individuals from this target group have an increased risk for developing problems related to SU and misuse and that the consequences for mental and somatic health are often detrimental. In this chapter, we have provided a brief overview of the literature of SU/SUD in IDD, identified gaps in the literature and clinical practice and provided recommendations for practice and care for individuals with IDD.

We stress that professionals working in the field of IDD need to (a) be aware of the possible co-occurrence of IDD and SU(D), especially in high-risk groups, (b) implement SU(D) screening in routine diagnostic procedures and pay extra attention to possible comorbid mental health and psychosocial problems, and (c) provide specialised and tailored treatment to clients with IDD and SUD, that matches the severity of SUD, includes biological, psychological and social interventions, and focuses on long-term management of SU according to the chronic care approach. To achieve these objectives, a close collaboration between the different sections of the mental health care system is vital.

References

American Psychiatric Association. (2013). *Diagnostic and statistical manual of mental disorders* (5th ed.). Washington DC: American Psychiatric Association.

Babor, T. F., Higgins-Biddle, J. C., Saunders, J. B., & Monteiro, M. G. (2001). *AUDIT the alcohol use disorders identification test, guidelines for use in primary care*. Geneva: World Health Organization.

Bravers, D., Bechara, A., Cleeremans, A., Komereich, C., Verbanck, P., & Noël, X. (2014). Impaired decision-making under risk in individuals with alcohol dependence. *Alcoholism, Clinical and Experimental Research, 38*, 1924–1931.

Carroll Chapman, S. L., & Wu, L.-T. (2012). Substance abuse among individuals with intellectual disability. *Research in Developmental Disabilities, 33*, 1147–1156.

Chester, V., Green, F., & Alexander, R. (2011). An audit of a smoking cessation programme for people with an intellectual disability resident in a forensic unit. *Advances in Mental Health and Intellectual Disabilities, 5*, 33–41.

Didden, R., Embregts, P., van der Toorn, M., & Laarhoven, N. (2009). Substance abuse, coping strategies, adaptive skills and behavioral and emotional problems in clients with mild to borderline intellectual disability admitted to a treatment facility: A pilot study. *Research in Developmental Disabilities, 30*, 927–932.

Donovan, D. M. (2005). Assessment of addictive behaviors for relapse prevention. In D. M. Donovan & G. A. Marlatt (Eds.), *Assessment of addictive behaviors* (2nd ed., pp. 1–48). New York: The Guilford Press.

Kerr, S., Lawrence, M., Darbyshire, C., Middleton, A. R., & Fitzsimmons, L. (2013). Tobacco and alcohol-related interventions for people with mild/moderate intellectual disabilities: A systematic review of the literature. *Journal of Intellectual Disability Research, 57*, 393–408.

Lindsay, W. R., Carson, D., Holland, A. J., Taylor, J. L., O'Brien, G., Wheeler, J. R., et al. (2013). Alcohol and its relationship to offence variables in a cohort of offenders with intellectual disability. *Journal of Intellectual and Developmental Disability, 38*, 325–331.

Lindsay, W., McPherson, F., Kelman, L., & Mathewson, Z. (1998). Health promotion and people with learning disabilities: The design and evaluation of three programmes. *Health Bulletin—Scottish Office Department of Health, 56*, 694–698.

Loeber, S., Duka, T., Welzel, H., Nakovics, H., Heinz, A., Flor, H., et al. (2009). Impairment of cognitive abilities and decision making after chronic use of alcohol: The impact of multiple detoxifications. *Alcohol and Alcoholism, 44*, 372–381.

Martin, C. S., Langenbucher, J. W., Chung, T., & Sher, K. J. (2014). Truth or consequences in the diagnosis of substance use disorders. *Addiction, 109*, 1773–1778.

McLaughlin, D. F., Taggart, L., Quinn, B., & Milligan, V. (2007). The experiences of professionals who care for people with intellectual disability who have substance-related problems. *Journal of Substance Use, 12*, 133–143.

McLellan, A. T., McKay, J. R., Forman, R., Cacciola, J., & Kemp, J. (2005). Reconsidering the evaluation of addiction treatment: From retrospective follow-up to concurrent recovery monitoring. *Addiction, 100*, 447–458.

Mendel, E., & Hipkins, J. (2002). Motivating learning disabled offenders with alcohol-related problems: A pilot study. *British Journal of Learning Disabilities, 30*, 153–158.

Rehm, J., Room, R., Van den Brink, W., & Jacobi, F. (2005a). Alcohol use disorders in EU countries and Norway: An overview of the epidemiology. *European Neuropsychopharmacology, 15*, 377–388.

Rehm, J., Room, R., Van den Brink, W., & Kraus, L. (2005b). Problematic drug use and drug use disorders in EU countries and Norway: An overview of the epidemiology. *European Neuropsychopharmacology, 15*, 389–397.

Reif, S., George, P., Braude, L., Dougherty, R. H., Daniels, A. S., Ghose, S. S., et al. (2014). Residential treatment for individuals with substance use disorders: Assessing the evidence. *Psychiatric Services, 65*, 301–312.

Room, R., Babor, T., & Rehm, J. (2005). Alcohol and public health. *The Lancet, 365*, 519–530.
Scott, S., & Kraner, E. (2014). Alcohol and public health: Heavy drinking is a heavy price to pay for populations. *Journal of Public Health, 36*, 396–398.
Singh, N., Lancioni, G., Myers, R., Karazsia, B., Winton, A., & Singh, J. (2014). A randomized controlled trial of a mindfulness-based smoking cessation program for individuals with mild intellectual disability. *International Journal of Mental Health and Addiction, 12*, 153–168.
Slayter, E. M. (2008). Understanding and overcoming barriers to substance abuse treatment access for people with mental retardation. *Journal of Social Work in Disability and Rehabilitation, 7*, 63–80.
Slayter, E. M. (2010). Disparities in access to substance abuse treatment among people with intellectual disabilities and serious mental illness. *Health and Social Work, 35*, 49–59.
Sterling, S., Chi, F., & Hinman, A. (2011). Integrating care for people with co-occurring alcohol and other drug, medical, and mental health conditions. *Alcohol Research & Health, 33*, 338–349.
Strack, F., & Deutsch, R. (2004). Reflective and impulsive determinants of social behaviour. *Personality and Social Psychology Review, 8*, 220–247.
Sturmey, P., Reyer, H., Lee, R., & Robek, A. (2003). *Substance-related disorders in persons with mental retardation*. Kingston: NADD Press.
Substance Abuse and Mental Health Services Administration. (2014). *The NSDUH report: Substance use and mental health estimates from the 2013 National Survey on Drug Use and Health: Overview of findings*. Rockville: SAMHSA.
Swendsen, J., Burstein, M., Case, B., Conway, K. P., Dierker, L., He, J., et al. (2012). Use and abuse of alcohol and illicit drugs in US adolescents: Results of the National Comorbidity Survey—Adolescent Supplement. *Archives of General Psychiatry, 69*, 390–398.
To, W. T., Neirynck, S., Vanderplasschen, W., Vanheule, S., & Vandevelde, S. (2014). Substance use and misuse in persons with intellectual disabilities (ID): Results of a survey in ID and addiction services in Flanders. *Research in Developmental Disabilities, 35*, 1–9.
Van Duijvenbode, N., Didden, R., Korzilius, H. P. L. M., & Engels, R. C. M. E. (under review). *The addicted brain: Cognitive biases in problematic drinkers with mild to borderline intellectual disability*.
Van Duijvenbode, N., VanDerNagel, J. E. L., Didden, R., Engels, R., Buitelaar, J., Kiewik, M., & De Jong, C. (2015). Substance use disorders in individuals with mild to borderline intellectual disabilities: Current status and future directions. *Research in Developmental Disabilities, 38*, 319–328.
VanDerNagel, J., Kemna, L., & Didden, R. (2013). Substance use among persons with mild intellectual disability: Approaches to screening and interviewing. *The NADD Bulletin, 16*, 87–92.
VanDerNagel, J. E. L., Kiewik, M., Buitelaar, J. K., & de Jong, C. A. J. (2011a). Staff perspectives of substance use and misuse among adults with intellectual disabilities enrolled in Dutch disability services. *Journal of Policy and Practice in Intellectual Disabilities, 8*, 143–149.
VanDerNagel, J. E. L., Kiewik, M., Dijk, M. van, Jong, C. A. J. de, & Didden, R. (2011b). *Handleiding SumID-Q, Meetinstrument voor het in kaart brengen van Middelengebruik bij mensen met een lichte verstandelijke beperking* [Manual of the SumID-Q. An instrument to assess substance use in individuals with a mild intellectual disability]. Deventer: Tactus.
Van Duijvenbode, N., Didden, R., Korzilius, H. P. L. M., & Engels, R. C. M. E. (submitted). *Does it take two to tango? The role of executive control and readiness to change in problematic drinkers with mild to borderline intellectual disability*.
Wiers, R. W., & Stacy, A. W. (2006). Implicit cognition and addiction. *Current Directions in Psychological Science, 15*, 292–296.
Wilson, C. R., Sherritt, L., Gates, E., & Knight, J. R. (2004). Are clinical impressions of adolescent substance use accurate? *Pediatrics, 114*, 536–540.

Chapter 11
Consultation with Medical and Healthcare Providers

Kimberly Guion, Erin Olufs and Kurt A. Freeman

Youth with intellectual and developmental disabilities (IDD) typically experience multiple health domains requiring intervention (e.g., medical health, behavior, developmental progress, motor development). Due to the complexity of their health care needs, primary care providers (PCPs) are in a position to support youth and families in these multiple domains and make referrals to subspecialists when needed. Effective management and referral requires PCPs to have expertise in multiple domains, many of which may fall outside the typical purview of medical providers. Thus, effective primary care for individuals with IDD may be best accomplished when PCPs access support from other providers with developmental and behavioral expertise.

This chapter details methods of behavioral consultation to medical and other healthcare providers in primary care settings, including methods to facilitate collaborative multidisciplinary decision-making and formulation of behavioral medicine protocols. This chapter also addresses issues about consultation specific to children with IDD. An overview of the history and models of integrating pediatric psychology into primary care settings is covered in a chapter written by Stancin and colleagues, which appears in the Handbook of Pediatric Psychology (Stancin et al. 2009). In the following sections, we define consultation along a continuum,

K. Guion · E. Olufs · K.A. Freeman (✉)
Division of Psychology, Institute on Development and Disability,
Oregon Health and Science University, Portland, USA
e-mail: freemaku@ohsu.edu

K. Guion
e-mail: guion@ohsu.edu

E. Olufs
e-mail: olufs@ohsu.edu

J.K. Luiselli (ed.), *Behavioral Health Promotion and Intervention in Intellectual and Developmental Disabilities*, Evidence-Based Practices in Behavioral Health,
DOI 10.1007/978-3-319-27297-9_11

and clarify that specific recommendations in the current chapter are based on a specific and narrow definition of consultation for clarity. Research in this area is limited, although several models of consultation that are previously described in the literature are summarized. However, given the state of literature on behavioral health consultation in a pediatric primary care setting, the chapter is primarily conceptual and provides an outline of domains and variables that one might consider for effective consultation. Finally, for definitional clarity, broad concepts within this chapter are written with the book's target population in mind: children with IDD of various kinds. Much of the research cited focuses on one or two specific populations, children with Intellectual Disability (ID), for example. Nomenclature throughout the chapter is specific to whether a particular population was included in a research study, and the term IDD is used when concepts are being addressed that are relevant to the larger population of children with IDD.

Why Behavioral Health Consultation?

The American Academy of Pediatrics' (AAP) has made the establishment of medical homes for all children one of its essential child health outcomes for the 21st century, where all children have a central source of health care (Sia et al. 2004). As the medical home model has gained prominence as the gold standard of care for children and their families, there has been an increased recognition that behavioral health may be most effectively addressed through family-centered, coordinated care that occurs in the medical home. Recognizing this need, pediatricians often express a strong interest in having a behavioral health provider integrated into their clinics (Williams et al. 2005). However, only 17 % of primary care providers identify having a behavioral health provider onsite (Guevara et al. 2009). Further, there continues to be a high degree of variability in how primary care clinics incorporate behavioral health services into their practices. This variation is largely based on what level of integration works best for each individual clinic and the needs of the patient population it serves.

One reason collaboration between providers has been promoted is due to the high demand of services for children identified as having behavioral health concerns. Parents raise concern regarding their children's behavioral health at approximately 25 % of all child primary care appointments (Cooper et al. 2006; Miranda et al. 1994). Approximately 15–18 % of children are identified by their PCP as having a behavioral health disorder (Costello and Pantino 1987; Wasserman et al. 1999), and a significantly greater percentage have emotional or behavioral issues that are challenging and concerning to parents yet are subclinical. These concerns are even more prevalent for children identified as having a developmental disability. Up to 40 % of children with an ID, for example, meet criteria for at least one behavioral health disorder, and for many these concerns severely impact their ability to function in everyday life (Dekker and Koot 2003; Einfeld and Tonge 1996).

Improving families' access to behavioral health providers increases the likelihood that families will utilize behavioral health services. Importantly, having behavioral health providers at the same site as PCPs increases the probability that families will follow through on referrals for behavioral health services (Valleley et al. 2007). Improved access to behavioral health providers is especially important for children with IDD, given that they often present with increased rates of comorbid behavioral and emotional concerns (Dekker and Koot 2003; Einfeld and Tonge 1996). Even with the complex biopsychosocial concerns of children with IDD, their access to behavioral health care may be limited. For instance, Dekker and Koot (2003) found that fewer than four in 10 children with intellectual disabilities will receive formal mental health care. Having a behavioral health provider embedded in a primary care clinic may help families establish with a specialist who can provide long-term support in addressing the challenges that often arise in raising a child with a developmental disability.

Beyond improving access and likelihood of following through with behavioral health care, having a behavioral health provider in primary care settings can help reduce the cost and time demands placed on PCPs. As most behavioral health visits are to PCPs rather than behavioral health providers (Miranda et al. 1994), a high demand is placed on PCPs to address both medical and behavioral concerns parents have regarding their children. Unfortunately, as a result pediatricians are often compelled to attempt to address a significant, often complex behavioral health concern in addition to addressing all other aspects of a child's health, wellness, and development in the same appointment. The result is longer appointments when parents raise a behavioral health concern spontaneously, with pediatricians spending half the appointment addressing these concerns (Cooper et al. 2006). Appointments made to specifically address behavioral health concerns with PCPs average 20 min in length, up to twice as long as other medical appointments (Cooper et al. 2006; Meadows et al. 2011). In addition, PCPs are often inadequately reimbursed for providing behavioral health services, receiving lower reimbursement per minute of service for addressing behavioral health concerns when compared to medication management (Cooper et al. 2006; Meadows et al. 2011). Fortunately, brief intervention with children and families provided in primary care by a behavioral health professional can result in attendance of fewer medical visits compared to children who do not receive behavioral interventions (Finney et al. 1991). Thus, providing behavioral health services within primary care environments has multiple potential benefits including improving working conditions for PCPs (Chomienne et al. 2011) and reducing the pressure on an already strained medical system, in addition to providing a valuable service to families.

Models of Consultation

While the benefits of integrating behavioral health services into medical care clinics are increasingly recognized, there is little agreement on the best way to accomplish this. There is also not a "one-size fits all" when it comes to what type of collaboration with a behavioral health provider will best serve the patients in a medical care clinic. Therefore, several models of integrated behavioral health care have been defined. Doherty and colleagues (Doherty 1995; Doherty et al. 1996) proposed a 5-level model articulating that collaboration between primary and behavioral health care falls on a continuum, ranging from minimal collaboration between providers to fully integrated health systems. While collaboration occurs to some extent at each level, it varies greatly between the two ends of the spectrum. At the most basic level, Minimal Collaboration (Level 1), providers rarely communicate and have separate systems and separate facilities. At the highest level of integration, Close Collaboration in a Fully Integrated System (Level 5), providers collaborate as members of the same care team, operating in the same system and within the same locations to develop comprehensive care plans and provide optimal patient care.

Building off the 5-level model (Doherty 1995; Doherty et al. 1996; Heath et al. 2013) developed a 6-level model of behavioral health and primary care collaboration and integration. Their model consists of three main categories (Coordinated Care, Co-Located Care, and Integrated Care) and two levels of degree within each category. In the Coordinated Care levels, providers operate within separate systems and in separate facilities. When communication occurs, it is rare and is focused on specific patient issues. Providers do not actively consult with one another, and as such there is no exchange of knowledge or ideas about medical and/or behavioral health concepts. Providers view themselves as individuals treating a shared patient rather than part of the same team, and decisions and treatment plans are made independent of one other. Moving from Level 1 to Level 2, providers begin to view each other as resources and behavioral health is considered specialty care. Patients connect with providers at this level either by seeking out services on their own or by being referred by an established care provider. An example of this is a private primary care clinic and a private mental/behavioral health center sharing patients through referrals or coincidence.

In the Co-Located Care category, providers practice at the same facilities but there continues to be separation of systems. Communication occurs more regularly due to close physical proximity, and may include occasional meetings to discuss specific patients. Consultation between providers may include topics not related to specific patients, but rather exchanges of information about common challenging childhood behaviors or how to implement brief interventions in a general pediatric appointment. While patient care decisions are made independently by each provider, they may begin to view each other as part of a larger care team. Providers often refer to each other based on their co-location and subsequent collaborative relationships, and there is a higher likelihood parents will follow through with referrals made by their PCPs to co-located behavioral health providers (Valleley et al. 2007). There may also be opportunities for "warm hand-offs" between providers (i.e., a physician facilitating a brief meeting between a patient and family and the behavioral health provider) due to their close proximity in the same clinic. Providers begin to have a better understanding of each other's roles in providing specialized care to families. Moving from Level 3 to Level 4, there begins to be some integration of care through shared systems and embedded practices. For example, an independent behavioral health provider may be a member of a private practice and rent office space in a primary care clinic to see patients. The front desk staff may assist the behavioral health provider with some administrative tasks, such as checking in patients and scheduling. However, the behavioral health provider would utilize their own resources to process billing and handle insurance claims and would likely maintain their own medical records separate from the PCP. This type of co-located behavioral health care is growing in popularity as the medical home model develops in tandem with insurance changes.

In the Integrated Care category, there is close collaboration between providers that approaches a fully integrated practice. At these levels, providers begin to function as members of an active, well-defined team. Collaboration and integration are evidenced by frequent personal communication and a team approach to seeking solutions and removing barriers to health care access. Members of the team operate in a dynamic system, where each provider changes how they practice due to the influence of those they work with to optimize patient care. Providers develop shared treatment plans and have regular discussions on how they can work together to help the patient achieve their wellness goals. Team members have regular conversations not just about specific patients but about a sharing of knowledge across specialty to better inform care across disciplines. Moving from Level 5 to Level 6, providers and patients experience a single, merged health system that is focused on treating the whole person. Patients are viewed as being "our" shared patients rather than "theirs" or "mine".

In the current chapter, we focus on the role of the Behavioral Health Consultant (BHC) integrated into a primary care clinic. The BHC operates in Level 5 and Level 6 of the Integrated Care category discussed by Heath et al. (2013). The BHC provides several services, including but not limited to conducting a brief assessment of a patient, providing brief behavioral intervention in the context of primary care visits, communication of suggested intervention routes to the patient and PCP, and communication of potential follow-up plans (e.g., additional referrals, when to re-consult). The BHC is available to the PCP to answer questions related to developmental and behavioral health concerns and to follow up with PCPs as needed. In this consultation model, the PCP maintains responsibility for the patient and their care, with the BHC being viewed as an integral provider in the primary care team. A BHC may also function effectively in other levels of the models of care, though the remainder of the chapter generally assumes a high level of integration of BHCs into the primary care setting.

Roles of a Behavioral Health Consultant

Brief Psychosocial Assessment

One of the roles of the BHC is to provide brief psychosocial assessments to patients seen in an outpatient pediatric primary care clinic. Screening of developmental and behavioral progress contributes to pediatric primary care in one of three ways, including assisting with the determination of whether more in-depth behavioral health assessment is needed, contributing to diagnostic decision making by the PCP, and/or determining appropriate type and frequency of interventions that are appropriate to address the child's behavioral health needs. Screening activities may occur at the request of the PCP, as follow-up to screening measures used in a clinic, or occur as a practice-based screening approach completed via the BHC's participation in well-child or other types of pediatric visits.

Specific assessment information can be gathered through interview-based screening or with screening tools, such as paper-pencil measures for parents. A BHC needs knowledge of the psychometric properties and clinical utility of such measures to use them as effective assessment tools. Using these methods, the BHC is able to define any behavioral concerns, obtain details about current intervention strategies, and determine whether the concern is isolated or related to a larger cluster of concerning behaviors. This may include an assessment of the function of a behavior and request the parent to track a behavior (e.g., bedtime, sleep initiation time) and related variables. The consultant should be clear with the family and with the PCP who will be receiving the tracked data, and who will be responding to the data. Based on the assessment of behavioral concerns, the BHC can determine whether appropriate treatment interventions are warranted, and if so what type.

Another domain in which a BHC may be a useful team member in assessment is if a BHC is upon to determine patients' and their families' understanding of a diagnosis made by their PCP and subsequent treatment recommendations. This may be particularly relevant when evaluating children's and adolescents' understanding of their own disability, treatment, or diagnosis, which will be dependent on their developmental level in multiple domains (e.g., language development, intellect, exposure and fluency with medical terminology). While a tailored approach to providing information is recommended for all families, children and adolescents with IDD often display uneven skill development (e.g., strong social skills, but delayed receptive language ability), which can make it difficult to assess whether they understand the medical information being given to them. The BHC can also assess a patient's perception of their medical treatment, and identify any barriers the family may be experiencing in following through with recommendations or accessing services. It can also be useful for the BHC to discuss a patients' motivation to implement intervention techniques and determine the likelihood an intervention will be successful. The BHC is then able to address adherence concerns with patients and families and engage in dialogue to increase their follow through with treatment recommendations.

Intervention

The BHC likely is often called upon to provide direct intervention in the primary care setting. Intervention may fall into one of three categories: reassurance and psychoeducation, prescriptive intervention, and referral to appropriate type and/or intensity of care.

One outcome of PCP or BHC assessment of behavioral status is that a child's behavioral presentation is developmentally typical (e.g., mild bedtime resistance in a 4 year old, nighttime wetting in a 4–6 year old). In such circumstances, effective intervention by the BHC includes affirming this for parents, providing psychoeducation about developmental trajectories, and offering assurance that current parenting approaches are appropriate and matched to the child's needs. BHCs can also provide education about behavioral red flags, or signs that a child's behavioral challenges are expanding beyond what is considered typical. Some minor modifications to existing approaches may also be offered to enhance the appropriateness and effectiveness of parental approaches. However, this type of intervention is largely focused on offering assurance and information.

Related, intervention may also focus on psychoeducation even when a youth has clinically relevant presenting concerns. For instance, the BHC may be asked to discuss the etiology of depression with an adolescent and how this informs treatment options. The BHC is not assuming the role of the ongoing treatment provider in such cases, but is helping educate youth and their families about behavioral health concerns.

If a child's behavior is determined to be outside the realm of typical development, then an intervention decision point exists based on presenting concerns, including a decision regarding whether intervention should focus on brief, evidence based strategies within the primary care environment or whether a referral to more comprehensive and intensive services is warranted. Prescriptive intervention in a primary care setting may be appropriate based on the assessment of the intensity, frequency, complexity and persistence of the child's behavioral health challenges and an assessment of a parent's readiness to benefit from brief intervention. This service is provided to the family either during their original appointment or during separate follow-up visits. Interventions are grounded in the BHC's theoretical orientation, informing case conceptualization and treatment recommendations. Common concerns that can be addressed with brief interventions include toilet training delays (Borowitz et al. 2002; Freeman et al. 2014), sleep concerns (Eckerberg 2002; Freeman 2006; Friman et al. 1999; Mindell et al. 2006), disruptive behaviors (Forehand and King 1977; Shaw et al. 2006), habit behaviors (Friman et al. 1986; Friman and Leibowitz 1990), and tic disorders (Azrin and Peterson 1990; Piacentini et al. 2010), as well as others that are outlined in this book.

Should it be determined the child and family need a higher level of services, then the BHC's intervention emphasizes assisting the PCP in making appropriate referrals to other service providers in the community. The BHC should be aware of the resources located in the medical system in which the BHC is operating, as well as those located in the community. This knowledge should extend beyond the BHC's own training background and area of expertise, and includes a familiarity with financial resources or support available from other disciplines or organizations, including state or county-based supports such as Developmental Disability Services and Social Security Income. The BHC should also be informed about how to make appropriate referrals to other disciplines or agencies in order to effectively support the families they serve. The BHC should be able to help families determine what services, providers, and community resources are covered by their insurance, or at least able to direct the family on how to find such information. Once an appropriate service provider is identified, the BHC can assist the PCP with making the referral. If this intervention emphasizing referral is pursued, the BHC may still provide some brief psych-education and/or intervention for the family to consider as they seek ongoing care. However, caution should be taken if doing so in such circumstances so as to avoid offering guidance without the proper ability to assist in follow-through and effective implementation.

Pre-Requisite Knowledge and Skills for Providing Behavioral Health Consultation

Although most clinicians providing behavioral health consultation for children with developmental disabilities are likely to be child or pediatric psychologists, providers in other disciplines can be a valuable source for consultation as well. In addition, some developing models include trainees at various levels, such as psychology doctoral interns or post-doctoral fellows. The following subsections outline several pre-requisite skill sets that will be essential for providers regardless of training level and discipline in order to provide effective behavioral health consultation for youth with IDD.

Developmental Understanding

An important role of a pediatric PCP is providing ongoing monitoring of developmental and behavioral progress of patients and to provide appropriate referrals for more in-depth assessment and/or intervention based on that monitoring (American Academy of Pediatrics 2006). Thus, in order for a BHC to be an effective team member within a medical home, s/he must have solid training in developmental norms and trajectories. This should be reflected in an ability to assess the developmental status of a child, including current abilities, skills, and skill deficits, as well as the ability to effectively communicate the outcome of such an assessment to families in a manner that is accessible and allows parents to act effectively on the information provided. For example, a child demonstrating difficult behaviors at bedtime may lack the foundational skills of self-soothing without a parent present or another variable (e.g., a sippy cup or bottle). This may be developmentally typical for an infant, or a child who is older than 1 year but who is experiencing developmental delays. On the other hand, the child may have the skill to put him/herself to sleep, but is struggling to perform this skill based on other factors (e.g., inconsistent scheduling, reinforcement of behaviors that delay bedtime). In all cases, it is critical for the BHC to have a clear understanding of developmental norms based on chronological age *as well as* the ability to assess the actual developmental level in various domains, regardless of chronological age.

Principles of Learning

Second, clinicians must have a firm grounding in the principles of learning (behavior change) and sufficient fluency to bring that knowledge to bear efficiently and succinctly. A foundational knowledge of learning principles will inform a clinician's conceptualization of a child's behavior as well as guide treatment recommendations. Principles of learning include a firm grasp of the role of operant and classical conditioning on human behavior, and child behavior in particular. Specifically, knowledge of strategies based in operant conditioning such as functional behavior assessment and managing contingencies will be important for understanding what functions certain behaviors play, variables that maintain certain behavior patterns, how to measure these variables, track them over time, and adjust them effectively. Additionally, concepts associated with classical conditioning can inform intervention approaches, for example, using knowledge about the role that fear-avoidance learning following a painful bowel movement may have in toileting training delays.

Systems

Third, it is expected that an effective BHC for children with developmental disabilities operating within pediatric primary care will have training and understanding in a systems perspective, described in numerous biopsychosocial models of health (Boyer 2008 for an overview). The overarching concept is that children with IDD (all humans, in fact) function within a complex system of individual, family, and broader social contexts and that variables in all of these levels may impact an individual's health and behavior. Children with IDD exist within a complex network of social systems including the family, the neighborhood and school context, the medical system (individual clinic, hospital, and national-level system), and inclusion of any other providers and supports that may be engaging with the child (e.g., Developmental Disabilities Services). At an even broader level, behavior concerns occur in the context of a financial system at multiple levels (e.g., family finances, SSI income, health care access) and policy (e.g., accessibility of Developmental Disability Services, accessibility of specialized health care in their community or region).

While general appreciation for and understanding of the various systems with which the child may interact is important when providing behavioral health consultation, direct assessment of certain systems is critical. Specifically, the BHC should have the skills to evaluate not only an individual child's behavioral presentation, but also the family system in which they occur. For example, the dynamics between parent and child, between two parents, and how daily schedules, siblings, and extended family interact can inform the emergence or maintenance of unhealthy behavior patterns. In addition, the BHC should be aware of the medical systems that are involved in a child's life, operating, as well as the community system in which children and their families live.

Professional Skills

Finally, BHCs should demonstrate a well-developed set of professional skills necessary for engagement within a primary care environment. This will include an ability to collaborate effectively with other professionals as well as patients and family members. It is important for BHCs to provide services and collaborate with other professionals in a manner that follows ethical guidelines. This can be difficult while in a consultative role, as ethical guidelines for mental health providers can differ from guidelines established for medical professionals. The BHC needs to find a balance between remaining true to ethical principles established by the field while maintaining positive, collaborative relationships with other professionals. The BHC will likely need to educate patients, their families, and other providers on the limits of confidentiality, for example, and how those limits may be different in a consultation situation than they would be in a traditional therapy setting. A BHC will need to demonstrate sophisticated professional skills in numerous domains in order to collaborate effectively and balance different training background, and these may include differences in case conceptualization, the role of medication versus non-medication treatment options, and styles of communication with families. It is also important for the BHC to understand the culture of the workplace in which they are operating and in some ways assimilate into that environment (Allen et al. 1993). Therefore, BHCs need to be flexible in their approaches to assessment and intervention while providing the best care possible to families.

Considerations for Consultants

In this section, we outline a series of domains, or questions, that the consulting and referring providers should consider when engaging in this type of collaboration. This section is meant to provide an outline of considerations a provider should make when developing a new or revising an existing collaborative model.

Communication and Collaboration

For a BHC to successfully integrate into a primary care clinic, it is of vital importance that the BHC be able to effectively communicate and collaborate with all providers and staff in the clinic. This includes medical providers, nurses, office staff, social workers, and other therapeutic providers. BHCs must exhibit their own skill set in communicating effectively with others, and an ability to help shape communication coming from others, such as the PCP. In all communications, it is most effective to be very clear about one's needs, to outline next steps, and to make the consultative process itself explicit. It is important for the BHC to understand one's unique role and role boundaries in a collaboration, handle disagreements diplomatically, and demonstrate flexibility in assessment and treatment planning as various players provide their own perspectives and information about a patient. The BHC should also look for opportunities to join in discussions with other providers on common challenges that patients and families experience. Through these conversations, providers can share knowledge of their area of specialization to assist in treatment planning to optimize patient care. These conversations help providers move beyond viewing each other as resources to appreciating each other as members of the same medical team.

Focusing on communication between the BHC and PCP, there are several points of contact at which explicit communication between the providers is critical. The first point of contact will usually be when the PCP initiates consultation from the BHC. During this interaction, it is important for a BHC to clarify not only the referral question, but also what specific goals the primary provider would like to accomplish with the consult. Is the consultation to confirm or provide a diagnosis, or to do in depth assessment of the contextual variable(s) impacting behavioral concerns? Many primary care providers may not have the specific training in these areas to define the assessment question clearly, and thus this is a prime opportunity for collaborative care and potentially providing training to one's colleagues. It is also critical to clarify the scope of the assessment question, rather than it being "assess everything", as the nature of a consultation is to be brief, limited in scope, and to provide specific feedback and suggestions for next steps to either the family or the PCP. For example, if receiving a consult requesting support "for repetitive skin picking", a BHC may need to ask questions and reflect back to the PCP a more clear consult request such as, "please evaluate skin picking and provide brief behavioral intervention strategies to family and myself (PCP) to intervene and determine whether more intensive behavioral services are warranted." Given that behavioral health care knowledge may be limited in some primary care settings, it may be an important role for the BHC to help define the referral question, goals, and scope of services that can be offered within the primary care environment. BHC's may also need to develop a system of asking PCPs to include information they already know or have about the child, the family, and the behavioral concern (e.g., explicit referral form). Finally, the primary care provider will need to be clear about what level of feedback is desired and how that will be transmitted. Following the consult, the BHC should discuss with the PCP his/her conceptualization of the case, recommendations provided to the family, and next steps in providing care to the patient.

Here is a summary of queries to ensure that a consult request and assessment are clear and complete:

- Is the referral question clear?
- What are the specific goals of this consult?
- What level of assessment is needed?
- Are data being tracked or collected from family?
  - If yes, who will receive data?
  - Who will interpret data?
  - Who will define next steps based on data?
- Will a second consult meeting occur?
- When and how will consult information be shared with the referring provider?
- Does the consultant have any additional steps or responsibilities?

Transfer of Responsibility

As noted above, it should be clear at all points during collaborative care with a particular patient which provider is responsible, or taking the lead, for addressing the patient's behavioral concerns. Given the consultative nature of the relationship between a PCP and BHC, the PCP will likely always be the primary point person. However, it should be clear which provider is (a) scheduling appointments with the patient, (b) following up regarding new interventions tried, and (c) determining if more intensive and/or different intervention is needed. Transferring responsibility from one provider to another can be as simple as stating it explicitly and charting it clearly. For example, "Dr. M, I have provided the family with two interventions and indicated that they will need to follow up with you in the next week. Please contact me again if you would like additional consultation."

Scope of Practice

Scope of practice issues should be considered at multiple levels. First, a BHC should always be clear about the type, frequency, and intensity of service s/he can provide to the patient in the context of pediatric primary care, and whether this is appropriate for the patient's needs. In some cases a client may need more intensive services than is appropriate in a consultation model. Such a scenario can be particularly tricky to navigate, as a BHC may have adequate skills and expertise to provide effective treatment for the youth's presenting concerns, but it may not be the best option for providing such care due to the nature of his/her consultative work within the primary care environment. Thus, the BHC will instead need to work within the shorter time frame of a consult or refer to a different clinic or provider. Further, for the BHC, referral for additional consultation from other providers can and is often very useful depending on the specialized nature of the referral question. For example, in many instances of children with feeding difficulties, it is critical that an appropriate medical and oral-motor evaluation be completed prior to engaging in behavioral intervention.

Scope of practice issues also apply to the referring PCP, and this is an especially sensitive consideration in the domain of consultation. There must be a clear and shared understanding of the level of expertise the PCP has in the assessment, conceptualization, and intervention domains being used for a particular case. In this way, the BHC can effectively recommend which portions of ongoing assessment or intervention are appropriate to continue with the PCP, and which require follow up with a different specialist or more intensive services. Further, developing open and collaborative discussion and relationships with members of the medical team is important so that all team members feel comfortable asking for additional support or explanation when needed. Direct and explicit communication over time will allow a BHC to learn whether a PCP may need more thorough explanation in some areas, compared to others. For example, some PCPs may feel very comfortable offering families follow up care related to disruptive sleep patterns, while being less comfortable doing the same in the domain of feeding.

Location, Location, Location

In order for a BHC to provide effective and integrated consultation, proximity to the PCPs is of critical importance. Close proximity (e.g., the same workroom) define and supports integrated, as opposed to co-located, care by fostering ongoing collaboration and conversation between the BHCs and PCPs. Our anecdotal observations as behavioral health consultants embedded within pediatric primary care suggests that sharing workspace increases the frequency of appropriate referrals, allows for more frequent warm hand-offs, and facilitates indirect consultation (that is, discussing with the PCP cases not seen by the BHC). PCPs, by nature of their role and also reimbursement models, are very busy, and having a BHC physically present and visible increases access to them. Further, when a BHC is present in a work room, brief discussions about patients may lead to "small" or seemingly inconsequential behavior challenges being caught early enough that a consultative model will be effective, rather than waiting until they become more complex problems requiring intensive follow up services.

Funding Considerations

Funding and reimbursement for a behavioral health psychologist who is providing consultative care has been a chronic barrier towards practices developing truly integrated medical and behavioral health care services (Duke et al. 2012; Fisher and Dickinson 2014; Lines et al. 2012; Talmi and Fazio 2012). One of the primary roadblocks to achieving financially sustainable integrated behavioral health care is the struggle to receive adequate reimbursement from 3rd party payers. While traditional medical care is covered under general health insurance, behavioral health care is often covered under mental health insurance carve-outs (Fischer and Dickinson 2014; Mauch et al. 2008). Given this separation, determining which insurance to bill for behavioral health services provided in a primary care clinic can be difficult, and reimbursement rates are often low (Kathol et al. 2010). In addition, traditional behavioral health payers are often reluctant to cover services focused on addressing adjustment to and management of medical conditions, which is frequently the focus of behavioral health consultation (Fischer and Dickinson 2014).

Mauch et al. (2008) identified several barriers to reimbursement of services provided through integrated health care systems. A significant barrier to reimbursement is the limitation placed by state Medicaid coverage on the same organization billing for both physical and mental health services on the same day. Similarly, collaborative care related to behavioral health concerns is rarely reimbursed. As Mauch and colleagues note, these restrictions often limit the opportunity for warm-handoffs from PCPs to behavioral health providers, the ability of providers to collaborate on shared patients, and the convenience of patients scheduling their behavioral health and medical appointments on the same day. The result is that the goals of integrated health care, including increased collaborative care, provision of consultative services, and ease of access to providers, are all too often hindered by insurance reimbursement policies and practices.

Several funding options are available for consultation services. Many providers use a fee-for-service (FFS) system to bill for services rendered. This includes the use of Current Procedural Terminology (CPT) codes. Behavioral health providers have traditionally used the mental health CPT codes (e.g. 90791, 90834) to bill for assessment and intervention services. However, these codes must be associated with an identified, diagnosed behavioral health condition (Noll and Fischer 2004). Therefore, their use can pose an ethical dilemma to BHCs who operate in a primary care setting. For instance, many children with developmental disabilities may benefit from behavioral health consultation and intervention, but do not qualify for a formal mental health diagnosis. In this case, providers may rely on Health and Behavior (H&B) CPT codes (e.g., 96150–96155) to bill for services.

H&B codes are billed under general medical health insurance rather than behavioral health carve-outs. The ability to bill for services as part of medical care rather than separate behavioral health care represents an important shift in how behavioral health provider's role in the medical setting is understood and appreciated (Noll and Fischer 2004). Due to the perceived benefits of using these codes, their use has increased in the past decade (Lines et al. 2012). One benefit of these codes is that they are billed in 15-min increments and thus feasibly apply to a consultative model. However, the reimbursement rates for services appropriately billed using H&B may be notably less than traditional psychological assessment and intervention codes (Duke et al. 2012) and thus may not (a) reflect the true value of the highly specialized service being provided and (b) be sustainable if only those codes are being billed on a regular basis. Due to the complexity of the use of H&B codes in billing for behavioral health services, hiring an insurance verification specialist may be a cost-effective way to improve reimbursement rates for services, primarily through educating insurance companies on the use of H&B codes and appealing when charges are denied (Brosig and Zahrt 2006).

As the FFS reimbursement model has been shown to inadequately reimburse for services rendered and results in a low reimbursement rate (Brosig and Zahrt 2006; Duke et al. 2012; Talmi and Fazio 2012), new models of reimbursement have been proposed. One emerging model has involved bundling payments for patients served (Cutler and Ghosh 2012; O'Donnell et al. 2013). There are two primary methods for combining FFS reimbursement into bundled payments from insurance companies. The first is patient-based bundling, whereby medical reimbursements are aggregated to the person-year level, and providers receive a single global payment for each patient's care. The second is episode-based bundling, whereby medical reimbursements are aggregated for specific medical conditions, such as diabetes mellitus (Cutler and Ghosh 2012).

Case Examples

Two case examples are provided to illustrate typical scenarios of behavioral health consultation in a primary care environment. While these examples do not address all issues pertinent to such care, they highlight different paths that may be taken when completing such work. These may be used for discussion and to explore methods of how to collaborate with other medical team members in some of the domains outlined in the sections above.

"Olivia" is a 3-year old female with cerebral palsy brought to clinic by her mother for a well-child check. As part of the appointment with her PCP, her mother raises concern with Olivia's behavioral development, specifically that

Olivia tantrums when given a parental direction or when she is denied access a preferred item or activity. Due to this concern, the BHC was called into discuss Olivia's behaviors. The BHC assesses the frequency, intensity, and length of Olivia's emotional outbursts, including contextual variables in the immediate environment that may be impacting her emotional outbursts. Olivia's mother reports that Olivia tantrums one to two times per day, each lasting less than 10 min. Olivia does not engage in physical aggression while she tantrums, or at other times. Olivia's mother reports that she and her husband place Olivia on the family couch when she tantrums and ignore her until she self-calms. Her parents report that following the tantrum they require Olivia to complete the original command given by them or continue to withhold access to her preferred item or activity. Her parents report they are concerned because prior to age two Olivia was a generally happy child who engaged in minimal emotional outbursts. Parents deny any other behavioral concerns.

Based on this information, the BHC determines that Olivia's behavioral presentation falls within the spectrum of developmentally appropriate behavior. Her parents are provided with psychoeducation about emotional and behavioral development in children, and the role tantrums play in development. Olivia's parents are reassured that their approach to Olivia's behavior is appropriate, and they are encouraged to remain consistent in their response to tantrums. They are educated about indicators that reassessment and/or active treatment may be warranted (e.g., worsening of tantrums, development of aggression), and affirmed for seeking guidance and support.

"Jack" is a 6-year-old male with Trisomy 21 brought to clinic by his mother and father for an appointment with his PCP to address toileting concerns. Due to the behavioral nature of the presenting concern, the BHC joins the PCP for conjoint assessment and decision-making. Jack's parents report they have encouraged Jack to use the toilet and have used "sticker charts" as motivation. His parents report that Jack is compliant with approximately one-half of parental commands for toilet sits. Jack's parents report they do not have scheduled times for implementing toilet sits with Jack. He currently wears pull-ups through the day. Of note, Jack has a history of constipation and currently takes stool softener as prescribed by his PCP. The PCP and BHC together assess toilet training readiness with Jack's parents, including a discussion about his motor abilities and proprioceptive awareness. Based on this discussion, it is determined that Jack is ready for toilet training, as the length of time between Jack's voiding have increased in length, he is able to tell his parents when he needs changing, and he is able to change is clothes independently. The BHC provides basic guidance to Jack's parents regarding general learning principles and how these principles can be applied to toilet training. Jack's parents express an understanding of the recommendations and intent to implement interventions. Jack's parents are directed to make an appointment with the BHC for a brief follow-up appointment in one month to assess Jack's progress in toilet training and determine if there are any barriers to the implementation of recommendations that would warrant further intervention or a higher level of care. Jack's parents are in agreement with the plan. This case highlights how the BHC can work with the PCP during an appointment to assess for medical and behavioral concerns and identify appropriate treatment interventions. In this situation, the BHC was able to provide the parents with a brief behavioral intervention for toilet training, with the plan to follow-up with the parents in one month.

Summary

Children with IDD are in a unique position to benefit from the medical home model due to the complexity of their health care needs. Whether or not a complete version of the medical home is available, the presence of a behavioral health consultant is an appropriate and valuable resource for this population. When developing a behavioral health consultation position within a primary care setting, several important considerations should be made to increase the likelihood of successful collaboration, which have been reviewed in this chapter. Specifically, (a) BHCs should be appropriately trained in principles of behavior change and systems to provide this level of care, (b) triage, scope of care, and communication skills are needed to work effectively in a collaborative setting, and (c) logistical considerations such as funding and location are important.

Despite some of existing barriers in the way of developing these types of consultative positions, within an integrated care, medical home model, it is possible to accomplish. Finally, we strongly suggest that programs and clinics that are beginning to engage to implement behavioral health consultation in primary care monitor their progress and collect outcome data to contribute to the growing evidence regarding integrated care models, and eventually render them easier to develop and be sustained.

References

Allen, K. D., Barone, V. J., & Kuhn, B. R. (1993). A behavioral prescription for promoting applied behavior analysis within pediatrics. *Journal of Applied Behavior Analysis, 26*(4), 493–502.

American Academy of Pediatrics (AAP). (2006). Infants and young children with developmental disorders in the medical home: An algorithm for developmental surveillance and screening. *Pediatrics 118*(1), 405–420. doi:10.1542/peds.2006-1231

Azrin, N. H., & Peterson, A. L. (1990). Treatment of Tourette sundrome by habit reversal: A waiting-list control group comparison. *Behavior Therapy, 21*, 305–318.

Borowitz, S. M., Cox, D. J., Sutphen, J. L., & Kovatchev, B. (2002). Treatment of childhood encopresis: A randomized trial comparing three treatment protocols. *Journal of Pediatric Gastroenterology and Nutrition, 34*, 378–384.

Boyer B. A., & Paharia, M. I. (Ed). (2008). Comprehensive handbook of clinical health psychology. (pp. 3–30). xxi, 482 pp. Hoboken, NJ, US: John Wiley & Sons Inc; US.

Brosig, C. L., & Zahrt, D. M. (2006). Evolution of an inpatient pediatric psychology consultation service: Issues related to reimbursement and the use of health and behavior codes. *Journal of Clinical Psychology in Medical Settings, 13*(4), 425–429.

Chomienne, M., Grenier, J., Gaboury, I., Hogg, W., Ritchie, P., & Farmanova-Haynes, E. (2011). Family doctors and psychologists working together: Doctors' and patients' perspectives. *Journal of Evaluation in Clinical Practice, 17*(2), 282–287.

Cooper, S., Valleley, R. J., Polaha, J., Begeny, J., & Evans, J. H. (2006). Running out of time: Physician management of behavioral health concerns in rural pediatric primary care. *Pediatrics, 118*(1), 132–138.

Costello, E. J. & Pantino, T. (1987). The new morbidity: Who should treat it? *Journal of Developmental and Behavioral Pediatrics, 8*(5), 288–291.

Cutler, D. M., & Ghosh, K. (2012). The potential for cost savings through bundled episode payments. *The New England Journal of Medicine, 366*(12), 1075–1077.

Dekker, M. C., & Koot, H. M. (2003). DSM-IV disorders in children with borderline to moderate intellectual disability: II. Child and family predictors. *Journal of the American Academy of Child and Adolescent Psychiatry, 42*, 923–931.

Doherty, W. (1995). The why's and levels of collaborative family health care. *Family Systems Medicine, 13*(3–4), 275–281.

Doherty, W. J., McDaniel, S. H., & Baird, M. A. (1996). Five levels of primary care/behavioral healthcare collaboration. *Behavioral Healthcare Tomorrow, 5*(5), 25–28.

Duke, D. C., Guion, K., Freeman, K. A., Wilson, A. C., & Harris, M. A. (2012). Health and behavior codes: Great idea, questionable outcome: Commentary. *Journal of Pediatric Psychology, 37*(5), 491–495.

Eckerberg, B. (2002). Treatment of sleep problems in families with small children: Is written information enough? *Acta Paediatrica, 91*, 952–959.

Einfeld, S. L., & Tonge, B. J. (1996). Population prevalence of psychopathology in children and adolescents with intellectual disability: II. Epidemiological findings. *Journal of Intellectual Disability Research, 40*, 99–109.

Fisher, L., & Dickinson, W. P. (2014). Psychology and primary care: New collaborations for providing effective care for adults with chronic health conditions. *American Psychologist, 69*(4), 355–363.

Forehand, R., & King, H. E. (1977). Noncompliant children: Effects of parent training on behavior and attitude change. *Behavior Modification, 1*, 93–108.

Finney, J. W., Riley, A. W., & Cataldo, M. F. (1991). Psychology in primary health care: Effects of brief targeted therapy on children's medical care utilization. *Journal of Pediatric Psychology, 16*(4), 447–461.

Freeman, K. A. (2006). Treating bedtime resistance with the bedtime pass: A systematic replication and component analysis with 3-year-olds. *Journal of Applied Behavior Analysis, 39*, 423–428.

Freeman, K. A., Riley, A., Duke, D. C., & Fu, R. (2014). Systematic review (and meta-analysis) of behavioral interventions for fecal incontinence with constipation. *Journal of Pediatric Psychology, 39*(8), 887–902.

Friman, P. C., Barone, V. J., & Christophersen, E. R. (1986). Aversive taste treatment of finger and thumb sucking. *Pediatrics, 78*, 174–176.

Friman, P. C., Hoff, K. E., Schnoes, C., Freeman, K. A., Woods, D. W., & Blum, N. (1999). The bedtime pass: An approach to bedtime crying and leaving the room. *Archives of Pediatric and Adolescent Medicine, 153*, 1027–1029.

Friman, P. C., & Leibowitz, J. M. (1990). An effective and acceptable treatment alternative for chronic thumb- and finger-sucking. *Journal of Pediatric Psychology, 15*, 57–65.

Guevara, J. P., Greenbaum, P. E., Shera, D., Bauer, L., & Schwarz, D. F. (2009). Survey of mental health consultation and referral among primary care pediatricians. *Academy of Pediatrics, 9*(2), 123–127.

Heath, B., Wise Romero, P., & Reynolds, K. A. (2013). *A standard framework for levels of integrated healthcare*. Washington, DC: SAMHSA-HRSA Center for Integrated Health Solutions.

Kathol, R. G., Butler, M., McAlpine, D. D., & Kane, R. L. (2010). Barriers to physical and mental condition integrated service delivery. *Psychosomatic Medicine, 72*(6), 511–518.

Lines, M. M., Tynan, W. D., Angalet, G. B., & Pendley, J. S. (2012). The use of health and behavior codes in pediatric psychology: Where are we now?: Commentary. *Journal of Pediatric Psychology, 37*(5), 486–490.

Mauch, D., Kautz, C., & Smith, S. A. (2008). Reimbursement of mental health services in primary care settings (HHS Pub. No. SMA-08-4324). Rockville, MD: Center for Mental Health Services, Substance Abuse.

Meadows, T., Valleley, R., Haack, M. K., Thorson, R., & Evans, J. (2011). Physician "costs" in providing behavioral health in primary care. *Clinical Pedaitrics, 50*(5), 447–455.

Mindell, J. A., Kuhn, B., Lewin, D. S., Meltzer, L. J., & Sadeh, A. (2006). Behavioral treatment of bedtime problems and night wakings in infants and young children. *Sleep: Journal Of Sleep And Sleep Disorders Research, 29*(10), 1263–1276.

Miranda, J., Hohmann, A. A., & Atkinson, C. C. (1994). Epidemiology of mental disorders in primary care. In J. Miranda, A. A. Hohmann, C. C. Atkinson, & D. P. Larson (Eds.), *mental disorders in primary care* (pp. 3–15). San Francisco: Jossey-Bass.

Noll, R. B., & Fischer, S. (2004). Commentary. Health and Behavior CPT Codes: An opportunity to revolutionize reimbursement in pediatric psychology. *Journal of Pediatric Psychology, 29*(7), 571–578.

O'Donnell, A. N., Williams, M., & Kilbourne, A. M. (2013). Overcoming roadblocks: Current and emerging reimbursement strategies for integrated mental health services in primary care. *Journal of General Internal Medicine, 28*(12), 1667–1672.

Piacentini, J., Woods, D. W., Scahill, L., Wilhelm, S., Peterson, A. L., Chang, S., et al. (2010). Behavior therapy for children with Tourette disorder: A randomized controlled trial. *JAMA, 303*(19), 1929–1937.

Sia, C., Tonniges, T. F., Osterhus, E., & Taba, S. (2004). History of the medical home concept. *Pediatrics, 113*, 1473–1478.

Shaw, D. S., Dishion, T. J., Supplee, L., Gardner, F., & Arnds, K. (2006). Randomized trial of a family-centered approach to the prevention of early conduct problems: 2-year effects of the family check-up in early childhood. *Journal of Consulting and Clinical Psychology, 74*(1), 1–9.

Stancin, T., Perrin, E., & Ramirez, L. (2009). Pediatric psychology and primary care. In M. Roberts & R. Steele (Eds.), *Handbook of pediatric psychology* (pp. 630–646). New York: The Guilford Press.

Talmi, A., & Fazio, E. (2012). Commentary: Promoting health and well-being in pediatric primary care settings: Using health and behavior codes at routine well-child visits. *Journal of Pediatric Psychology, 37*(5), 496–502.

Valleley, R. J., Kosse, S., Schemm, A., Foster, N., Polaha, J., & Evans, J. H. (2007). Integrated primary care for children in rural communities: An examination of patient attendance at collaborative behavioral health services. *Families, Systems, & Health, 25*(3), 323–332.

Wasserman, R. C., Kelleher, K. J., Bocian, A., Baker, A., Childs, G. E., Indacochea, F., et al. (1999). Identification of attentional and hyperactivity problems in primary care: A report from pediatric research in office settings and the ambulatory sentinel practice network. *Pediatrics, 103*(3), 38.

Williams, J., Palmes, G., Klinepeter, K., Pulley, A., & Foy, J. M. (2005). Referral by pediatricians of children with behavioral health disorders. *Clinical Pediatrics, 44*(4), 343–349.

Chapter 12
Parent Training and Support

Jonathan Tarbox, Monica L. Garcia and Megan St. Clair

Introduction

Parenting a child with intellectual and developmental disabilities (IDD) presents a unique set of challenges and rewards. Parents of children with disabilities often report that they have a renewed perspective on what really matters and, accordingly, parenting a child with special needs can be tremendously rewarding in many ways. At the same time, parenting a child with special needs can be challenging, overwhelmingly so for many. Parents often report that, when their child was first diagnosed, it was the most traumatic and stressful event in their life. In addition to the shock and dismay of the initial diagnosis, caring for a child with developmental or intellectual disabilities presents continuous sources of financial and psychological stress for parents. These elevated levels of stress take a toll on parents. For example, 23 % of marriages of parents raising children with developmental disabilities end in divorce versus 13 % of marriages of parents raising children without disabilities (Baeza-Velasco et al. 2013; Hartley et al. 2010). In addition, research has shown that parenting a child with developmental disabilities, low adaptive skills, or severe problem behaviors is related to higher depression, anxiety, and stress levels than those parents raising typically developing

J. Tarbox (✉)
FirstSteps for Kids, 2447 Pacific Coast Highway, Suite 111,
Hermosa Beach, CA 90254, USA
e-mail: jtarbox@firststepsforkids.com

M.L. Garcia
Center for Autism and Related Disorders, Woodland Hills, USA

M.S. Clair
The Help Group, San Marino, USA

J.K. Luiselli (ed.), *Behavioral Health Promotion and Intervention in Intellectual and Developmental Disabilities*, Evidence-Based Practices in Behavioral Health,
DOI 10.1007/978-3-319-27297-9_12

children (Rivard et al. 2014; Hayes and Watson 2013). To put it simply, parenting a child with developmental or intellectual disabilities is difficult and parents therefore need and deserve support.

The purpose of this chapter is to summarize existing research on parent support and training that has relevance for promoting health and caring for health related problems in children who have IDD. Heath issues, for example, require that parents learn how to apply specialized symptom-focused protocols, implement preventive strategies, establish compliance with prescribed methods, and intervene to prevent and reduce challenging behavior that is often occasioned by invasive medical procedures. Parents are also responsible for adhering to physician ordered regiments such as administering medications and following therapeutic routines with their children. Our descriptions of parent training approaches further include recommendations for practitioners and as well, we refer the reader to other recent, good quality chapters on the topic (Najdowski and Gould 2014; Schaffer and Minshawi 2014).

For the sake of simplicity, we choose to use the word "parents" throughout the chapter to refer to primary caregivers who live with the child with intellectual or developmental disability. We acknowledge that, quite frequently, the primary persons responsible for such care are not the child's birth parents, but rather, grandparents, adopted parents, guardians, foster parents, aunts, uncles, older siblings, step-parents, same-sex partners of parents, and so on. We advise that the reader keep all possible formats of families in mind while reading the chapter and to remember that we use the term "parent" merely for simplicity and readability.

Importance of Supporting and Training Parents

Parent training and support is not only important because parents need and deserve it. It is also important because it is critical to the success of the child's treatment. No matter how intensive the treatment format might be, the child's parents are still with him/her for more hours than the professional clinician. Even in situations where the child is hospitalized and receives 24/7 professional support, hospitalization will not last forever. The parents will ultimately be the ones whose behavior most impacts the child's outcome. Furthermore, for parents of many children with IDD, parenting does not end when the child turns 18 years old. Many individuals with developmental disabilities continue to live with their parents well into adulthood, often until their parents are deceased or need to move into supported living, themselves. Therefore, parenting habits (be they adaptive or maladaptive) can literally last a lifetime. And the stakes are high. For parents who do not develop effective behavior management skills, for example, they may continue to deal with their son or daughter's behavioral emergencies for decades, and such emergencies become much more serious when children become adults and are larger and stronger. Often, if such problems are not solved through effective behavioral parenting, the only remaining alternatives are over-medication or institutionalization, both of which can have devastating effects on the whole family.

Priority Concerns

The primary job of the parent trainer is to provide training and support that will empower the parent by giving them new repertoires of behavior that will enable them to be more effective with their children. Parenting is an incredibly complex and stressful experience and parent behaviors are influenced by multitudinous factors, both directly and indirectly related to their child with a disability. From the standpoint of the parent trainer, it is easy to make the error of believing that the only relevant variables in the parent's environment are the ones directly related to their child and his/her behavior. But the reality is that parenting behavior occurs in the context of relations with siblings, significant others, grandparents, financial stressors, and myriad other factors that can complicate even the simplest parent training process. For example, parents may actively disagree with one another about how to respond to challenging behavior and child misbehavior may therefore be an occasion for conflict between parents. For parent training to be successful, it is critical for the trainer to consider the many potential functions of the parent's behavior, in the broader context in which it occurs.

Environmental Factors Influencing Child and Parent Behavior

In order to best establish effective parenting behaviors, it is important to analyze and understand the contingencies that support the behaviors of both parent and child. A delicate and yet critically important dance plays out in the interactions between parents and their children with developmental disabilities on a daily basis. A classic example is that of child misbehavior. When a child misbehaves, it is virtually always because the misbehavior results in some type of desired outcome for the child. The most common desired outcomes include getting attention from others, escaping or postponing a demand the child does not want to do, or getting access to desired items or activities (Hanley et al. 2003). Depending on the function of the child's misbehavior in the moment, the parent's reaction to that misbehavior plays a critical role in either increasing or decreasing the likelihood of the child repeating similar behavior in the future. Classic examples include a parent giving their child candy when the child engages in a tantrum to get it, or giving their child a break from cleaning their room when the child protests the demand by screaming or throwing objects, or a parent yelling at their child when the child hits them, when in fact the child hit the parent in order to get their attention. These and similar situations are particularly concerning in caring for children who have health problems.

The effect of parent reaction to child behavior is perhaps most clear when the behavior is misbehavior, but parents' reactions to appropriate child behavior are equally critical. A classic example is a family wherein the parents are very busy and only pay attention to a particular child when that child misbehaves. Initial appropriate behaviors on the part of the child, such as attempts to communicate, often produce no reaction from parents who are busy, stressed, and trying to attend to many other tasks at the same time. Consequently, it is a simple matter for the child to engage in destructive behavior if he/she wants attention.

In recent years, the proliferation of electronic devices that display videos and video games, such as smart phones, tablets, and laptops, has created a new source of temptation for parents. It is often the case that giving a child with a developmental disability access to electronic devices produces an immediate improvement in their mood and/or cessation of challenging behavior. It is no wonder, then, that many parents give their children access to multiple hours of electronics per day. Of course, providing access to electronics as a consequence of challenging behavior may inadvertently reinforce the behavior. But another potential negative effect of prolonged "screen time" is less obvious: It decreases the opportunities for interaction with caregivers, peers, and others. Frequent, upbeat, reciprocal interactions with between parent and child are critical in order to maximize language and social development, decrease challenging behavior and promote healthy living. Extended periods of time where a child independently consumes electronics inevitably decreases these critically needed interactions. And, of course, the same may be said of us parents. When parents are stressed-out and tired, it can be very tempting to spend time engaging in social media on smart phones or watching television. Small amounts of these activities are not a problem, but extended periods of time spent engaged in electronic devices, even for parents, reduces opportunities for positive interpersonal interactions with children.

Short-Term Versus Long-Term Contingencies for Parent Behavior

The unfortunate reality is that the natural tendencies for the vast majority of parents are not what is necessarily in their own or their child's best interests. It is natural for humans to respond to immediate, short-term contingencies. In all of the examples of problematic parent-child interactions described above, parents are responding to short-term contingencies. The immediate effect of giving-into problematic behavior is usually that the behavior goes away in the short-term. If a child is having a tantrum to get candy, then giving him/her candy usually makes the tantrum stop. Therefore, the short-term effect for the parent reinforcing the tantrum is to receive negative reinforcement in the form of making the tantrum stop. However, the tantrum may stop, but it does not go away in the long run. The next time the child wants candy he/she will be even more likely to have a tantrum. That is, the long-term effect is to strengthen tantrums, which should be a punishment effect for the parent's behavior of reinforcing the tantrum, but it is not an effective punishment for the parent because it is too delayed. If the parent chooses the more behaviorally sound reaction to the tantrum and does not give candy in the moment, the short-term effect could be to worsen the tantrum, as in an extinction burst, thereby potentially punishing the parent's good behavior in the short-term. So, unfortunately, the situation that many parents find themselves in is immediate punishment for doing the right thing and immediate reinforcement for doing the wrong thing.

A very large part of parent training involves orienting parents to this problem in order to bring their parenting behavior under the influence of long-term contingencies and thereby making it less susceptible to influence by short-term contingencies that prevail in the moment in which misbehavior is occurring. Interestingly, it is helpful for both clinicians and parents to notice how many other behavioral decision points share very similar features throughout life and to note that those who are successful are often those who choose to work toward longer-term consequences. Consider eating and exercising, two dominant health related topics. The short-term consequences of eating junk food (pleasurable eating experience) and not exercising (avoiding effort) are almost always more reinforcing than eating healthy (less pleasurable) and choosing exercise (more effort). However, the long-term consequences of doing so such as obesity, diabetes, heart disease are exponentially more terrible than the short-term reinforcers were good. Studying in school is nearly identical. In summary, choosing to eschew the smaller reward now (e.g., stopping the tantrum immediately) in order to get the much larger reward later (e.g., tantrums go away completely in the future) and effective parent training almost always involves orienting parents to help them commit to decisions such as these.

Research Review

A significant amount of research has been published on training and supporting parents of children with developmental disabilities. A comprehensive review is far beyond the scope of this chapter. Instead, this section provides an overview of some of the main areas of research, with descriptions of key studies in each area, in order to set the stage for practice recommendations later in the chapter. To reiterate, the research we describe covers several areas of behavioral parent training that have relevance for families with a child who has IDD and health concerns.

Management of Challenging Behaviors

Many studies have shown that parents of children with developmental disabilities can be successfully trained to manage a variety of challenging behaviors. For example, Tarbox et al. (2007) used behavioral skills training (BST) to train parents to implement three-step prompting with their children with autism and other disorders. Results showed that, for all parents, excessive prompting decreased and child compliance increased. Similarly, Miles and Wilder (2009) used BST to train parents to implement guided compliance using three caregiver-child pairs. The children each had high frequency non-compliance and one child having a diagnosis of autism, one child with a diagnosis of unidentified learning disorder, while the third child had no diagnosis. Results of the study showed that caregivers' ability to implement guided compliance increased and child compliance increased.

Wacker et al. (1998) trained parents of 28 young children with developmental disabilities to conduct functional analyses and treat their child's behavior through functional communication training (FCT). On average, treatment resulted in an 86 % decrease in challenging behavior across children. In addition, appropriate social behavior increased an average of 69 % across children. The researchers also assessed parent treatment acceptability and, on a scale from 1 (least acceptable) to 7 (most acceptable), the average rating obtained was 6.35, indicating that the approach was highly acceptable to parents.

Feeding Challenges

Feeding issues and associated health complications are common among children with IDD (Gulotta and Girolami 2014). Research indicates that parents can be effectively trained to implement both functional assessment and treatment procedures for treating feeding disorders in children with IDD. For example, Najdowski et al. (2008) trained parents to conduct experimental functional analyses of mealtime misbehavior. Training consisted of a one-hour session, during which the experimenter used BST, consisting of verbal explanation, modeling, and role play to train the parents on functional analysis procedures. After training, parents implemented functional analyses with their children, with occasional live verbal feedback from experimenters. Parents achieved high procedural fidelity and the functional analyses produced clear results for all six children.

Najdowski et al. (2010) trained parents to implement evidence-based feeding intervention procedures, consisting of escape extinction and positive reinforcement, as well as collecting data on their child's eating behaviors. Training occurred in the home and followed a BST format, consisting of 10 min of verbal explanation, modeling, and role play. Parents then implemented feeding sessions with their child and were given live feedback by experimenters. After a parent achieved 90 % treatment integrity across three consecutive sessions, they began to implement treatment sessions with the experimenter absent. Parents were then asked to videotape one session per week to review at a later time with the experimenter. All parents achieved high treatment integrity within the minimum amount of time allowable and maintained high integrity at up to 12 weeks follow-up.

Tarbox et al. (2010) trained a mother of a child with autism to implement a non-intrusive form of escape extinction for treating her child's food selectivity. The mother implemented all sessions in her home and a behavioral consultant was present only to answer questions, give feedback, and provide emotional support. The mother successfully implemented the procedures and at the conclusion of the study, her son successfully consumed whatever normal family meals she chose to cook.

Skill Acquisition

Research has shown behavioral training procedures have been effective in training parents of children with IDD to implement a wide variety of skill acquisition procedures to teach their children a wide variety of skills.

Language. Specific language development procedures include incidental teaching, Pivotal Response Training (PRT), the Picture Exchange Communication System (PECS), and enhanced milieu teaching (EMT), among others. For example, Symon (2005) evaluated the effects of an intensive clinic-based program that trained parents of children with ASD on the implementation of PRT procedures with their children. Experimenters used a BST format, consisting of verbal explanation, modeling, and in vivo feedback, for 5 h per day, across five consecutive days, constituting 25 h of one-to-one training for each parent. The purpose of the training program was to directly train the parents who were present; however, the program also encouraged the parents to then train other significant caregivers (e.g., spouses) who were not present, after the training program was complete. The results of the study showed that parents successfully trained other significant caregivers after returning to their homes in other states, that child behavior changed in a positive direction during the same period, and that these improvements were maintained at three-month follow-up. This study is compelling because, although the direct training was labor and time-intensive, the effects were maintained at long distances, across three months, and generalized to other caregivers who were not able to be present for training.

Chaabane et al. (2009) trained mothers of two children with autism to implement PECS with their children. The researchers used a BST training format, including written instructions, verbal explanation, modeling, practice, and feedback to train the mothers. The procedure was effective in training the mothers and mother implementation of PECS resulted in increased independent child mands (i.e., requests) and generalization was observed for both children. Similalry, Park et al. (2010) trained mothers of three children with ASD to implement PECS with their children. All three children successfully learned independent requests, generalization was observed across caregivers, and effects maintained at one month follow-up.

Kaiswer et al. (2000) studied the effectiveness of parent implemented EMT on social communication skills in children with autism. Experimenters conducted 25 (2 per week) clinic-based parent training sessions. During the first 15 min of each session, the trainer met separately with the parent (child absent), reviewed videotapes, and gave feedback from the previous session, introduced new information, set goals for the current session, and engaged in modeling and role play. During the second 15 min, the parent worked directly with the child and the trainer was present to provide live coaching and feedback. During the last 15 min, the trainer reviewed that session and provided the parent with feedback and helped him/her generate ideas for generalizing what was learned to the home environment. The results demonstrated that parents were able to learn EMT, their children's language improved across multiple measures, and improvements generally maintained at follow-up, although to a slightly lesser degree.

Daily living skills. Research has shown that parents can be effectively trained to teach their children a variety of important daily living skills. For example, Kroeger and Sorensen (2010) trained parents of two boys with autism to implement a modified version of the Azrin and Fox rapid toilet training method. Each parent received 6 h of training on a single day, consisting of verbal instruction, modeling, and then practice with their child, with live feedback from the trainer. Parents were then given written instructions on how to proceed and the opportunity to contact the trainers via telephone to ask questions, which they both did five times over the next several days. Data revealed that both boys were continent in under 2 days from the beginning of training, fully toilet trained within 10 days, and maintained continence at three-year follow-up.

Tekin-Iftar (2008) trained four parents of children with autism to implement prompting strategies to teach their children with developmental disabilities skills to access the community (e.g., ordering bread in a bakery, ordering dry cleaning at a launder, purchasing food at a grocery store). Parents were trained using a BST format, consisting of verbal instruction, modeling, and role-play with feedback in a small group setting. All four parents successfully trained their children to display the community skills in the settings in which they were trained and all four children displayed the trained skills in other sites that were not used in training, thus demonstrating generalization across settings.

Imitation. The ability to imitate others is a critical foundational skill for learning more complex skills because imitation allows the child to learn through observing peers. In addition, modeling prompts is a key teaching procedure in intervention programs for individuals with IDD. However, modeling prompts cannot be effective if the learner does not have the ability to imitate. Ingersoll and Gergans (2007) trained parents to implement reciprocal imitation training (RIT) with their children with autism. Parents used RIT to train their children in object imitation and/or imitation of language gestures. Parents successfully learned to implement RIT and the rates of imitation improved for all three children with autism to a small but significant degree.

Social skills. Parents of children with IDD have also been trained to teach their children social skills. For example, Stewart et al. (2007), used BST to train a mother how to teach her son with Asperger's disorder a variety of social skills, including eye contact, asking his conversational partner if he/she was bored, asking if they would like to change topics, and decreasing perseverating on his favorite conversational topics. The results demonstrated significant improvements in the child's social skills following his mother's training.

Reagon and Higbee (2009) used BST to train mothers of children with autism to implement script-fading procedures to increase their children's vocal initiations during play. Specifically, mothers were trained to create their own scripts for increasing their child's initiations, to implement those scripts during play, and to fade them out. The mothers successfully implemented the procedures with their children in their homes. In addition, both targeted initiations and untargeted initiations (i.e., generalization) increased during intervention and at follow-up.

Discrete trial training. DTT is a procedure that is typically implemented by professionals working with children with ASD, and may not be the first target for parent training that many would consider. However, the vast majority of families living with ASD around the world today still have little or no access to qualified professionals who are trained in applied behavior analysis (ABA) techniques and who are available to deliver therapy directly. Therefore, many families are forced to take on the responsibility of delivering most or all of their child's treatment and DTT is a critical piece of that process. Several studies have demonstrated effective procedures for training parents in accurate DTT implementation. For example, Crockett et al. (2007) used BST, consisting of instruction, modeling, role-play, and practice with feedback to train two mothers of children with ASD to implement DTT with their children. Both mothers achieved large improvements in implementing DTT to teach skills that they were trained to teach, as well as demonstrating generalization of DTT ability to new skills.

Ward-Horner and Sturmey (2008) combined behavioral skills training with general case instruction to help parents generalize their learned DTT skills such that they could teach their children with autism skills that the trainers had not taught the parents directly. Three parent-child dyads were included in training. Training resulted in substantial increases in accuracy for all parents, as well as generalization to untrained skills.

The two studies described above demonstrated that behavioral skills training can be used to teach parents to implement DTT. In a more recent study, Young et al. (2012) tested a self-instructional training package for teaching parents to implement DTT, in order to decrease the amount of time required of professionals. In the first experiment, they evaluated a self-instructional manual combined with a self-instructional video and observed a substantial increase in accuracy of DTT implementation for three of five parents; however, the procedure was not sufficient for two of five parents. In a second experiment, the authors combined the self-instructional video and manual with brief role-playing implemented by professional trainers. Parents received an average of only 4.68 h of training in the second study and all five parents implemented DTT with high accuracy with their children after training. The results of this study suggest that some parents may require only self-instructional training to learn DTT skills, while some may still require at least a minimal amount of direct instruction from a professional.

Intensity and Duration

Although there is some research on the intensity (frequency of training) and duration (length of training) of parent training, this information varies significantly between effective studies, therefore ideal intensity and duration of parent training have yet to be identified by research (Najdowski and Gould 2014). However, many parent-training studies have demonstrated positive outcomes, irrespective of intensity and duration training specifics (Schultz et al. 2011). For example, Symon (2005) obtained substantial treatment effects after 25 h of training, whereas Young et al. (2012) produced substantial effects after only 4.68 h of training, thereby demonstrating both high and low intensity formats can be effective. Future research should attempt to identify what levels of intensity may be required to train which particular skills and for which particular populations.

Trainee Characteristics

Research on trainee variables that may impact parent-training outcomes is significantly lacking in the literature. Nevertheless, studies have noted that culture, socioeconomic status, history of mental health, and available resources may be potential factors influencing parent-training outcomes (Schultz et al. 2011; Steiner et al. 2012). In addition, research on parent training has primarily used mothers to implement treatment–more research is needed on whether mothers or fathers (or a combination) produce the best outcomes (Najdowski and Gould 2014; Steiner et al. 2012). Furthermore, in families where only one parent is available for training, it is unknown what training procedures produce best generalization across parents.

Trainer Characteristics

There is little research that has evaluated which trainer variables ensure optimal parent training outcomes. However, studies have highlighted some prerequisite trainer characteristics, such as fluency in presentation, a solid understanding of program procedures, providing effective feedback, organizational skills, and rapport-building skills as potentially critical trainee characteristics (Najdowski and Gould 2014). Individual funding agencies often have their own policies or traditions regarding who is considered competent to train (e.g., BCBA certification), however little research has directly evaluated the effects of trainer education, certification, number of years of experience, age, gender, or other variables. Additional research is needed to identify specific trainer variables that predict optimal parent training outcomes.

Training Formats

Given the steady increase in the number of children diagnosed with ASD, the extensive clinical attention this population demands, and the numerous constraints to accessing treatment (e.g., geographic, financial, educational, etc.), it is imperative that several training formats are readily available to effectively, efficiently, and flexibly meet the needs of each individual family. Fortunately, empirical support has been found for a variety of training formats. The most traditional format consists of training a parent in-person, on a one-to-one basis. This interaction can occur in the clinic or in the home, with the child present, in the child's absence, or a combination of both. Training can also be conducted in groups (Anan et al. 2008), across geographical distances using Web tools such as FaceTime, in self-directed programs such as e-Learning modules (Jang et al. 2012), through "three-tier" models, and in a "train the trainer" or pyramidal format (Symon 2005). Many different formats have been shown to work, and yet, it also seems plainly apparent that the format used with any particular family could critically impact the success of the training program. Therefore, more research is needed that helps identify which formats are likely to be optimal for which particular families.

Training Procedures

Behavioral skills training. As has been described thus far, BST is a multicomponent training procedure, consisting of (1) verbal or didactic instruction, (2) modeling, and (3) role-play or rehearsal with feedback. BST is among the most empirically validated package procedures for training many skills in children, parents, staff, and others. Most evidence-based parent training procedures implement some version of BST and have shown that it can be effective for training parents to improve a wide variety of child skills, including compliance (Tarbox et al. 2007), conversation (Stewart et al. 2007), independent vocalizations (Reagon and Higbee 2009), and as noted previously, health intervention and health promoting activities (Luiselli 2015).

A small amount of research has found individual component procedures to be at least somewhat effective. Lerman et al. (2000) evaluated verbal and written instruction alone and found that some parents acquired skills using only these training procedures, but the results varied across parents and skills being trained. Although some research suggests that individual components, such as verbal instruction, can be effective alone, the vast majority of research has shown that parent skill acquisition is effective when parents are given the opportunity to actually do the skills they are being trained on and then directly receive feedback, rather than merely hearing the trainer talk about the skills.

Technology. In recent years, researchers have begun to explore the vast potential of technology for parent training. For example Jang et al. (2012) used a randomized trial to evaluate the effects of a web-based eLearning module for training parents of children with autism in the principles and procedures of applied behavior analysis. Results showed that parents acquired the knowledge being trained, however, the study did not attempt to assess real-life implementation of procedures.

Wacker et al. (2013) evaluated the effects of a telehealth model for training parents of children with developmental disabilities and challenging behavior to conduct brief functional analyses and functional communication training treatments. Parents attended local (average 15 miles away from home) clinics, where they teleconferenced with expert behavioral consultants (average 222 miles away). Consultants trained parents and gave them direct, live instruction while they implemented assessment and treatment procedures. Results demonstrated an average reduction in problem behavior of 93.5 %, suggesting that telehealth-based behavioral parent training can be highly effective.

Wainer and Ingersoll (2014) evaluated the effects of a hybrid telehealth system for training parents of children with autism on RIT. The hybrid system consisted of web-based self-instruction and distance coaching. Self-instruction consisted of five web-based learning modules. Coaching consisted of three, 30-min coaching sessions, wherein coaches watched videos of parent implementation and gave parents specific feedback on their performance. Five parents participated and all five demonstrated substantial improvements in the fidelity of their treatment implementation.

Overall, although interest and productivity in research on the role of technology in parent training is increasing dramatically, a great deal is still unknown. For example, it is still not known how, if ever, web-based or other types of eLearning training can replace live instruction (be it in-person or via video conference) by an expert trainer. It seems unlikely that expert trainers will ever be replaced entirely but a great deal more research is needed on how live training by an expert might be made more efficient or more cost-effective through means such as eLearning or videoconferencing. Continued advancements in training technology will make automated training more interactive. For example, enhancements in virtual or augmented reality may make computer-based training much less distinguishable from real-life than it currently is today. Thus, through continued development, it seems likely that parents will be able to be active participants in technology-based training, rather than passive recipients.

Future Research

The vast differences among parent training approaches illustrates the importance of future research for informing practitioners about which particular approach/duration/intensity/format will be most effective. Toward this end, research that evaluates the relation between particular parent/family characteristics and comparative effectiveness between different approaches would be particularly valuable.

For example, perhaps parents with different numbers of children or different levels of familial support or different degrees of socioeconomic resources might benefit from different types or intensity or formats of parent training. Unfortunately, research that addresses such questions will likely require large groups of parents assessed on a number of characteristics and then randomly assigned to two or more different approaches. Such research is inherently costly and labor-intensive and is therefore less likely to be accomplished, but it would be valuable, nonetheless.

One exciting area for future research is in the application of Acceptance and Commitment Therapy (ACT) to training and support for parents of individuals with IDD. As discussed in the introduction and priority concerns sections above, parenting an individual with IDD can be highly challenging, resulting in feelings of guilt, stress, inadequacy, and desperation. It is common for humans to believe that they are being controlled, and even "imprisoned," by their thoughts and feelings. Therefore, when under stress, most people spend much of their time and energy trying to avoid negative thoughts and feelings. Unfortunately, when caring for children with IDD, health problems, and behavioral challenges, many parents may understandably avoid situations that cause them distress.

Research on ACT has found that it is possible to empower people to accept difficult thoughts and feelings and "hold them more loosely," while making space for choosing overt actions, other than those aimed at reducing negative feelings. In other words, ACT empowers people to experience their negative emotions and at the same time make choices that allow them to lead fuller, more effective lives. ACT is a behavioral approach to psychotherapy that now has over 100 published randomized controlled trials, resulting in ACT being recognized as a "well-established" treatment for chronic pain and a "probably efficacious" treatment for depression, mixed anxiety, obsessive compulsive disorder, and psychosis (http://www.psychologicaltreatments.org/). Researchers have only just begun to apply ACT to supporting parents of individuals with IDD but the initial research is encouraging (Blackledge and Hayes 2006; Whittingham et al. 2014) and we advise researchers and practitioners to learn more about this promising approach (http://contextualscience.org/). Mindfulness caregiving and support is a similar strategy worthy of consideration (Singh et al. 2014).

Practice Recommendations

In this section of the chapter, we provide concrete recommendations for how to successfully train parents in your practice. The vast majority of recommendations come directly from the peer-reviewed literature. However, where research is lacking, best-practice recommendations are given that, generally speaking, are supported by a broad consensus among the IDD treatment and support community.

Building the Relationship with Parents

Building a productive, positive, upbeat relationship with the parents you are going to train is the first task of parent training and is among the most important. Establishing rapport with parents is the foundation upon which successful parent training depends. In effect, most parent training efforts, regardless of how adept, are likely to fail if this first step is not executed effectively. Trainers must present themselves as professional, knowledgeable, effective, competent, and confident. However, merely being perceived as an expert is not enough to build a productive relationship with parents. It is just as important for the trainer to demonstrate to parents that he or she is dedicated to the wellbeing of the child and parents, is sensitive to the challenges they are facing, and is willing to work hard to help them achieve their goals.

Goals. The trainer must identify the parents' values and align the goals and processes of training accordingly. Ultimately, the trainer cannot make the parents do anything because the trainer is not in control of the vast majority of contingencies that matter to parents—they cannot hire or fire them, they cannot give them a raise if they perform well, and so on. Therefore, if parent commitment and follow-through is desired, the trainer must find a way to clarify how compliance with the training program moves the parents closer to the parents' values. A good way to do this is to begin by identifying what the parents' values and desired outcomes are (more on outcomes in the next section below). Then, the processes and goals of training should be discussed in terms of those values and outcomes. This approach is much more likely to result in parent buy-in than simply telling parents that they need to do what the trainer wants them to do. Consider the following two hypothetical explanations for why a parent who wants their child to properly follow a medication-taking regimen without resistance should implement extinction:

1. "I need you to ignore your child's tantrums from now on. I know it's hard but you just need to do it. When you don't give a child what he wants when he tantrums, that's called putting the behavior on extinction. Tons of research has shown that putting a behavior on extinction is the most effective way to decrease the behavior."
2. "We talked about how being able to take his medication without displaying a tantrum. If you really want your child to benefit from the medication he was prescribed, the best step you can take in that direction is to no longer react to his tantrums, because that will help decrease the behavior. The sooner we decrease his tantrums, the more compliant he will be with your medication administration."

In the first explanation, the trainer emphasizes important, valid points but fails to address what matters most to the parent. Behavioral parent trainers often talk about what matters most to *them* (e.g., research, behavioral principles, etc.), rather than what matters most to parents. In the second explanation, the rationale for compliance with the training program is framed wholly in terms of the outcome *that particular parent values*. The goal is to transform the function of parent compliance from "doing what the trainer wants" to "doing what will help my child attain goal X."

Talk like a normal person. It is very common for behaviorally trained clinicians to talk to parents in overly technical, dry-sounding jargon. It makes sense that, after spending so much time and effort to learn to talk in technical terms in graduate school, that the professional would then use that newly learned skill frequently. This is certainly also common in medical doctors. However, just as in medicine, parents generally do not appreciate being talked to in technical jargon that can be difficult to understand, off-putting, and pedantic. You should remember how you talked before you became an expert and speak in that language when instructing parents.

Training Outcomes

Defining behavior change goals. Behavior change goals for both the parent and child should be beneficial in the daily life of the family, measurable, achievable, and should produce clinically meaningful behavior change.

Quality of life. A good focus for goal setting is improving the quality of life of the child and those most impacted by the child's health condition and behavior. Beneficial goals typically involve increasing the feasibility of day-to-day routine completion, as well as improving the family's ability to manage social and community activities together. Child specific goals should increase overall independence and reduce problematic behavior. For example, a child's quality of life suffers when he resists every health promoting opportunity presented to him. Parental goals should enhance parents' current skills, reduce stress, and maximize success without a trainer present. Using the latter example, a parental goal may include training parents in skill acquisition techniques that conveniently fit into their daily routine and problem behavior management techniques that may result in decreased stress. In general, goals should benefit both the parent and child in ways that improve their overall quality of life.

Measurable. Behavior change goals should also be measurable. Goals that are objectively defined provide a detailed measure of the overall outcome desired for both the parent and child. Clear goals provide a coherent and unambiguous outline of the plan to reach success, helping to prevent ambiguity and miscommunication. Goals that are comprehensively stated help establish mutual agreement and understanding between parent and trainer. An example of a measurable child goal is: Susie will complete her prescribed nebulizer treatment each evening without pulling away, screaming, or throwing materials. An example of a measurable parent goal is: Mom will monitor Susie's targeted behaviors during nebulizer treatment each night by placing a tally mark on the corresponding date on the calendar.

Challenging but achievable. Understandably, parents often have very high expectations for what their children should achieve as a result of training. Aiming high is good but goals must also be achievable. For example, for a child who makes almost no eye contact under any circumstances, establishing appropriate eye contact across all peers and adults and in all socially appropriate contexts would be an ideal outcome. However, a more achievable goal might be to make eye contact when his name is called, during at least 80 % of opportunities, within three months. Similarly, an ideal goal for a parent might be to establish effective prompting procedures during all interactions with their children but a more achievable goal might be for a parent to implement prompting procedures with 90–100 % accuracy when calling their child's name to occasion eye contact. Goals that are challenging but achievable set the occasion for trainer, parent, and child success by specifying a high standard while still ensuring success at achieving the goals. Particularly during the early stages of parent training, parental success is crucial because it helps establish the overall process of training as a source of positive reinforcement for the parent and trainer alike.

Data collection. Collecting data provides a way to evaluate progress and provides rationale for treatment change if necessary. For the parent, data collection should be effective and easy to implement into a daily routine. For example, tallying the frequency of bites consumed each meal is a relatively simple data collection procedure for parents implementing a feeding intervention at home. For the trainer, data collection should be more detailed and comprehensive based on direct observations, graphical displays of data, and assessment of interobserver agreement, when possible.

Trainer and Trainee Characteristics

Trainee. Although trainee/parent characteristics cannot be controlled and training should be provided to all who need it, there are many trainee characteristics that should be considered when developing and implementing a parent-training program. In addition to caring for a child with IDD and health related concerns, parents may be experiencing other stressors which interfere with their commitment to training. Such stressors could be depressive symptoms, lack of resources and services (child care, transportation, etc.), marital conflict, limited family and social support, scheduling/time conflicts, mental health or medical issues, and caring for multiple children. Practitioners should assess what stressors are most prominent in the family's life and individualize training by minimizing or at least not adding to present family stressors. Other trainee features to consider are those relating to educational background, culture, and language. Parents with lower educational backgrounds may need extra training in understanding and implementing treatment techniques (Steiner et al. 2012). The family's cultural attitudes and practices and the trainer's own cultural biases should be assessed before developing and implementing a parent training program in order to ensure that the training program encompasses the family's cultural needs, values, and beliefs (Najdowski and Gould 2014). Language barriers may also influence the success of parent training. The family's primary language should be used throughout training, as well as non-jargon language and appropriate reading level materials, at least as much as possible (Najdowski and Gould 2014). Where it is not possible to implement the parent's first language on an ongoing basis, consider hiring an interpreter to at least attend the most critical planning meetings. Parent genders, parenting styles, parent preferred setting and format of training, and potential resistance to training are additional trainee characteristics that should be considered. In particular, patterns of parenting behavior often differ considerably between mothers and fathers within the same family. Therefore, training programs need to be customized to accommodate both parents (Schreibman et al. 2011). Because resources such as child care, transportation, or an optimal training setting may be limited, parents may prefer one teaching strategy over another, for example, in vivo versus video modeling, group versus one-on-one, or in-home versus clinic settings (Steiner et al. 2012). Practitioners must consider these factors to ensure successful training outcomes. While taking all of these variables into consideration, trainers should build rapport and develop a training program that is the best contextual fit for the family to encourage compliance and active participation.

Trainer. Critical trainer characteristics include thorough knowledge of the intervention procedures, collaborating with parents, being fluent in providing effective feedback (Najdowski and Gould 2014), and having rapport-building, empathy, and organizational skills. Trainers should also have demonstrated the ability to train at an excellent level with other families in the past. All other things being equal, trainers with higher graduate degrees (e.g., masters and PhDs) and with professional certifications (e.g., Board Certified Behavior Analysts) are preferred, but such credentials, by themselves, do not ensure competence. Many experienced clinicians who lack those credentials can still be highly effective trainers.

Intensity and Duration

Although research has not yet identified an optimal level of intensity or duration of parent training, several critical factors appear to be family goals, expectations, needs (Najdowski and Gould 2014), resources, preferred training formats, and practitioner accessibility. Intensity and length of training should also be based on goals being met and the most practical outcomes reached. Ideally, the duration of parent training should be dictated by how long it takes for parents to achieve the goals of training.

Setting

Given that training has been shown to be effective across many different settings, the trainer should consider multiple variables when choosing an appropriate setting for training, notably the availability of the parent and child, the feasibility of training itself in relation to parent resources, and cost-effectiveness for the clinic. School, home, and/or community goals may require training to occur in their corresponding setting. Trainers should also consider the benefits and drawbacks of each setting. For example, home-based parent training may provide a more natural environment where acquired skills need to be displayed. Home settings may also lead to better generalization of acquired skills. However, home-based parent training may contain more distractions or less controlled environments. Clinic-based parent trainings on the other hand control for distractions, but may require additional effort to ensure generalization to home. Thus, collaboration with parents is a necessity in order to select a mutually agreed upon setting that ensures optimal success.

Parent Homework

Assigning homework for parents may assist in the success of a parent-training program. Homework assignments are in-between training sessions when the trainer is absent. Homework should require low-response effort to complete, should be understandable and achievable, and should produce small, but meaningful behavior change. Trainers should ensure that homework aligns with the family's current goals, daily routine, availability, and current training topics and targets. For example, with a parent whose initial goal is to teach his child to mand, an appropriate assignment would be one simple mand (such as "break") to teach his child in between training sessions.

Behavioral Skills Training

As described earlier, much research has documented the effectiveness of BST for training parents. In what follows, we review each of the major components of BST and offer several practice recommendations.

Defining the target. Both parent and child targets should be clearly identified and defined. Effective operational definitions facilitate understanding, both between the trainer and parent, as well as between parents. The characteristics of an adequate operational definition are objectivity, clarity, and completeness (Cooper et al. 2007). An objective definition breaks down all non-observable features of a skill or behavior into its directly observable counterparts, such that each individual can reliably identify and record an instance. A clear definition is one that is unequivocal, easily read, and clearly understood. Finally, a complete definition discriminates what will be classified as an occurrence and non-occurrence of the skill or behavior on the basis of strict inclusion and exclusion criteria. In this way, potential moment-to-moment subjective judgments are eliminated.

Written instruction. Following the development of operational definitions of the parent and child behaviors of interest, trainers should prepare written instructions as supplementary materials for later verbal didactic instruction. Written instructions should provide both a visual aid that can be referenced and notated throughout training and a permanent reminder of how to practice and perform the procedures in the trainer's absence. Therefore, such instructions should be easily accessible at all times, given to each caregiver expected to have involvement in the implementation of the intervention, and clearly delineate respective performance responsibilities. Lastly, when writing these written instructions, it is important to remember that the ultimate goal is to effectively divide complex interventions to be trained into concise and consumable steps.

Didactic instruction. Didactic or verbal instruction should include a thorough review of the target child and parent behaviors, intervention procedures, prompting strategies, fading criteria, and rationale for the entire plan. Clinician's should take the necessary precautions by pacing themselves in accordance with each parent's learning curve and by strategically linking parent values with training objectives. In addition to speaking directly and openly, it is essential to welcome questions and concerns.

Modeling. Modeling allows the parent to observe the trainer directly demonstrate how to perform each component of the intervention described in the written instructions. First, trainers should announce which procedure they are going to demonstrate. Throughout the course of modeling, trainers should explain why they are engaging in each behavior that they are demonstrating. During and following modeling, trainers should encourage questions and comments from parents. In addition, it may be helpful to model examples of incorrect implementation of the intervention and ask parents to identify what about the model was incorrect and why. Finally, it may be necessary for trainers to model a particular procedure more than once, or even one time at the beginning of each training session.

Role Play Rehearsal. During role-play, the parent takes the role of him or herself and the trainer takes the role of the child. Roles can switch back and forth until proficiency is observed. Throughout role-play, trainers should provide just enough verbal prompting and feedback for parents to be successful, but not so much that they do not have the opportunity to demonstrate skills independently. Sometimes, parents have difficulty implementing a procedure accurately and the trainer may need to shape successive approximations by praising one small piece of the procedure demonstrated correctly before asking the parent to demonstrate other components. During and immediately after each role-play, the trainer should engage parents in self-evaluative dialogue by asking questions such as, "What did you like about your performance?", "What didn't you like?", "What about this works for you?", and "What about this do you think is not going to work?" These questions provide an open, non-judgmental context for parents to give input and often help identify ways in which the intervention may need to be adjusted or customized to fit the family's individual context or needs. Overall, keep in mind that role-playing can be awkward and stressful, for both parent and trainer, alike. It is often helpful to use humor to make the experience less stressful and more fun for everyone. Good trainers model flexibility and creativity during role-play, not rigid insistence on rules or dogma.

Feedback. Effective role-playing is dependent on trainers giving immediate and specific feedback to parents. There are two forms of feedback, praise and corrective. While both should be frequent, descriptive, and contingent, praise should significantly outnumber corrections. Praise should be genuine and not "patronizing." Corrective feedback should be clear and frank but not harsh. It is important to emphasize that errors are expected and acceptable–they are merely opportunities to learn. A good motto for parents when learning a new intervention is that "it's best to fail early and fail often," that way they become experts while they still have the support of the trainer. Positive feedback should always outnumber corrective feedback, ideally on at least a 2:1 or 3:1 ratio. "Sandwiching" can also be useful by presenting corrective feedback between one prior and one later piece of positive feedback. For example, "Okay, the way you delivered the instruction was perfect! Now, try to give praise even faster after I comply with the instruction. Also, you are doing a great job at remaining positive even though it can be so frustrating when your child is resisting." Overall, trainers must remember to be respectful, patient, and sensitive throughout the training process. If you as a trainer notice that the training session is becoming tense or uncomfortable, that is a red flag that should indicate to you that you need to "throttle back" a little bit and reestablish a positive and upbeat context with the parent.

In Vivo. Once parents have demonstrated proficiency in role-play rehearsals, training sessions can be extended to the natural environment. This will involve each parent practicing implementation of the trained interventions in vivo with their child, in the trainer's presence, and with his or her continued guidance, assistance, and constructive feedback. As proficiency is observed, the trainer gradually fades him or herself out. However, even after complete fading, the trainer should conduct occasional competency checks in order to ensure that the treatment plan continues to be carried out as planned and that the trained intervention skills remain firmly within each parent's repertoire.

Group Training

Training parents of children with IDD on behavioral procedures in a group format has many benefits, such as cost-effectiveness (for both the provider and consumer), efficiency, behavior change gains, and parental social support (Childres et al. 2012; Ingersoll and Wainer 2013; Minjarez et al. 2011; Steiner et al. 2012). Group parent training typically begins by identifying shared goals among the families, as well as individual family goals facilitated by a qualified professional (Minjarez et al. 2011; Steiner et al. 2012). Once these goals have been identified, an intervention may be selected for parents to begin training. The dissemination of training may be assisted by the use of slideshow lectures, videos, intervention manuals, group discussion, and homework assignments (Childres et al. 2012; Minjarez et al. 2011). Group parent training programs often involve education on behavior principles and procedures, followed by instruction on how to implement interventions (Dempsey et al. 2013). Next, demonstrations of the interventions are provided through modeling and role-play, often with the larger group of parents breaking into smaller groups for role-play and feedback (Dempsey et al. 2013). The larger the group is, the less individual training can occur, so adding some amount of one-on-one training (in person or over live video chat) with a qualified professional is suggested (Minjarez et al. 2011).

Technology

Providing technology-based training on evidence-based principles and procedures to parents of children with IDD has many advantages. This method of training is cost-effective by eliminating travel or reducing the need of a qualified professional's physical presence. Technology-based training also benefits families in rural areas or families that may not have access to trained professionals. Furthermore, some families are unable to attend in-person trainings due to personal availability, costs, long waitlists, lack of child care, and/or distance of travel (Heitzman-Powell et al. 2014; Jang et al. 2012; Wainer and Ingersoll 2014). Note, too, that technology-based trainings are used to replace some or all of traditional lecture/classroom didactic trainings (Jang et al. 2012; Wainer and Ingersoll 2014) and typically involve selecting a program that consists of an overview of the intervention and procedures (i.e. eLearning program, Web-based workshops, DVD treatment manuals, video modules, online teaching websites, etc.) (Heitzman-Powell et al. 2014; Jang et al. 2012; Vismara et al. 2013; Wainer and Ingersoll 2014). Parents are then trained to use the equipment required to participate in the program, for example, navigating the site, updating/using computer, and accessing Internet. Usually, parents are required to meet a mastery criterion on program information. Another critical procedure is providing parents with live video conferencing or in person trainings after tech-based training to deliver feedback, answer any unanticipated questions, and/or to provide more opportunities to enhance training (Heitzman-Powell et al. 2014; Vismara et al. 2013; Wainer and Ingersoll 2014). Little or no research has shown that technology can completely replace training by a live trainer, so technology should be considered a valuable supplement to live training, not a replacement. When used optimally, it seems likely that technology can increase the efficiency of live training by decreasing the total number of hours required of a live trainer.

Generalization and Maintenance

Generalization strategies and tactics for promoting generalized behavior change for both the parent and child should be included from the onset of training. Training parents to implement procedures across multiple settings (different rooms, home vs. community, etc.), implementing skill acquisition techniques across multiple targets, and training parents to implement behavior management strategies across multiple different challenging behaviors, are all effective strategies to promote generalization. Generalization should not be considered an important potential side effect of training, but rather, some demonstration of generalization should be criteria for deciding that parents have mastered the trained material. For example, a parent should be trained to implement a particular procedure across multiple different settings but should not be considered to have mastered that procedure until they can demonstrate it in a new setting in which it was not directly trained. It is also very helpful to train parents in the overall process of identifying how to apply their newly learned skills to new problems that may arise. For example, by the time training is done, parents should be able to tell the trainer three new challenges that may arise in the future and how they might address them.

In addition to generalizing, it is critical that parents' newly learned skills maintain across time. Therefore, trainers should include a maintenance plan in their program from the start. Trainers should also select targets that are the most useful for both the parent and child in their daily life to ensure continued demonstration of targets by the child and utilization of treatment strategies by the parent (Najdowski and Gould 2014). Ideally, these targets will be maintained by naturally occurring reinforcement contingencies in everyday life. However, when natural consequences may not be sufficient to ensure maintenance, the trainer would be wise to schedule regular follow-ups with the parent in order to provide additional reinforcement for the parent's behavior. Measurement of parent and child behavior and check-ins should continue as needed so that procedural integrity is maintained (Najdowski and Gould 2014).

Conclusion

A large amount of research has shown that parents can be effectively trained to manage their children's challenging behavior, in addition to teaching them new skills and improving quality of life. Good parent training programs have the features that we have described thus far, including defining challenging but achievable parent and child goals, as well as establishing data collection systems that accurately represent target behaviors for parents and trainers to use. In addition, trainers should consider parent and family variables that may impact training and adjust the program accordingly. Intensity and duration of training should be based on family goals, learning rate, and practical outcomes being reached. Settings can impact training effectiveness, so trainers should evaluate the advantages and disadvantages of each potential setting, as well as transportation, family availability, family goals, and cost-effectiveness when choosing a setting for training. Parents and trainers may have preferences for particular training formats and these should be considered when designing training programs. The most research-proven training strategy is BST, so trainers are most likely to be successful if they implement some or all elements of BST while training. Trainers should consider supplementing BST with group trainings, homework, and technology-based approaches. Finally, training is incomplete if procedures to generalize and maintain desirable training outcomes are not identified from the outset of training.

References

Anan, R. M., Warner, L. J., McGillivary, J. E., Chong, I. M., & Hines, S. J. (2008). Group intensive family training (GIFT) for preschoolers with autism spectrum disorders. *Behavioral Interventions, 23*(3), 165–180.

Baeza-Velasco, C., Michelon, C., Rattaz, C., Pernon, E., & Baghadadli, A. (2013). Seperation of parents raising children with autism spectrum disorders. *Journal of Developmental and Psysichal Disabilities, 25*, 613–624.

Blackledge, J. T., & Hayes, S. C. (2006). Using acceptance and commitment training in the support of parents of children diagnosed with autism. *Child & Family Behavior Therapy, 28*, 1–18.

Chaabane, D. B. B., Alber-Morgan, S. R., & DeBar, R. M. (2009). The effects of parent-implemented PECS training on improvisation of mands by children with autism. *Journal of Applied Behavior Analysis, 42*(3), 671–677.

Childres, J. L., Shaffer-Hudkins, E., & Armstrong, K. (2012). Helping our toddlers, developing our children's skills (hot docs): a program-solving approach for parents of young children with autism spectrum disorders. *Journal of Early Childhood and Infancy Psychology, 8*, 1–19.

Cooper, J. O., Heron, T. E., & Heward, W. L. (2007). *Applied behavior analysis*. Upper Saddle River, NJ: Pearson.

Crockett, J. L., Fleming, R. K., Doepke, K. J., & Stevens, J. S. (2007). Parent training: Acquisition and generalization of discrete trials teaching skills with parents of children with autism. *Research in Developmental Disabilities, 28*, 23–36.

Dempsey, J., Kelly-Vance, L., & Ryalls, B. (2013). The effect of a parent training program on children's play. *International Journal of psychology: A Bi psychosocial Approach, 13*, 117–138.

Gulotta, C. S., & Girolami, P. A. (2014). Food selectivity and refusal. In J. K. Luiselli (Ed.), *Children and youth with autism spectrum disorder: Recent advances and innovations in assessment, education, and intervention* (pp. 163–173). New York: Oxford University Press.

Hanley, G. P., Iwata, B. A., & McCord, B. E. (2003). Functional analysis of problem behavior: A review. *Journal of Applied Behavior Analysis, 36*, 147–185.

Hartley, S. L., Erin, T. B., Seltzer, M. M., Floyd, F., Orsmond, G., & Greenberg, J. (2010). The relative risk and timing of divorce in families of children with an autism spectrum disorder. *Journal of Family Psychology, 24*, 449–457.

Hayes, S. A., & Watson, S. L. (2013). The impact of parenting stress: A meta-analysis of studies comparing the experience of parenting stress in parents of children with and without autism spectrum disorder. *Journal of Autism and Developmental Disorders, 43*(3), 629–642.

Heitzman-Powell, L. S., Buzhardt, J., Rusinko, L. C., & Miller, T. M. (2014). Formative evaluation of an ABA outreach training program for parents of children with autism in remote areas. *Focus on Autism and Other Developmental Disabilities, 29*, 23–38.

Ingersoll, B., & Gergans, S. (2007). The effect of a parent-implemented imitation intervention on spontaneous imitation skills in young children with autism. *Research in Developmental Disabilities, 28*(2), 163–175.

Ingersoll, B. R., & Wainer, A. L. (2013). Pilot study of a school-based parent training program for preschoolers with ASD. *Autism, 17*, 434–448.

Jang, J., Dixon, D. R., Tarbox, J., Granpeesheh, D., Kornack, J., & de Nocker, Y. (2012). Randomized trial of an eLearning program for training family members of children with autism in the principles and procedures of applied behavior analysis. *Research in Autism Spectrum Disorders, 6*, 852–856.

Kaiser, A. P., Hancock, T. B., & Nietfeld, J. P. (2000). The effects of parent-implemented enhanced milieu teaching on the social communication of children who have autism. *Early Education and Development, 11*, 423–446.

Kroeger, K., & Sorensen, R. (2010). A parent training model for toilet training children with autism. *Journal of Intellectual Disability Research, 54*(6), 556–567.

Lerman, D. C., Swiezy, N., Perkins-Parks, S., & Roane, H. S. (2000). Skill acquisition in parents of children with developmental disabilities: Interaction between skill type and instructional format. *Research in Developmental Disabilities, 21*(3), 183–196.

Luiselli, J. K. (2015). Health and wellness. In N. N. Singh (Ed.), *Clinical handbook of evidence-based practices for individuals with intellectual disabilities*. New York: Springer (in press).

Miles, N. I., & Wilder, D. A. (2009). The effects of behavioral skills training on caregiver implementation of guided compliance. *Journal of Applied Behavior Analysis, 42*(2), 405–410.

Minjarez, M. B., Williams, S. E., Mercier, E. M., & Hardan, A. Y. (2011). Pivotal response group treatment program for parents of children with autism. *Journal of Autism and Developmental Disorders, 41*, 92–101.

Najdowski, A. C., & Gould, E. R. (2014). Behavioral family intervention. In J. K. Luiselli (Ed.), *Children and youth with autism spectrum disorder (ASD): Recent advances and innovations in assessment, education, and intervention* (pp. 237–253). New York, NY, US: Oxford University Press.

Najdowski, A. C., Wallace, M. D., Penrod, B., Tarbox, J., Reagon, K., & Higbee, T. S. (2008). Caregiver-conducted experimental functional analyses of inappropriate mealtime behavior. *Journal of Applied Behavior Analysis, 41*, 459–465.

Najdowski, A. C., Wallace, M. D., Reagon, K., Penrod, B., Higbee, T. S., & Tarbox, J. (2010). Utilizing a home-based parent training approach in the treatment of food selectivity. *Behavioral Interventions, 25*, 89–107.

Park, J. H., Alber-Morgan, S. R., & Cannella-Malone, H. (2010). Effects of mother-implemented picture exchange communication system (PECS) training on independent communicative behaviors of young children with autism spectrum disorders. *Topics in Early Childhood Special Education, 31*, 37–47.

Reagon, K. A., & Higbee, T. S. (2009). Parent-implemented script fading to promote play-based verbal initiations in children with autism. *Journal of Applied Behavior Analysis, 42*(3), 659–664.

Rivard, M., Terroux, A., Parent-Boursier, C., & Mercier, C. (2014). Determinants of stress in parents of children with autism spectrum disorders. *Journal of Autism and Developmental Disorders, 44*, 1609–1620.

Schaffer, R. C., & Minshawi, N. F. (2014). Training and supporting caregivers in evidence-based practices. In J. Tarbox, D. R. Dixon, P. Sturmey, & J. L. Matson (Eds.), *Handbook of early intervention in autism spectrum disorders: Research, policy, and practice*. NY: Springer.

Schreibman, L., Dufek, S., & Cunningham, A. B. (2011). Identifying moderators of treatment outcome for children with autism. In J. L. Matson & P. Sturmey (Eds.), *International handbook of autism and pervasive developmental disorders* (pp. 295–305). New York, NY, US: Springer Science + Business Media. doi:10.1007/978-1-4419-8065-6_18

Schultz, T. R., Schmidt, C. T., & Stichter, J. P. (2011). A review of parent education programs for parents of children with autism spectrum disorders. *Focus on Autism and Other Developmental Disabilities, 26*, 96–104.

Singh, N. N., Lancioni, G. E., Winton, A. S. W., Singh, J., Singh, A. N. D., & Singh, A. D. A. (2014). Mindful caregiving and support. In J. K. Luiselli (Ed.), *Children and youth with autism spectrum disorder (ASD): Recent advances and innovations in assessment, education, and intervention* (pp. 207–221). New York: Oxford University Press.

Steiner, A. M., Koegel, L. K., Koegel, R. L., & Ence, W. A. (2012). Issues and theoretical constructs regarding parent education for autism spectrum disorders. *Journal of Autism and Developmental Disorders, 42*(6), 1218–1227. doi:10.1007/s10803-011-1194-0

Stewart, K. K., Carr, J. E., & LeBlanc, L. A. (2007). Evaluation of family-implemented behavioral skills training for teaching social skills to a child with Asperger's disorder. *Clinical Case Studies, 6*(3), 252–262.

Symon, J. B. (2005). Expanding interventions for children with autism: Parents as trainers. *Journal of Positive Behavior Interventions, 7*, 159–173.

Tarbox, J., Schiff, A., & Najdowski, A. C. (2010). Parent-implemented procedural modification of escape extinction in the treatment of food selectivity in a young child with autism. *Education and Treatment of Children, 33*(2), 223–234.

Tarbox, R. S., Wallace, M. D., Penrod, B., & Tarbox, J. (2007). Effects of three-step prompting on compliance with caregiver requests. *Journal of Applied Behavior Analysis, 40*(4), 703–706.

Tekin-Iftar, E. (2008). Parent-delivered community-based instruction with simultaneous prompting for teaching community skills to children with developmental disabilities. *Education and Training in Developmental Disabilities, 43*, 249.

Vismara, L. A., McCormick, C., Young, G. S., Nadhan, A., & Monlux, K. (2013). Preliminary findings of a telehealth approach to parent training in autism. *Journal of Autism and Developmental Disorders, 43*, 2953–2969.

Wacker, D. P., Berg, W. K., Harding, J. W., Derby, M. K., Asmus, J. M., & Healy, A. (1998). Evaluation and long-term treatment of aberrant behavior displayed by young children with disabilities. *Journal of Developmental and Behavioral Pediatrics, 19*(4), 260–266.

Wacker, D. P., Lee, J. F., Dalmau, Y. C. P., Kopelman, T. G., Lindgren, S. D., Kuhle, J., et al. (2013). Conducting functional communication training via telehealth to reduce the problem behavior of young children with autism. *Journal of developmental and physical disabilities, 25*(1), 35–48.

Wainer, A. L., & Ingersoll, B. R. (2014). Increasing access to an ASD imitation intervention via a telehealth parent training program. *Journal of Autism and Developmental Disorders*,. doi:10.1007/s10803-014-2186-7

Ward-Horner, J., & Sturmey, P. (2008). The effects of general-case training and behavioral skills training on the generalization of parents' use of discrete-trial teaching, child correct responses, and child maladaptive behavior. *Behavioral Interventions, 23*, 271–284.

Whittingham, K., Sanders, M., McKinlay, L., & Boyd, R. N. (2014). Interventions to reduce behavioral problems in children with cerebral palsy: An RCT. *Pediatrics, 133*, e1249–e1257.

Young, K. L., Boris, A. L., Thomson, K. M., Martin, G. L., & Yu, C. T. (2012). Evaluation of a self-instructional package on discrete-trials teaching to parents of children with autism. *Research in Autism Spectrum Disorders, 6*, 1321–1330.

Index

J.K. Luiselli (ed.), *Behavioral Health Promotion and Intervention in Intellectual and Developmental Disabilities*, Evidence-Based Practices in Behavioral Health,
DOI 10.1007/978-3-319-27297-9

The manufacturer's authorised representative in the EU is Springer Nature Customer Service Centre GmbH, Europaplatz 3, 69115 Heidelberg, Germany. If you have any concerns regarding our products, please contact ProductSafety@springernature.com

Printed and bound by CPI Group (UK) Ltd, Croydon, CR0 4YY
22/09/2026
02221061-0009